CURRENT CONCEPTS IN PLASTIC SURGERY

Edited by **Francisco J. Agullo**

Current Concepts in Plastic Surgery
Edited by Francisco J. Agullo

Published by InTech
Janeza Trdine 9, 51000 Rijeka, Croatia

Publishing Process Manager Romana Vukelic

Technical Editor Teodora Smiljanic

Cover Designer InTech Design Team

Additional hard copies can be obtained from orders@intechopen.com

Current Concepts in Plastic Surgery, Edited by Francisco J. Agullo
p. cm.
ISBN 978-953-51-0398-1

For EU product safety concerns:
IN TECH d.o.o., Prolaz Marije Krucifikse Kozulić 3, 51000 Rijeka, Croatia,
info@intechopen.com or visit our website at intechopen.com.

Meet the editor

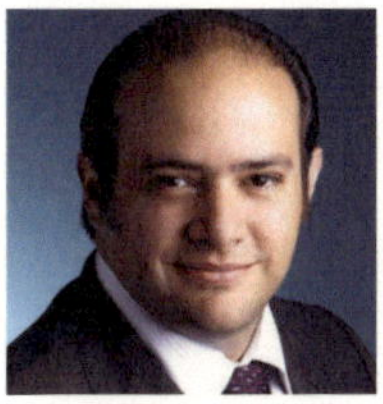

Francisco J. Agullo, MD, FACS is a board certified Plastic Surgeon based in El Paso, Texas. He holds the title of Clinical Associate Professor of Plastic Surgery at the Texas Tech University Health Sciences Center, Paul L. Foster School of Medicine, as well as Affiliate Professor at the University of Texas at El Paso. His private practice is primarily based at El Paso Cosmetic Surgery. Dr. Agullo graduated from Universidad Anahuac in Mexico City, and trained in general surgery at Texas Tech University. He then completed plastic surgery training at the Mayo Clinic in Rochester, Minnesota. He is a Fellow of the American College of Surgeons and member of the American Society of Plastic Surgery. He has also become a member of the International Society of Aesthetic Plastic Surgery. Dr. Agullo has an extensive number of publications and presentations to his name at both national and international levels.

Contents

Preface

Plastic surgery continues to be a rapidly growing field in medicine. There have been multiple recent advancements in the field. Specifically, there has been a continuously growing interest in fat grafting, body contouring, minimally invasive surgery, and plastic surgery education. At the same time, there have been continued advances and modifications in surgical techniques, which translate into improved results for our patients while increasing safety and efficacy.

The title of the book is *Current Concepts in Plastic Surgery*, and, as such, it highlights some of the "hot topics" in recent years. Some of the topics continue discussion on controversial issues such as fat grafting for breast reconstruction and the combination of liposuction and abdominoplasty. Other topics offer reviews of and refinements in techniques of head and neck, breast, aesthetic, and microsurgical procedures.

We have invited renowned specialists from around the world to share their valued expertise and experience. Most of the chapters will expose the reader to multiple techniques for achieving desired results, with emphasis on the author's preferred methodology. This book is a brief snapshot of plastic surgery today, and does not attempt to cover its entirety, as we acknowledge the immense depth of the field and its ongoing improvement.

Francisco J. Agullo
Texas Tech University Health Sciences Center – El Paso, TX
El Paso Cosmetic Surgery Center – El Paso, TX
USA

Part 1

Head and Neck

1

Minimal Invasive Surgery in Head and Neck Video-Assisted Technique

Jorge O. Guerrissi
Department of Plastic Surgery,
Argerich Hospital, Buenos Aires,
Medicine Faculty of Buenos Aires University (UBA)
Plastic Surgery Academic Unit Buenos Aires University
Argentina

1. Introduction

The recent advent of endoscopic procedures has compelled to plastic surgeons to reconsider the conventional methods by which the excision different type of head and neck tumors are classically achieved. Endoscopic resection is a safe and minimally invasive approach and spares unnecessary discomfort to the patient.

The introduction of endoscopy into surgical practice is one of the biggest successes in the history of medicine; the recent advents of endoscopic procedures have revolutionized the practice of surgery in many specialties.

The outcome achieve with endoscopic techniques in other surgical areas has permitted to considerer this technique in head and neck offering more advantages than the classic approaches. (1)(2)(3)(4)(5).

Plastic surgeons have been compelled to consider the video-assisted surgical technique as a safe and effective technique in the treatment of benign tumor in head and neck.

This technique has many advantages as minimal morbidity; significantly decreased scarring and it also enhance the surgeon´s ability to view the area decreasing the danger of injuring anatomical structures.

In Department of Plastic Surgery at Argerich Hospital in Buenos Aires, Argentina from 1999 to 2007 video-assisted approaches were used in the treatment of 108 patients whom presented: 1. Frontocygomatic cysts; 2. Benign subcutaneous tumors in frontal, nasal and facial areas; 3. Benign tumors and sialolithiasis of submandibular gland; 4. Wharton duct obstruction by sialolith; 5. Benign tumors in sublingual gland, and 5. Branchiogenic cervical cysts and 6. Cervical lipomas.

In this paper to be described not only endoscopic techniques for several diseases in head and neck , but also project the use of natural orifice surgery (NOS) as a procedure with spectrum of innovative operations .(5)

2. Material and method

One hundred eight patients were operated from August 1999 to September 2007 in the Department of Plastic Surgery at Argerich Hospital of Buenos Aires, Argentine using video-assisted surgery.

Of the 108 patients 19 (18%) were more than 55 years old and the other 89 remaining patient's ages range from 11 to 55 years old (82%).

Seventy eight patients were female (70%) and 30 (30%) were males.

Thirty-six patients (20 %) presented branchiogenic cysts; 18 (50%) found 14 on the right and the remains 18 on the left; 2 lateral cervical cystic hygromas were found in the right upper third of the neck. (Figs. 1 and 2)

In the frontal area were located thirty-two tumors (18%); 16 of them were (50%) frontocygomatic cysts (Figs. 3 and 4); 8 lipomas (12,5%) and 8 osteomas (12,5%).

Three nasal epidermic cysts (4%) were detected in the middle line of the upper nasal dorsum; a transnasal approach was used as a rhinoplasty, using natural orifice surgery (NOS) (Figs. 5 and 6)

Transoral technique was used as a basic approach in Wharton obstruction, submandibular and sublingual glands tumor resections.

Wharton lithiasis was operated en 12 cases and 12 adenomas of the submandibular gland were resected 7 in right gland and 5 in left one.

Two ranulas and 1 benign adenoma were resected in sublingual gland.

In all 108 cases no severe complications were observed; in 4 cases (4,3 %) were detected hematomas, in other 2 cases wound infection and in other 2 transitory disestesis of lingual nerve. (Table 1)

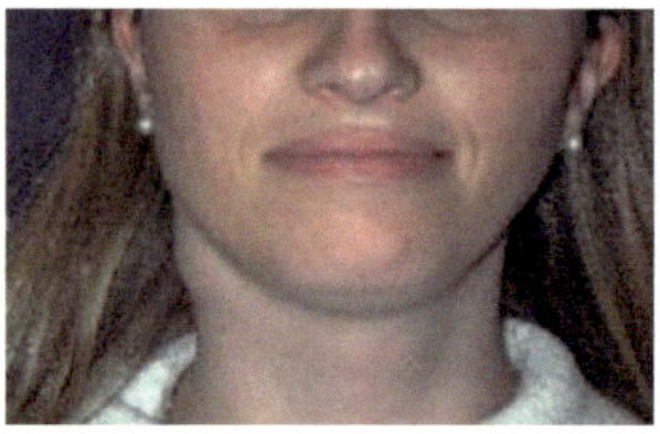

Fig. 1. Preop. Branchial cyst in right side of the neck

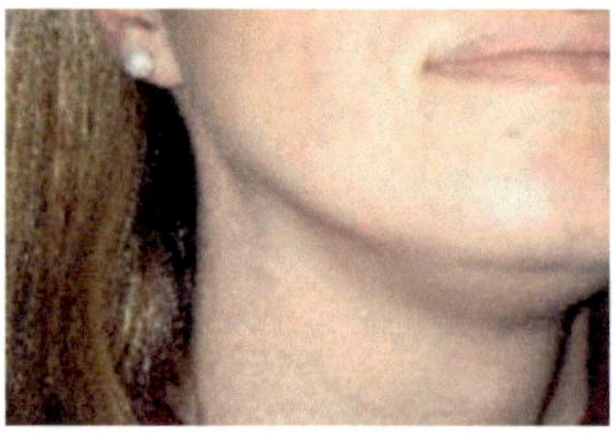

Fig. 2. Postop. Six months after surgery: Inconspicuous scar
The incision is planned on domes of the cyst in natural wrinkle.

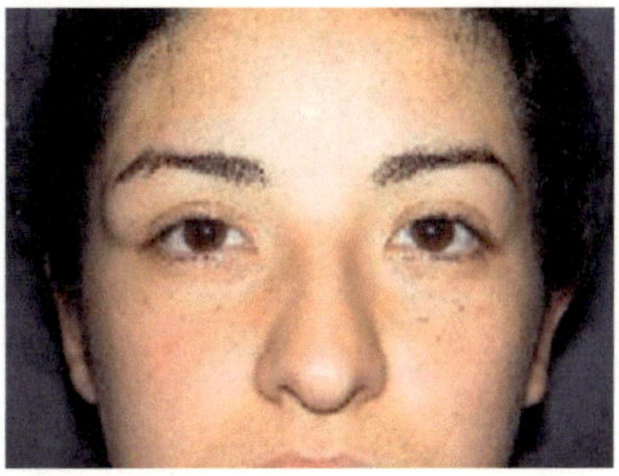

Fig. 3. Preop. Left frontocigomatic cyst

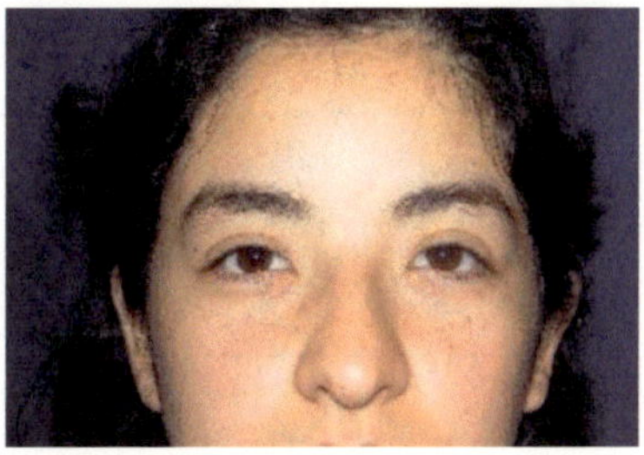

Fig. 4. One year postoperative.

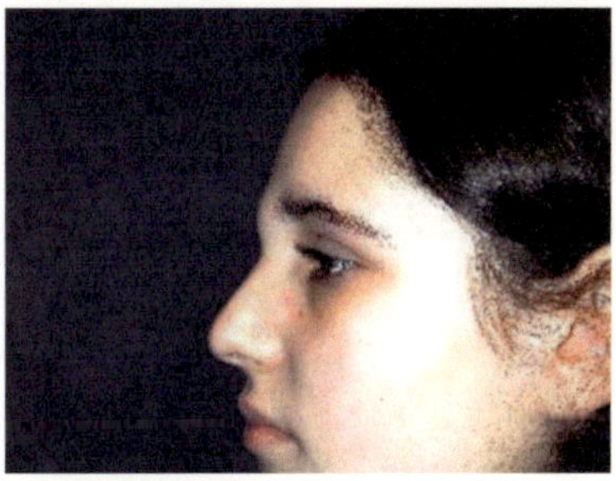

Fig. 5. Epidermic congenital nasal cyst located in the middle line

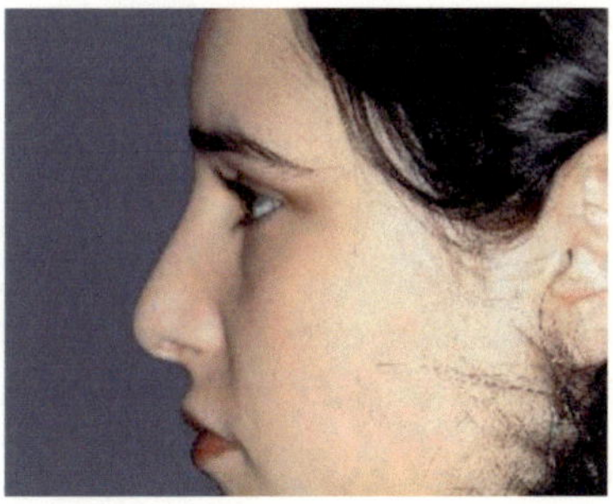

Fig. 6. After 18 months

PATHOLOGY	CASES	TECHNIQUE	NOS *	COMPLICATIONS
CERVICAL CYSTS	36	VIDEO-ASSISTED		YES WOUND INFECTION (2) HEMATOMA (1)
CERVICAL LIPOMAS	8			
HYGROMA NECK	2	IDEM		NO
FRONTOCYGOMATIC CYSTS	16	IDEM		YES HEMATOMA (2)
FRONTAL LIPOMAS	8	IDEM		NO
FRONTAL OSTEOMAS	8	IDEM		NO
NASAL CYSTS	3	IDEM	YES	NO
SUBMANDIBULAR GLAND TUMOR	12	IDEM	YES	YES HEMATOMA. (1) DISESTESIS LINGUAL NERVE (2)
SUBLINGUAL GLAND TUMOR	3	IDEM	YES	NO
WHARTON LITHIASIS	12	IDEM	YES	NO

*NOS: Natural Orifices Surgery

Table 1. Clinic Clases

3. Surgical endoscopic techniques

In all cases three basic endoscopic surgical steps were planned: 1. Incision; 2. Exposure of the tumor and 3.Resection.

An endoscope of 20 cm long with a diameter of 4 mm and vision angle of 0° and 30° was used.

A subcutaneous endoretractor permitted the stabilization of endoscope, maintaining the optical cavity and subcutaneous retraction. Special dissectors were used, as also delicate conventional or endoscopic scissors, clamps and forceps.

3.1 Branchiogenic cysts

Incision was placed in a natural wrinkle, over the middle of the protruding dome of the cyst; not more than 1,5 cm of length. The exposure of the cyst was made whit concave blades retractors placement over both cyst walls and anatomical elements around of the cyst, permitting liberation of adherences round of the cyst. (Fig. 7) Resection of cysts was carried out after liberation of carotid and internal jugular vein. (Fig. 8) (6)

In large cysts a complete aspiration was made to facilitate not only the dissection but also the extirpation.

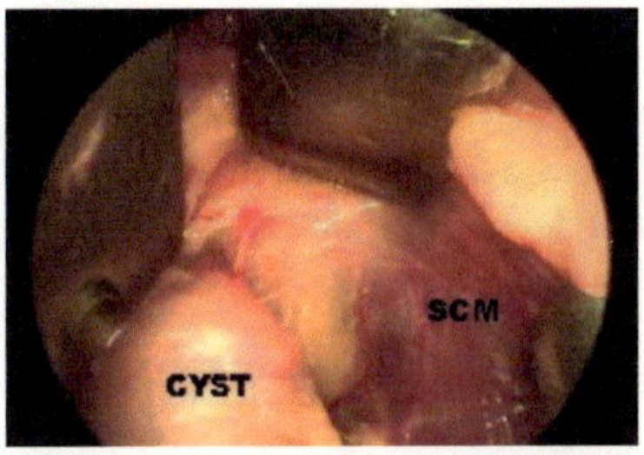

Fig. 7. Exposition and liberation of the sternocleidomastoid muscle

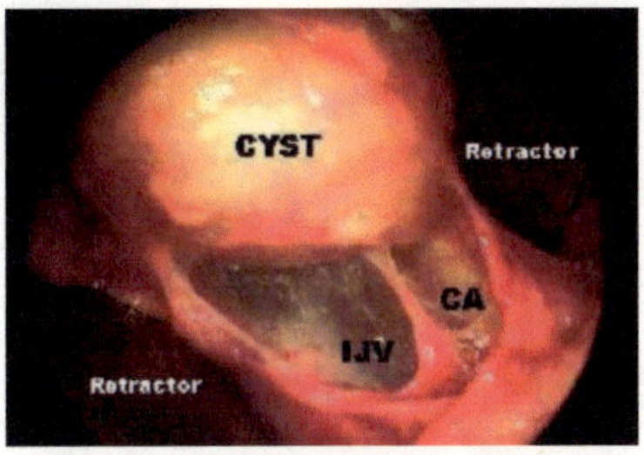

Fig. 8. Endoscopic view: Great vessels with IJV (Internal Jugular Vein) and CA (Carotid Artery) are separated of the external layer of the cyst.

3.2 Frontal tumors

Incisions (1 or 2) were placed behind of hair line (Fig 9). A subperiostic dissection was carried out in the frontal area from incisions to the tumor; tumor resection was carefully performed avoiding the injury frontal nerve. In frontocygomatic cyst resection an additional dissection on superficial temporal fascia was necessary widening operative field; the cystic liberation was carried out from orbicularis oculis muscle and the supraorbitary nerve. (Fig. 10)

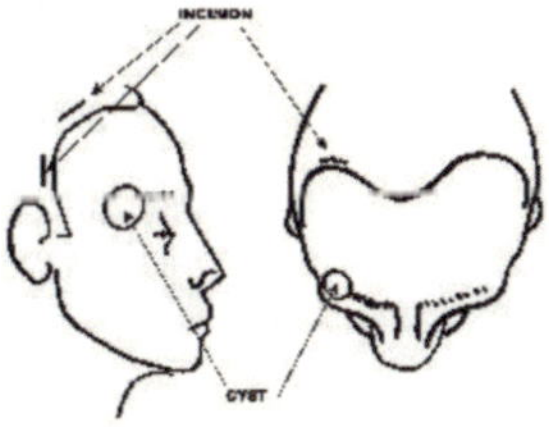

Fig. 9. Incisions placement behind of hairline.

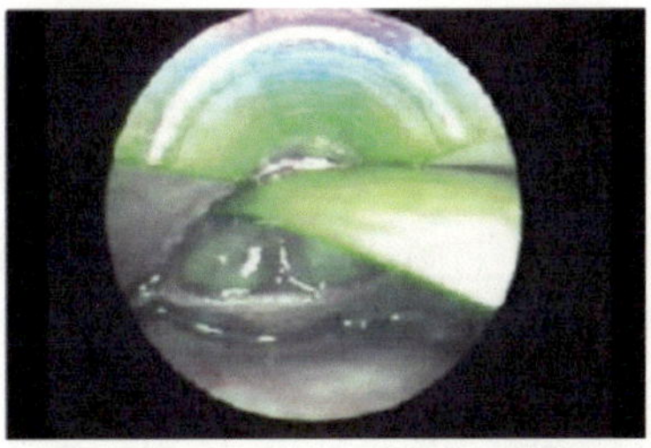

Fig. 10. Intraoperative view shows exposition and resection of the cyst.

3.3 Nasal cysts

In all 3 cases of congenital epidermic nasal cysts, a transnasal approach as a rhinoplasty was used.(Fig. 11) Cysts were exposed and resected after conventional subperiosteal skeletonizing of the nose was carried out (Fig 12).

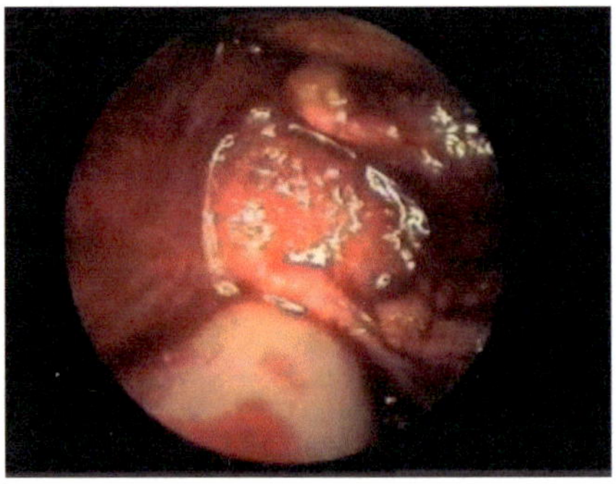

Fig. 11. Endoscopic exposition of the nasal congenital cyst.

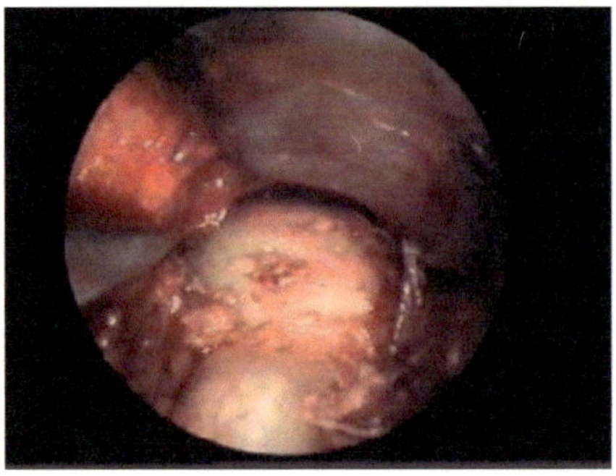

Fig. 12. After cystic resection a tumor impress on nasal bone can be observed.

3.4 Submandibular tumor resection

An incision in mandibular-lingual sulcus was preferred, after were exposed: the sublingual gland; the Wharton duct; the lingual nerve and the mylohyoid muscle.

Two oblique retractors placement over mylohyoid muscle and lingual nerve allowed the creation the "new" space with excellent submandibular gland visualization (Fig. 13). This technique had two principal "surgical key"; the first is the anatomical relation between Wharton duct and lingual nerve and the second is the posterior pole of the gland where facial vessels running.

The sublingual gland can be excised to provide optimal exposure; another useful maneuver is the digital elevation of the gland from skin to surgical field permitting an intraoral gland exposition. (Fig. 14)

Either complete gland or isolated tumor exceresis was made.

Sublingual Gland resection and Wharton sialolithiasis

Better visualization and magnified view of the sublingual gland and Wharton duct were the more important advantages. Both structures are widening exposed and surrounding anatomical landmark was protected while exceresis is carried out.

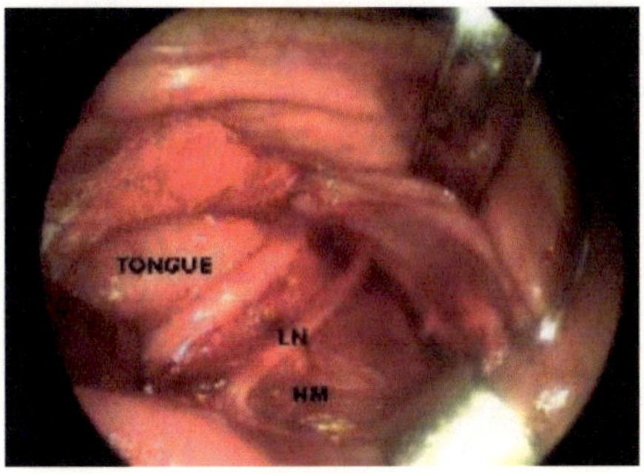

Fig. 13. "New space" where anatomical elements as lingual nerve and hypoglossal muscle are identifies.

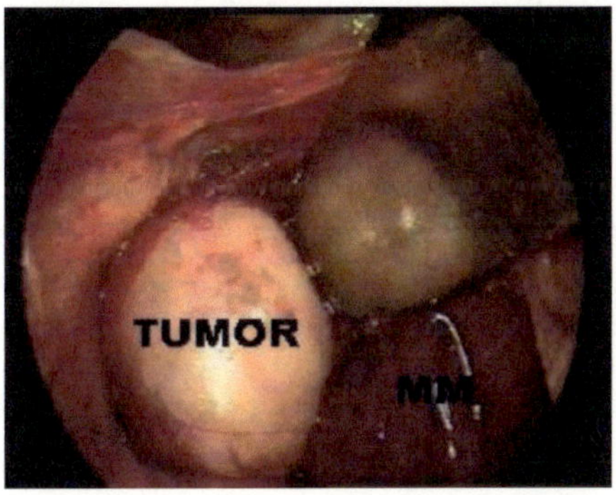

Fig.14. The mylohyoid muscle is retracted and the gland tumor is clearly exposed into surgical field.

4. Discussion

The recent advent of endoscopic procedures has compelled to plastic surgeon to reconsider the conventional methods of excision of different type of tumors placed in head and neck areas are classically achieved. (5) In head and neck areas the use of transnasal and transoral areas are the most feasible approaches of NOS.

Benign tumors, sialoadenitis and sialolithiasis of submandibular gland are current pathologies which can be successfully treated by endoscopic surgery.

The surgery of this gland has been traditionally, performed through a cervical incision; this is a safe procedure, but some complications such a pathologic scarring and injury of the marginal mandibular nerve can occur between 1 to 7 % of cases (7) (8). Conventional intraoral approach was described in 1960 by Dawnton and Qvist (9) and Yoel in 1961. (11). In 2001 was described the use of video-assisted surgery of the submandibular gland using a transoral approach. (11). Principal advantages are good illumination and magnification providing clear and sharply vision permitting safe anatomical dissections. Technical difficulties are a reduced operative field between the tongue and mandible and a hardly dissection of the facial vessels in "posterior pole" of the gland. Three complications (25 %) were detected in all 12 patients operated with this technique: 1 hematoma and 2 transitory lingual nerve disestesis with spontaneous recuperation 6 months later.

In the cases of the tumors located in frontal region as lipomas, osteomas and principally frontocygomatic cysts, the use of video-assisted techniques avoid visible fontal scars, hidden behind of hairline. An excellent visualization permits a dissection in avascular planes avoiding injuries of frontal nerve; subperiosteal plane provides the necessary optical cavity for operation.

In all frontocygomatic cysts additional dissection on anterior third of the temporal muscle must be performed widening surgical field. (11).

The anatomy of the nasal area is ideally suited for application of endoscopic principles; it is an expandable cavity with avascular planes of dissection and direct visualization. Hide intranasal incision is the most important advantages this technique.

According to conventional rhinoplasty technique the skeletonizing permits to achieve to cyst after scoring the periosteum over dorsum as high as nasofrontal area; a compression dressing prevent formation of a hematoma and facilitate tissue adhesion.

The ideal treatment of a branchial cleft cyst is the complete resection. One of the most evident advantages of the endoscopic resection is the use of a small incision onto a natural wrinkle; the length of it is no more than 1,5 cm.

This incision permits to introduce both endoscope and surgical instruments.

The identification and protection of nerves and vessels around cysts is most important surgical maneuver. While a concave retractor is placed on the cyst wall, another retractor is in front of it protecting identified anatomical elements.

In large cysts, the content must be partially aspired to facilitate the surgical maneuvers of dissection and exceresis. In all 35 cases of branchiogenic cysts, no severe complications were observed.

Two patients (13%) presented partial wound infections, which healed leaving a more evident scar.

In 32 patients (90%), the final scars were inconspicuous and remain occluded in a natural cervical fold.

In all 108 patients minimal or no pain was reported, and analgesic drugs were only necessary in the first postoperative hours; any kind of discomfort was claimed by patients.

The anatomy of the head and neck areas is ideal for application of endoscopic principles; its soft tissues can transform in an expandable cavity with avascular planes of dissection.

5. Conclusion

Advantages of endoscopic resection are: 1. Better visualization and magnified view of the dissection areas: as a consequence the injury of important anatomical landmark, nerves and vessel can be avoided; 2. Small incision; 3. Inconspicuous or hide scar; 4.Excellent postoperative comfort; and 5. Short hospital stay.

Disadvantages are: 1. It is necessary to have an endoscope and special instruments and 2. Specific surgical training must be made by surgeons.

With the arrival the new surgical techniques, surgeon experience and advanced endoscopic instruments, the video-assisted surgery can be a safe method of choice in the treatment of the several diseases of head and neck

6. References

[1] Mangnan J, Chays A, Lepetre C et al. Surgical perspective of endoscopic of the cerebellopontine angle Am. J. Otol 1994;15: 366-370.
[2] Breant AS. Endoscopic approach to benign tumors of the paranasal sinuses. In Wackym PA, Rice DH and Schaefer SD (eds) In Minimally Invasive Surgery of the Head and Neck and Cranial Base. Philadelphia, Lippincott Williams & Wilkins. 2002: 297-310.
[3] Litynski GS. Endoscopic surgery: the history, the pioneers. World J Surg 1999; 23:745-753.
[4] Davis CJ. A history of endoscopic surgery. Surg. Laparosc Endosc. 1992; 2: 16-23.
[5] Benhidjeb T, Witzel K, Barlehner E, et al. The natural orifice surgery concept. Vision and rationale for a paradigm shift. Chirurg. 2007; 78: 537-542.
[6] Guerrissi JO. Innovation and Surgical Technique. Endoscopic Resection of Cervical Branchiogenic Cysts. J. Craniofac. Surg. 2002; 13: 478-482.
[7] Goh YH, Sethi DS Submandibular gland excision: 5 years review. J Laryngol Otol 1998; 112: 269-272.
[8] Ellies M, laskawi R, Aregeble C at al. Surgical management of nonneoplastic diseases of the submandibular gland. Int J Oral Maxillofac Surg 1996; 35: 285-289.
[9] Downton D, Qvist G. Intra-oral excision on the submandibular gland. Proc R Soc Med 1960; 53: 543-546.
[10] Guerrissi JO, Taborda G. Endoscopic excision of the submandibular gland by an intraoral approach. J Craniofac Surg 2001; 13: 299-303.

[11] Rhee JS, Gallo JF, Constantino PD. Endoscopic facial rejuvenation. In Wackym PA, Rice DH and Schaefer SD.(eds) In Minimally Invasive Surgery of the Head and Neck , and Cranial Base. Philadelphia, Lippincott Williams & Wilkins. 2002: 356-366.

2

Basal Cell Carcinoma

Tomasz Dębski, Lubomir Lembas and Józef Jethon
Department of Plastic Surgery,
The Medical Centre of Postgraduate Education in Warsaw
Poland

1. Introduction

Neoplastic lesions of the skin are among the most common human malignancies. They originate from different skin tissues and structures such as:

- epidermis
- skin appendages (hair follicles, sebaceous glands, eccrine sweat glands, apocrine sweat glands)
- pigment cells (melanocytes)
- mesenchymal structures (fibrous tissue, fatty tissue, blood and lymphatic vessels, muscles)
- nerves and APUD cells of the neuroendocrine system
- lymphatic system cells.

The vast majority of neoplasms originating from the above skin structures are benign neoplasms. They are characterised by slow local growth and lack of intensive tissue damage.

The remaining part of neoplastic lesions consists of skin malignancies including carcinomas (originating from the epidermis and skin appendages), melanomas (originating from pigment cells), lymphomas (originating from the lymphatic system cells) and sarcomas (originating from other skin cells) Other classification of malignancies is as follows:

Non-Melanoma Skin Cancer (NMSC) and Melanoma Malignum (MM.) NMSC include skin cancers (96% of skin malignancies), lymphomas and sarcomas (1% of skin malignancies.) The remaining 3% is MM which is characterised by high malignancy and accounts for 75% of all deaths due to skin neoplasms (Kordek et al., 2004 ; The Burden of Skin Cancer, 2008).

Despite the fact that there are different classifications available in literature, one thing that does not change is that cancer is the most common histopathological form of malignancies. Almost all skin cancers originate in the epidermis. Cancers arising in the skin appendages constitute a very low per cent. From a histological point of view the epidermis is stratified epithelium with several layers of cells. Depending on an epidermal layer (the basal cell or squamous cell layer) skin cancers are divided into:

- Basal Cell Carcinoma (BCC) originating from the basal cell layer of the epidermis and sheaths of hair follicles. It constitutes 80% of all skin cancers.

- Squamous Cell Carcinoma (SCC) originating from cells in the Malpighi layer and it accounts for 20% of skin cancers (Kordek et al.,. 2004).

Although both BCC and SCC originate from the epidermis, their biology is completely different and therefore they cannot be discussed together. For that reason the authors of this review have decided to present problems associated only with one of them, namely BCC.

BCC is of the most common human malignancies, and its incidence has been rising within the last decade (Preston & Stern, 1992). Although it is not life-threatening, its local malignant features, especially in the area of the face may cause significant functional and aesthetic disturbances what has a profound effect on the quality of life of patients. If BCC is left untreated, it can infiltrate not only adjacent tissues but also bones and even deeper structures like brain (Franchimont, 1982). Moreover, extremely rare distant metastases of this neoplasm have been described (Lo et al., 1991).

BCC diagnostics and treatment is managed by physicians of different specialities (dermatologists, plastic surgeons, general surgeons, oncologists, ophthalmologists, ENT specialists, and even general medicine specialists) who promote therapeutic options which are closely related to their specialities and are often controversial. Available literature reports different therapeutic methods including non-invasive techniques such as local application of Imiquimod-containing ointments (Mark et al., 2001), photodynamic therapy (Clark et al., 2003), radiation therapy (Kwan et al., 2004), CO_2 laser ablation (Nouri et al., 2002), cryosurgery (Giuffrida et al., 2003), cautery (Spiller WF & Spiller RF, 1984) and curettage (Reyman, 1985) or surgical excision of a lesion with a margin of clinically normal surrounding tissues (Walker & Hill, 2006).

Functional and aesthetic results, treatment efficacy, side effects and effects on the quality of life are different and depend on the method that has been used.

Method selection depends on lesion morphological features and patient's condition and preferences. The majority of methods to treat BCC described so far may be used only in some, highly selected cases. The only universal method that can be used to treat all cases of BCC is surgical excision with a margin of clinically normal surrounding tissues.

Due to high efficacy of this method, its versatility, good functional and aesthetic results, low risk of complications, availability, low costs, and what is the most important, the ability of postoperative histological assessment of excision completeness, surgical treatment is currently the most common method to treat BCC.

2. Epidemiology

Among all human malignancies skin cancer occurs the most frequently and it accounts for almost 1/3 of all detectable neoplasms (Kordek et al., 2004). Despite the fact that since the early 1990s the global incidence of neoplasms has been decreasing the rate of incidence of skin cancer has been rising and it is estimated to be 10-15% annually, what is almost ten times higher than the population growth rate (Cole & Rodu, 1996; Kordek et al., 2004; Parkin et al., 1999). It has to be emphasised that there are no precise records especially with regard to BCC and therefore epidemiological data are often understated and not included in global lists of incidence rates of neoplasms (Kordek et al., 2004).

Only in the USA, more than one million cases of skin cancers are detected every year (American Cancer Society, 2008). It is the number almost equal to the number of all other cancers detected annually in this country (American Cancer Society, 2006). It is estimated that one out of five Americans will develop skin cancer (American Cancer Society, 2008), and in almost half of 65-year-olds this cancer will occur at least once in their lives (Robinson, 2005).

Although the data presented above regard all cases of skin cancers it can be assumed that they reflect BCC epidemiology to a large extent, as BCC accounts for almost 80% of all cases of skin cancers (Kordek et al., 2004).

Global statistics unanimously indicate that BCC is one of the most common neoplasms in Europe, Australia and the USA (Miller & Weinstock, 1994), and the number of new cases is increasing every year (Table 1.)

Country	Non-melanoma skin cancers (w/m)	Lung cancer (w/m)	Colon cancer (w/m)	Breast cancer (w)
Finland	399 / 416	20 / 55	43 / 41	137
Switzerland	433 / 560	26 / 78	54 / 75	137
Netherlands	402 / 470	29 / 92	57 / 62	130
United Kingdom	458 / 471	51 / 83	55 / 66	135
USA	459 / 534	59 / 84	55 / 60	144
Australia	403 / 483	27 / 57	58 / 67	114
Poland	320 / 382	23 / 104	40 / 41	73

Table 1. Incidence rate for selected neoplasms based on Globocan 2002 (number of detected cases/year/100 000 citizens) (Global Cancer Statistics Globocan, 2002).

Epidemiology of skin cancer unanimously indicates that it is a significant global problem. However, this problem is not noticed and is underestimated especially because of the fact that mortality related with these neoplasms is low (in the USA 1000-2000 patients/year) (Jemal et al., 2003) and that this neoplasm is not listed in incidence records (data are not complete.) The importance of this problem is mainly affected by the number and dynamics of new cases, a high recurrence rate (even 18%) (Silverman et al., 1991) and generally high costs of treatment (in the USA the costs of treating skin cancers were more than one billion dollars in 2004) (Bickers et al., 2006).

3. Etiopathogenesis

Although currently several factors are suspected to be responsible for BCC the most important roles in cancerogenesis are played by UV radiation and advanced age of patients. They account for more than 90% of neoplastic lesions (Taylor, 1990).

3.1 Aetiological factors

Solar radiation (UV) can be divided into three parts depending on the wavelength: UVA (wavelength of 320-400 nm), UVB (wavelength of 280-320 nm) and UVC (wavelength of 200-280 nm) (Kordek et al., 2004).

The majority of radiation emitted by the Sun is absorbed by the ozone layer of the atmosphere, and consequently, only a low amount reaches the Earth. As due to atmosphere pollution the thickness of the ozone layer is gradually reduced, more and more UV radiation reaches the Earth, therefore the incidence of BCCs can increase (Goldsmith, 1996). This phenomenon may also explain the fact that this neoplasm occurs in younger and younger patients as they earlier achieve a cancerogenesis threshold of Average Accumulated Exposure (The Skin Cancer Foundation, 2008).

Exposure to UVB radiation contributes to the BCC development the most (Boukamp, 2005).

Contrary to common opinions short-term but intensive and long-term but less-intensive exposure are equal (Marks et al., 1990). The dose of UV absorbed in the childhood does not contribute significantly to neoplasm pathogenesis according to the latest reports (Godar et al., 2003).

Long-term UVB actions lead to the formation of mutagenic photoproducts that damage DNA chains in skin cells. DNA damaged in this way is repaired within 24 hours as a result of the effective repair system called NER (nucleotide excision repair system) (Szepietowski et al., 1996). Impairment of this system present in patients with xeroderma pigmentosum inevitably leads to multifocal skin cancer and death at a young age.

Apart from damage to DNA of skin cells UV radiation also causes mutations in a suppressor gene of the p-53 protein. The protein coded by this gene has anti-oncogenic properties as it induces apoptosis in the cells with damaged DNA. As a result of a mutation in this gene the anti-oncogenic properties of the p-53 protein are turned off, therefore the cells with damaged DNA proliferate without control. The presence of a mutation in the p-53 gene is found in 60-100% of cases of skin cancer (Marks, 1995).

The skin inflammatory response induced during the exposure to UV also participates in the process of damaging DNA (Maeda & Akaike, 1998) inducing disturbances of division and mutations in newly produced cells (Hendrix et al., 1996).

The sources of UV radiation include not only solar radiation but also PUVA lamps used to treat psoriasis and albinism as well as tanning lamps.

Due to the fact that tanning lamps are widely accessible and due to fashion trends they have become especially important in BCC etiopathogenesis in the last years. Some of these modern tanning lamps may emit radiation doses which are even 12 times higher than the ones emitted by the Sun (11th ROC: Ultraviolet Radiation Related Exposures, 2008). The risk of BCC in subjects using tanning lamps regularly is twice the risk observed in the general population (Karagas et al., 2002).

The significance of solar radiation in BCC pathogenesis is emphasised by the fact that this neoplasm is found on the skin areas with the most exposure to sunlight, such as the head and neck (85% of all lesions, including 30% within the nose (DeVita et al., 2001; McCormack et al., 1997).

It is claimed that such substances as arsenic, wood tar, gas pitch, synthetic antimalarial agents or psoralens participate in BCC cancerogenesis (Kordek et al., 2004).

3.2 Risk groups

Age. A peak in the incidence is between 60 and 80 years of age. More than 95% of patients are patients above 65 years old (Kordek et al., 2004) although recently it has been observed that the incidence in the population below 40 years old is growing (The Skin Cancer Foundation, 2008). With age the total period of UV radiation exposure (Average Accumulated Exposure) increases, therefore when a given threshold is exceeded cancerogenesis processes are initiated. Moreover, the reduced immunity and reduced DNA repair and regeneration properties occurring in the elderly also contribute to the increasing incidence of BCC in this age group (Pietrzykowska-Chorążak, 1978).

Sex. Men slightly more frequently suffer from BCC (M/F ratio 1.2) (Brodowski & Lewandowski, 2004). It is probably associated with higher exposure to UV radiation what is a result of different working conditions (usually outdoors) and rarer use of sun screens in the case of men (McCarthy et al., 1999). It should be noted that during the last 30 years the rate of women below 40 years of age suffering from BCC has tripled (The Burden of Skin Cancer, 2008).

Race. People with fair skin type, light blue and grey eyes and with light red and fair hair suffer from BCC more frequently than people with dark skin (Gloster & Neal, 2006; Jabłońska & Chorzelski, 2002; McCarthy et al., 1999).

Fair hair, frequent sunburn and freckles in the childhood are features which are especially associated with BCC development (Bouwes et al., 1996).

Previous BCC treatment. After the first case of BCC in one's life the probability of the second one increases ten times (Marcil & Stern, 2000). In 50% of patients with previously diagnosed BCC other foci will form within 5 years since the first manifestation (Brodowski & Lewandowski, 2004). It is estimated that the likelihood of BCC in such patients is almost 140 times higher that the one in the general population (Aston et al., 1997)

Post-organ transplant patients. In post-organ transplant patients BCC is the most frequent neoplasm and accounts for 35% of all neoplasms occurring in this group of patients. It is estimated that post-organ transplant patients suffer from BCC 65-250 times more frequently than the general population. BCC most frequently occurs in patients after heart and renal transplantation (Jensen et al., 1999).

Higher incidence of BCC in this group is associated with long-term immunosuppressive therapy that reduces the number of CD4+ cells (Viac et al., 1992).

The pharmacological immunosuppression combined with UVB radiation that additionally reduces the number of Langerhans cells (immune properties) leads to increased immunosuppression in the skin and increases the risk of neoplasm (Parrish, 1983).

Leukaemic patients due to immune system dysfunctions are the next group at a risk. BCC most frequently occurs in patients with chronic lymphocytic leukaemia (8-13 times more frequently than in the general population) (Manusow & Weinerman, 1975).

Other risk groups. According to recent opinions risk factors that have not been so widely studied include genetic predisposition (Gailani et al., 1996; Gilbody et al., 1994; Schreiber et al., 1990), freckles (Gilbody et al., 1994) and rich-fat diet (Zak-Prelich et al., 2004) which is low in antioxidants and vitamins (Jeacock, 1998).

3.3 Precancerous lesions

Precancerous lesions are morphologically changed tissues (a pathological process) on the basis of which neoplasm develops more frequently than in other unchanged tissues (Kordek et al., 2004).

BCC most frequently develops in the skin without previous lesions. It can significantly more rarely (contrary to SCC) develop on the basis of precancerous lesions. Precancerous lesions leading to BCC development include:

- post-radiation dermatitis is most frequently induced by X-ray radiation and is characterised by irregular skin thickening accompanied by discolouration, hyperpigmentation, teleangiectasia and scared atrophy (Jabłońska & Chorzelski, 2002).
- It is estimated that in 60% of cases it transforms into BCC (Aston et al., 1997).
- nevus sebaceous of Jadassohn is a superficial, protruding, yellow-pink, irregular nonhairbearing lesion on the head or neck. Its diameter rarely exceeds 3 cm. It is very frequently present since birth or early childhood and the likelihood of its transformation into BCC is 15% (Aston et al., 1997) .
- actinic keratosis is characterised by multifocal, dry, yellow-brown, slightly protruding keratic build-up, sometimes brown spots are present, they are often numerous on the forehead and temples (Jabłońska & Chorzelski, 2002). The risk of neoplastic transformation into BCC is 10% (1/1000/year) (Chicheł & Skowronek, 2005).
- chemical keratosis is a result of exposure to arsenic or wood tar.
- xeroderma pigmentosum is present in patients with a defective system of DNA repair (NER) what leads to the development of multifocal skin cancer and death at a young age (Marks, 1995). Lesions resemble intensified freckles and the skin shows atrophy, discolouration and teleangiectasia (Jabłońska & Chorzelski, 2002).
- other rarer precancerous lesions include inflammatory changes with scars and hypertrophied scars after burn injuries (Jabłońska & Chorzelski, 2002).

Although in the majority of patients with BCC it is possible to find at least one of the above factors it has to be remembered that the risk of BCC development increases in proportion to the number of existing risk factors.

For example, in Australia the incidence of this neoplasm is the highest. The reason for that is the fact that this continent is located close to the equator (much sunlight and UV radiation), its population has fair skin type (emigrants from England and Scotland) and the ozone layer above Australia is gradually decreasing (Marks et al., 1993).

4. Clinical picture

Diagnosis of BCC basing on the clinical picture is associated with many problems. Diagnosis precision among experienced dermatologists ranges from 50% to 70% (Kricker et al., 1990; Presser & Taylor, 1987). The sensitivity of a clinical test is estimated to be 56-90%, and its specificity 75-90% depending on physician's experience (Mogenses & Jemec, 2007). Diagnostic accuracy is enhanced by good lightning, magnification and dermatoscope (Costantino et al., 2006).

Based on the data presented above it can be concluded that BCC diagnosis basing only on a clinical picture is difficult and depends on physician's experience to a large extent. It is often the case that a lesion previously diagnosed as a benign lesion turns out to be BCC following a biopsy and the reversed situation is also common. BCC diagnosis basing on the clinical picture is not of significance in the diagnostic process. A histopathological examination is the only test that can verify and complete the BCC diagnosis.

Several clinical forms of BCC are traditionally distinguished due to various clinical pictures and biological features.

It has to be emphasised that the awareness of their existence may only help distinguish oncologically suspicious lesions, and not diagnose them.

4.1 Clinical forms of BCC (pict. 1)

Nodular BCC (BCC nodosum) (pict. 1a)- This is the most common form of BCC. Its dimensions may range from several millimetres to 1 cm. It is mainly present in the elderly and develops for years. It has a form of a non-inflammatory, glistening nodule or papule with pearly appearance. The bigger it is, the more pearly it becomes and present capillaries are more and more visible, their layout is radial and they form telangiectasias. The skin covering a nodule is very often so thin that even the smallest trauma causes bleeding and ulceration. Repetitive ulceration leads to the formation of a basin in the middle (BCC partim exulcerans) surrounded by an edge consisting of transparent nodules similar to pearls.[44] In its central part clusters with discolouration suggesting melanoma may be visible. In rare cases tenderness occurs. Small nodules that are difficult to distinguish from seborrhoeic warts, moles or psoriasis are a diagnostic problem. Differential diagnosis has to take SCC into account; however, it is darker and lacks a pearly edge, horizontally branching telangiectasias and clusters with discolouration. Lupus tuberculosis is different from nodular BCC in that it has lupus nodules in a scar and lacks a pearly edge; whereas chronic lupus erythematosus can be distinguished by the presence of more advanced inflammation, perifollicular hyperkeratosis and lacks disintegration (Bers & Berkow, 2001; Jabłońska & Chorzelski, 2002).

Pigmented BCC (BCC pigmentosum) - it is an intensely pigmented variant of a nodular form. Differential diagnosis should consider pigmented naevus which is different in that its dimensions do not grow and it lacks a characteristic edge. On the other hand, melanoma grows faster and more frequently occurs in young patients, with dark hair and dark eyes. (Jabłońska & Chorzelski, 2002; The Skin Cancer Foundation)

Ulcerating BCC (BCC exulcerans, ulcus rodens) (pict 1c, 1d) is an ulcer with prominent, heaped-up edges, that tends to bleed and infiltrate stroma. It may penetrate deeply and cause damage to the muscles, cartilage, bones or even eye protective apparatus (rodent ulcer.) It is distinguished from SCC by the presence of a pearly fold and slower course (Jabłońska & Chorzelski, 2002; Raasch & Buettner, 2002).

Morphoeic or sclerosing BCC (BCC morpheiforme) (pict. 1f) is an aggressive variant of BCC and resembles foci of systemic sclerosis. It is most frequently located on the face and has a form of a yellow-white lesion not subject to disintegration, with ill-defined borders. In its central part sclerosis, scarring and telangiectasias are often present. It may grow fast and reach several centimetres within a few months or remain unchanged for many years. Due to ill-defined borders and infiltrations reaching even 7 mm outside a macroscopic border this type of BCC is often resected incompletely and is associated with a high risk of recurrence (Jabłońska & Chorzelski, 2002, Wagner & Casciato, 2000).

Cystic BCC (BCC cysticum) (pict. 1 b) has a form of small, transparent nodules located on the eyelids (Jabłońska & Chorzelski, 2002)

Superficial BCC (BCC superficiale) (pict. 1 e)is a type of BCC that grows especially slowly (months and years, often regression.) It occurs more often in young patients and its form includes numerous, flat, glistening, light pink lesions with well-defined borders, surrounded by a slightly prominent edge. Recent studies regarding a microscopic 3D analysis indicated that different lesions are connected what proves their origin from one focus (Wade & Ackerman, 1978).

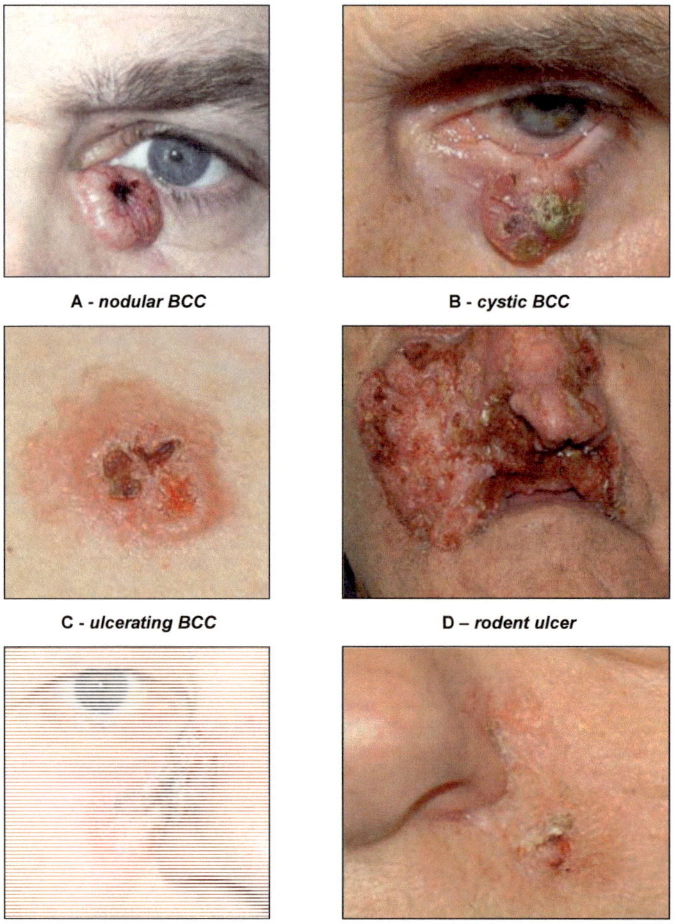

A - *nodular BCC* B - *cystic BCC*

C - *ulcerating BCC* D – *rodent ulcer*

E - *superficial BCC* F – *morphoeic BCC*

Photo 1. Clinical forms of BCC

Photo 1. Clinical forms of BCC

Contrary to other variants this type of BCC is not located on the face, but mainly on the trunk and limbs, what suggests that its cancerogenesis threshold due to UV radiation is lower (McCormack et al., 1997). Its characteristic feature is the fact that the intensity of reddening increases when a lesion is stretched and rubbed. When a lesion is stretched, its glistening surface is visible, and it may show a peripheral, pearly ring or pearly islets inside a lesion. Such lesions are rarely itchy, they rarely bleed or form ulcers. They may be formed after arsenic intoxication and coexist with other types of BCCs. Frequently they are mistaken for Bowen's disease and they can be distinguished from it by the presence of glistening surface, lack of hyperkeratosis and a lighter shade. Some lesions may be similar to psoriasis, pigmented lichen planus, eczema, fungal infections, solar keratosis or even amelanotic melanoma (Australian Cancer Network Management of Non-Melanoma Skin Cancer Working Party, 2002; Jabłońska & Chorzelski, 2002; The Skin Cancer Foundation)

Fibroepithelial BCC (fibroepithelioma) is single or multiple reddish nodules, often pedunculated, located mainly on the back. They resemble fibroma from a clinical point of view (Aston et al., 1997; The Skin Cancer Foundation).

Basal cell nevus syndrome (Gorlin syndrome) is an autosomal dominant hereditary disorder the mutation of which is located in the chromosome 9. Its characteristic features include multiple BCCs coexisting with such abnormalities as palmoplantar pits, skin cysts in the mandible, bifid ribs, calcification of the dura, mental impairment (Aston et al., 1997).

Linear basal cell nevus occurs in the form of several streaks consisting of brownish nodules. Contrary to Gorlin syndrome which is clinically similar this disorder is not hereditary and not associated with abnormalities. It is the rarest variant of BCC (Aston et al., 1997).

In conclusion, the diagnosis of BCC based on the clinical picture is not an easy task, therefore each skin lesion exhibiting some dynamic features, namely growing when compared to adjacent structures, with inflammatory changes, bleeding or crusted should be treated as potentially neoplastic and requires further diagnostics.

4.2 Clinical course

The clinical course of BCC is not characteristic and cannot be predicted: a lesion may not change for years, it may grow slowly or extremely fast, infiltration area may enlarge or recede, it may also ulcerate or tend to heal (Franchimont, 1982). The tendency to heal may lead to decreased vigilance of a physician and their patients, what can be the reason why patients with advanced neoplasia (Table 2.) often report at clinics.

BCC is a locally malignant neoplasm and infiltrates tissues in a three-dimensional fashion, forming fingerlike outgrowths not visible to a naked eye originating from the central part of a tumour (Braun et al., 2005). Their course and range are unpredictable, therefore it is extremely difficult to excise a lesion completely (Raasch & Beuttner, 2002). In the most dangerous cases the infiltrate may spread to the dura, bones, nerves and vessels (Franchimont, 1982).

BCC metastasises really rarely as a result of developed extracellular matrix and preserved epithelial basement membrane (Jabłońska & Chorzelski, 2002). In 1894-2004 only 268 such cases were described, what is less than 0.1% (Ionesco et al., 2006; Weedon & Wall, 1975). Metastases were mainly in patients with a long medical history and after radiation therapy

(Domarus & Stevens, 1984), with histopathologically aggressive BCC located in the central face or near the ear (Randle, 1996) and lesions were larger than 2 cm (>3 cm -2% risk of metastases, >5 cm - 25 %, >10 cm-50%) (Snow et al., 1994) BCCs the most frequently spread along lymphatic vessels and its metastases were mainly observed in the lymph nodes, lungs, bones, pleura, spleen and brain (Safai & Good, 1977).

Mortality due to BCC is low and mainly regards people older than 85 years and patients who did not consent to surgical treatment (Weinstock et al., 1991).

TNM Staging System for Non-melanoma Skin Cancer			
T0	No evidence of primary tumour	**Nx**	Regional lymph nodes cannot be assessed
Tis	Carcinoma in situ	**N0**	No regional lymph node metastasis
T1	Tumour 2.0 cm or less in greatest dimension	**N1**	Regional lymph node metastasis
T2	Tumour more than 2.0 cm but not more than 5.0 cm in greatest dimension	**Mx**	Presence of distant metastasis cannot be assessed
T3	Tumour more than 5.0 cm in greatest dimension	**M0**	No distant metastasis
T4	Tumour infiltrating anatomical structures located under the skin such as bones, cartilage, skeletal muscles etc.	**M1**	Distant metastasis present (includes distant lymph nodes)

Staging			
	T	**N**	**M**
0	Tis	N0	M0
I	T1	N0	M0
II	T2 or T3	N0	M0
III	T4 Each T	N0 N1	M0 M0
IV	Each T	Each N	M1

Table 2. Classification TNM and stages of skin cancers based on AJCC 2002 (AJCC, 2002)

5. BCC diagnostics

5.1 Invasive diagnostics (biopsy)

Despite the fact that clinical features are well described and relatively specific, it should be emphasised that only a result of a histopathological examination can confirm the diagnosis and a biopsy is the gold standard in BCC diagnostics. Some specialists recommend to perform a biopsy in all cases when BCC is suspected. Others recommend it only in diagnostically doubtful cases or when a histological type can affect the choice of a therapeutic method and prognosis (Costantino et al., 2006). There are following types of a biopsy:

Curettage – involves removing neoplastic tissue using a special spoon. Due to the fact that the internal structure of curetted tissues is lost this method is not reliable and currently not recommended (Australian Cancer Network Management of Non-Melanoma Skin Cancer Working Party, 2002).

Shave biopsy – involves cutting the half-thickness skin at a tangent to the skin. It is recommended for superficial BCC, especially if a tumour is multifocal, is present in regression areas and in the case of recurrent disease. A shave biopsy allows for collecting material from a large area. The wound heals fast and leaves no secondary deformations, therefore it can be difficult to locate when a patient returns to continue treatment (a biopsy site should be marked and photographed.) (Australian Cancer Network Management of Non-Melanoma Skin Cancer Working Party, 2002).

Punch biopsy (trepanobiopsy) – a full-thickness skin fragment with the diameter of 4-5 mm is removed with a punch consisting of a metal tube with a sharp edge and a handle.

It is recommended in diagnostics of lesions located in aesthetically and functionally important skin regions (e.g. face.) The repetitive 2-mm punch biopsy may be used to determine poorly demarcated neoplasms (Australian Cancer Network Management of Non-Melanoma Skin Cancer Working Party, 2002).

Incisional biopsy – involves removing a lesion fragment with a healthy skin fragment of usually about 3-4 mm. It is recommended in highly advanced cases and in recurrent disease. It allows for the estimation of infiltration depth, which is of special importance before radiation therapy (Australian Cancer Network Management of Non-Melanoma Skin Cancer Working Party, 2002).

Excisional biopsy – is a diagnostic and therapeutic method. It is recommended in all cases where a defect formed after lesion excision can be sutured without leaving deformities (trunk, limbs.) Not only does it provide information regarding final diagnosis but also informs about the treatment efficacy (completeness). It involves primary excision of a lesion with a margin of clinically normal surrounding tissues. The recommended margin ranges from 2 to 8 mm. Unfortunately, it occurs quite often that clinically normal surrounding tissues are saved to too large an extent and excision is not complete, and as a result neoplastic recurrence is observed (Australian Cancer Network Management of Non-Melanoma Skin Cancer Working Party, 2002).

5.2 Imaging diagnostics

Dermatoscopy includes observing the skin with a dermatoscope consisting of a microscope with 10-100x magnification. In addition, a dermatoscope is equipped with an internal light source that illuminates the skin at an angle of 20°, therefore the picture is enlarged and its resolution is higher. This method is of the greatest importance in the diagnostics of pigmented lesions and melanoma. It makes it possible to distinguish melanoma from pigmented BCC. According to the Monzi criteria pigmented BCC has the following features: lack of pigment network and the presence of one of the following features: maple leaflike areas, spoke wheel areas, large gray-blue ovoid nests, large gray-blue globules, telangiectasias with arborisation and ulceration (Menzies et al., 2000). In the case of nodular BCC in 82% it is possible to observe branching vessels, and the superficial form has delicate and short telangiectasias (Argenziano et al., 2004).

Imaging tests such as computed tomography or magnetic resonance imaging are used to determine the extent of neoplastic infiltration when cartilage, bone, large nerve (Williams et al., 2001), eyeball (Leibovitch et al., 2005, Meads & Greenway, 2006) or parotid gland (Farley et al., 2006) involvement is suspected.

Other modern methods are only of academic interest and do not play important roles in clinical diagnostics. They include:

High resolution ultrasound examination (20-100 Hz) allowing for imaging the skin up to the depth of even 1.1 mm which may be helpful during evaluation of the depth of lesion infiltration (Vogt & Ermert, 2007).

Optical coherence tomography (OCT) (Olmedo et al., 2006) – the mechanism of action is similar to the ultrasound examination; however, infrared light is used instead of ultrasounds – it is possible to visualise skin layers, appendages and vessels (Welzel et al., 1997) ; nevertheless, it is not possible to see the basement membrane or to evaluate the depth of infiltration (Welzel et al., 2003).

Confocal microscopy (RCM, reflectance confocal microscopy and FLSM, fluorescence confocal laser scanning microscopy) (Ulrich et al., 2008)- involving the detection of endogenous (RCM) or exogenous (FLSM) dye with special light, what makes it possible to visualise cells and cell structures with the precision nearly as good as the one of a histopathological examination (Swindle et al., 2003a; Swindle et al., 2003b).

Photodynamic diagnostics (PDD) involves the detection of light (using electromagnetic waves) emitted from tissues after fluorescence excitation (Morawiec et al., 2004).

Spectrometric diagnostics involves differentiation and evaluation of the excitation spectrum of healthy tissue and tissues with dysplastic or neoplastic lesions (Sieroń et al., 2007).

Fluorescence lifetime imaging methods (FLIM) - this time is different for healthy tissues and neoplastic tissues (Galletly et al., 2008).

6. BCC: Therapeutic options

BCC treatment is managed by physicians of many specialities. Dermatologists often use cryotherapy and remove small lesions located on the face and trunk, small eyelid neoplasms belong to ophthalmologists, lesions on the nose and ear are resected by ENT specialists, whereas dental surgeons remove lesions located in the area of the mouth cavity. Lesions the size of which makes it possible to direct closure are also excised by general surgeons and even by general practitioners in some countries (Australian Cancer Network Management of Non-Melanoma Skin Cancer Working Party, 2002). In the treatment of more extensive and advanced BCC cases in order to cover a defect after neoplasm excision it is necessary to use different reconstruction methods, what is possible only in specialist centres of plastic, maxillary or oncological surgery.

As there are many specialists managing BCC treatment, there are also numerous and different therapeutic options. They can be divided into destructive methods where neoplastic tissue is destroyed and it is not possible to evaluate a histopathological type or procedure completeness, and surgical methods involving the excision of neoplastic tissue with a margin of clinically normal surrounding tissues.

Destructive methods include:

- local immunotherapy using imiquimod-containing ointment that stimulates and intensifies a local anti-inflammatory reaction what leads to BCC regression (Marks et al., 2001).
- photodynamic therapy, which uses the fact that some photosensitive substances, namely substances absorbing light of specific wavelength accumulate in neoplastic tissues. When they are selectively accumulated in the neoplastic tissue the lesion is exposed to laser light at the wavelength absorbed by a given photosensitive substance. Consequently, the high levels of radiation energy are accumulated in the neoplastic tissue and it becomes destroyed (Morawiec et al., 2004).
- radiation therapy, combining many methods starting from superficial radiation (up to 170 kV) in the case of lesions with the depth up to 6 mm, to electron beam radiation and brachytherapy (Telfer et al., 2008).
- curettage, which is often combined with other methods such as: coagulation (Reymann, 1985), imiquimod (Wu et al., 2006), photodynamic therapy (Soler et al., 2001), cryosurgery (Nordin & Stenquist, 2002) or surgery (Chiller et al., 2000; Johnson et al., 1991).
- cryosurgery, which involves the destruction of neoplastic tissue during one or several cycles of freezing using liquid nitrogen (Graham, 1983).
- CO_2 laser is a new therapeutic option still studied in clinical trials (Telfer et al., 2008).
- local application of fluorouracil (5-FU)-containing ointment, which is a classic cytostatic. Further studies are necessary to evaluate its long-term efficacy (Telfer et al., 2008).

The destructive methods presented above may be used only in some highly selected cases. Appropriate patient qualification combined with experience of a specialist using a given therapeutic method may provide good therapeutic effects.

As BCC, contrary to other malignant neoplasms, is rarely responsible for patient's death, 5-year survival as an outcome measure is not justified. For that reason, in order to assess the efficacy of BCC treatment the recurrence rate during a 5-year follow-up period is used. Moreover, it is necessary to take cosmetic and functional results and treatment comfort into account.

Currently it is difficult to evaluate unanimously which destructive method is the best. It is a result of the fact that current literature lacks in prospective trials comparing different methods and that the criteria of patients' qualification are extremely narrow and suitable only for individual methods, therefore it is not possible to compare them objectively. It is commonly thought that each method is good if it is applied in an appropriate case by an experienced specialist.

Surgical methods include classic excision of a lesion with a margin of clinically normal surrounding tissues and Mohs micrographic surgery that involves staged resection of a lesion with intraoperational histopathological evaluation of its edges.

6.1 Selecting a therapeutic method

In order to determine the indications for different methods, prognostic factors predicting BCC with a high-risk of recurrence have been identified.

6.2 Prognostic factors

Tumour site - a significantly higher risk of recurrence compared to the trunk and neck (recurrence in 0.5%) was observed for BCC located on the face (lateral canthal region – 43% of recurrence, upper lid and eyebrow 33%, nose 19%), ear (24%) and scalp. Some specialists think that it is associated with a specifical anatomical structure of the subcutaneous tissue of these areas, which creates a risk of deeper invasion (Monney & Parry, 2007).

Other specialists make attempts to explain a higher risk of recurrence in the central face (17.5% of recurrence vs 8.6% for other parts of the face) by the fact that a neoplasm changes its way of spreading from horizontal to vertical, what is reflected by the fact that infiltration spreads along embryonic connections between facial buds (Włodarkiewicz & Muraszko-Kuźma, 1998; Wronkowski et al., 1978).

Based on the risk of recurrence, the following areas can be distinguished: high risk of recurrence (H), middle risk of recurrence (M) and low risk (L) (Figure 1.).

However, it has to be emphasised that the above division into risk areas is based on a series of retrospective studies that analysed recurrence sites following surgical treatment. The margin of a clinically normal surrounding tissues resected with a lesion was not taken into account.

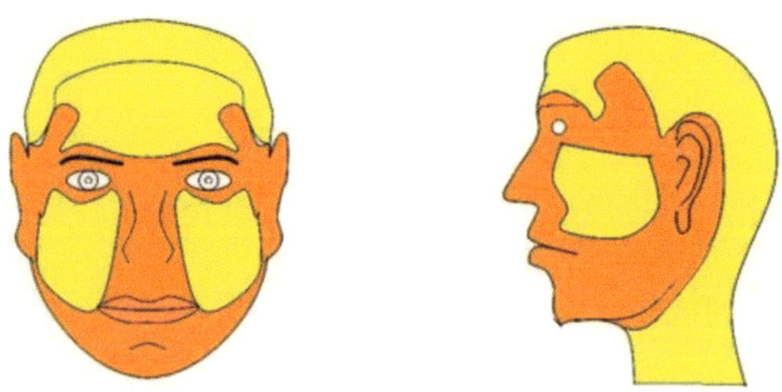

- H area (high risk) - "mask area" (central face, eyelids, eyebrows, periorbital area, nose, lips, chin, mandible, temples, preauricular and postauricular area, ear), genitalia, hands, feet.

- M zone (middle risk) – cheeks, forehead, scalp, neck

- L zone (low risk) – trunk and extremities

Fig. 1. Recurrence risk areas (Swanson, 1983)

According to the authors more frequent recurrences in the H zone may be associated with the fact that a smaller margin of clinically normal surrounding tissues is applied in these face areas. It is a result of the fact that operators are afraid of poor aesthetical and functional effects. For example, applying a larger margin in the medial canthal region could deform and disturb the functions of the eye protective apparatus. In other risk areas (M or L area) e.g. on the neck or the trunk it is possible to resect lesions with larger margins of clinically normal surrounding tissues, what has no significant effects on aesthetical and functional results; however, it will significantly increase completeness of excision.

Tumour size and depth of invasion – the recurrence rate increases with the increasing size of a tumour. Depending on a diameter the recurrence rate in a 5-year follow-up period is as follows for the following tumour sizes: <1.5cm-12%, >3cm-23.1% (Dubin & Kopf, 1983). In other studies: <1cm-3.2%, 1-2cm–8%, >2cm recurrence in almost 1/3 of cases (Włodarkiewicz & Muraszko-Kuźma, 1998; Wronkowski et al., 1978).

Moreover, invasion of structures lying under the skin such as cartilages and bones is associated with a higher risk of recurrence.

The guidelines of National Comprehensive Cancer Network (NCCN), an American organisation studying therapeutic algorithms for treatment of neoplasms, combine tumour site and size in order to assess the recurrence risk (Diagram 2.)

Definition of clinical margins – the recurrence risk for lesions with ill-defined clinical tumor borders is higher than for lesions with well-defined borders (Rowe et al., 1989).

Histological subtype of BCC – for some morphological subtypes, e.g. morpheaform, infiltrating, micronodular or mixed types, the recurrence risk is higher (Table 3.) (Costantino et al., 2006 ; Włodarkiewicz & Muraszko-Kuźma, 1998).

Lesion excision with a classic margin is incomplete in 6.4% for a nodular lesion, for a superficial lesion – 3.6%, for a micronodular lesion – 18.6%, for an infiltrating lesion - 26%, for a morpheaform lesion – 33.3% (Mooney & Parry, 2007). Moreover, histological features of infiltration, especially perineural and perivascular involvement, are significant risk factors of recurrence (Costantino et al., 2006).

Non-aggressive growth pattern (well circumscribed, low recurrence rate)	**Aggressive growth pattern (poor circumscribed, high recurrence rate)**
Nodular subtypes (approx. 50%): - nodular-solid (nodularis-solidum) - nodular-adenoid (nodularis adenoides, nodularis cribriforme) - nodular-cystic (nodularis – cysticum)	Infiltrating (5-20%) (infiltrativum, infiltrative non-sclerosing, styloides) Morpheaform (approx.5%) (sclerodermiforme, morpheiforme, morphea-like, sclerosans, sclerotic, cicatrisans, infiltrative sclerosing)
Keratotic (keratoticum)	Micronodular (micronodulare)
Pigmented (pigmentosum)	Metatypic (matatypicum, baso-spinocellulare)
Fibroepithelial (fibroepithelioma, Pinkus tumour)	Superficial multifocal (15%) (superficiale multicentricum, Arning)

Table 3. Clinical-pathological classification of BCC (WHO 2006) and classification based on the recurrence risk (Bieniek et al., 2008; Kossard et al., 2006).

Recurrent BCC - treatment of recurrent BCC is associated with a significantly higher recurrence rate than treatment of primary lesions (Australian Cancer Network Management of Non-Melanoma Skin Cancer Working Party, 2002).

Immunosuppression - is associated not only with a higher risk of BCC in general, but also with a higher recurrence rate.[39]

BCC in patients after organ transplantation and leukaemic patients constitute a special problem.

Other prognostic factors, which are mentioned more rarely: age <35 years (Boeta-Angeles & Bennet, 1998), a reconstruction method after surgical excision (recurrent disease within the first year when full-thickness skin is grafted, after two years when split-thickness skin is grafted and within 4 years after local tissue transfers) (Koplin & Zarem, 1980; Richmond & Davie, 1987). Prognosis for Gorlin syndrome treatment is also poor (Gorlin, 1995).

The presence or lack of such features makes it possible to divide all types of BCC into high or low-risk lesions, therefore it is possible to select an appropriate therapeutic method. The latest guidelines for BCC treatment suggested by the British and American Scientific Societies are outlined (Diagram 1 and 2).

As it can be concluded from the guidelines, all high- and low-risk BCC as well as recurrent BCC may be surgically treated.

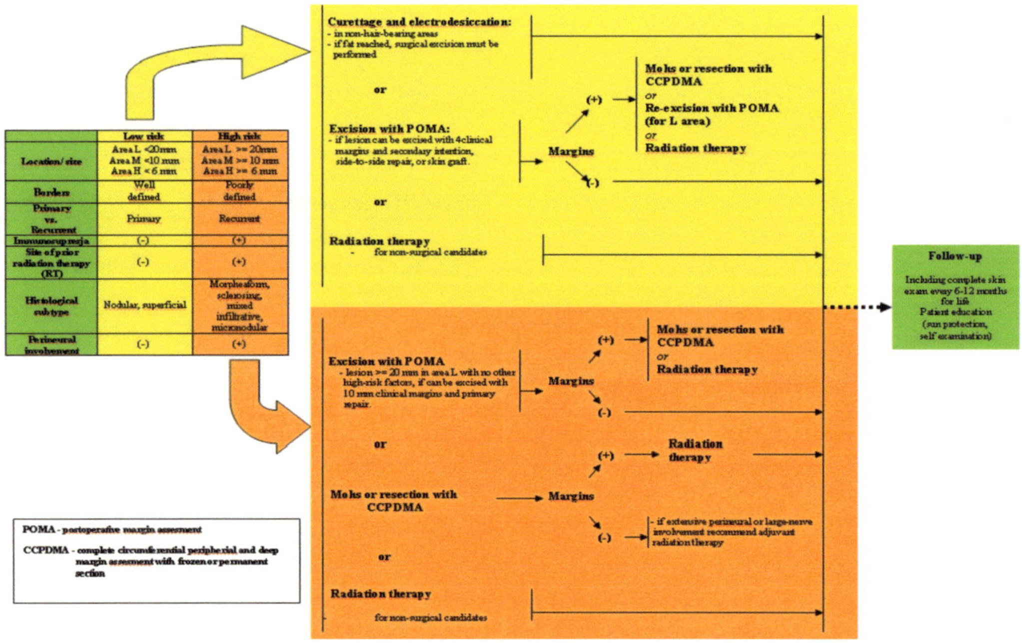

Diagram 1. Guidelines for BCC treatment based on *NCNN Clinical Practice Guidelines in Oncology: Basal Cell and Squamous Cell Skin Cancers* (USA, 01.2009)

Surgery is currently the gold standard for BCC treatment because of high efficacy, its versatility, fast results, good aesthetical and functional outcome, low risk of complication, availability (the majority of mentioned destructive methods can only be applied in highly specialized clinics), low costs of treatment and what is even more important, the possibility to evaluate procedure completeness (Bath-Hextall et al., 2007).

PRIMARY BCC

BCC type: histology, size*, site**	PDT	Imiquimod	Curettage and cautery	Radiation therapy	Cryosurgery	Excision	Mohs surgery
Superficial, small and low-risk site	++	++	++	?	++	?	X
Nodular, small and low-risk site	+	-	++	?	++	+++	X
Infiltrative, small and low-risk site	X	X	+	+	+	+++	?
Superficial, large and low-risk site	+++	++	++	+	++	+	?
Nodular, large and low-risk site	-	-	++	++	++	+++	?
Infiltrative, large and low-risk site	X	X	-	+	+	+++	++
Superficial, small and high-risk site	+	+	+	++	+	++	+
Nodular, small and high-risk site	-	-	+	++	++	+++	++
Infiltrative, small and high-risk site	X	X	-	+	+	++	+++
Superficial, large and high-risk site	+	+	-	+	+	++	++
Nodular, large and high-risk site	-	X	X	-	+	++	++
Infiltrative, large and high-risk site	X	X	X	X	X	+	+++

RECURRENT BCC

BCC type: histology, size*, site**	PDT	Imiquimod	Curettage and cautery	Radiation therapy	Cryosurgery	Excision	Mohs surgery
Superficial, small and low-risk site	++	+	+	+	++	++	-
Nodular, small and low-risk site	-	X	++	++	++	+++	-
Infiltrative, small and low-risk site	X	X	-	++	++	+++	+
Superficial, large and low-risk site	++	+	+	++	++	+	+
Nodular, large and low-risk site	X	X	-	+	+	+++	+
Infiltrative, large and low-risk site	X	X	-	+	+	++	++
Superficial, small and high-risk site	?	X	+	+	+	++	++
Nodular, small and high-risk site	X	X	+	+	+	+++	++
Infiltrative, small and high-risk site	X	X	X	+	+	++	+++
Superficial, large and high-risk site	?	X	X	+	-	++	++
Nodular, large and high-risk site	X	X	X	-	-	++	+++
Infiltrative, large and high-risk site	X	X	X	-	-	+	+++

+++ *probable treatment of choice,* ++ *generally good choice,* + *generally fair choice,* ? *reasonable, but not often needed,* - *generally poor choice,*
X *probably should not be used*

* *size: small <2cm, large >2cm*
** high-risk site *(central face, especially around the eses, nose, lips and ears), low-risk site (other sites)*
PDT – *photodynamic therapy*

Diagram 2. Treatment of BCC based on *Guidelines for the Management of Basal Cell Carcinoma* (UK, 07.2008 r.)

7. Surgical treatment

7.1 Surgical excision with a margin of clinically normal surrounding tissues

Surgical treatment is the simplest, the most effective and nowadays the most popular method of treatment. Its efficacy evaluated as the recurrence rate in a 5-year follow-up is 2-10% (Cullen et al., 1993; Goldberg et al., 1989; Griffiths et al., 2005; Silverman et al., 1992; Walker et al., 2006). So far only few prospective studies comparing surgical excision with other methods have been published in the literature.

Thissen compared cryosurgery (spray technique and double cycle of freezing) with surgical treatment of nodular and superficial BCC of the head and neck with the diameter of <2cm and observed better therapeutic outcomes in surgically treated patients; however, the differences were not statistically significant (Thissen et al., 2000).

On the other hand, Rhodes compared surgical treatment of nodular BCC located on the face with photodynamic therapy (PDT.) He did not observe significant differences in recurrence rates during the first 3 months; however, in 12- and 24-month follow-up he observed a statistically significant increase in the recurrence rate and worse cosmetic results in the case of PDT (Rhodes et al., 2004). Taking into account long-term results (after 60 months), recurrence occurred in 14% after PDT and only in 4% after surgical treatment (Rhodes et al., 2007).

Moreover, another study where surgical excision of primary BCCs with the diameter below 4 cm was compared with radiation therapy indicated that during a 4-year follow-up a lower recurrence rate was associated with surgical excision (0.7% vs 7.5%.) Moreover, cosmetic results after surgical excision were more acceptable than the ones after radiation therapy (79% vs 40%), which were associated with discolouration and telangiectasia in more than 65% and radiodystrophy in 41% of cases (Avril et al., 1997; Petit et al., 2000).

An important stage in surgical excision of a lesion is the determination of a macroscopic (clinical) lesion border. It can be done using magnification (3x at least), Wood's lamp or dermatoscope (Costantino et al., 2006). Applying curettage before excision may increase the completeness of a procedure because it may be possible to determine real borders of a tumour more precisely (neoplastic tissues are more curettable) (Chiller et al., 2000; Johnson et al., 1991). When lesion borders have been precisely determined a margin (range) of clinically normal tissue is planned, and they are removed together with a lesion en-block. The specimen resected in this way is subject to histopathological evaluation during which a histopathological subtype of BCC is confirmed as well as procedure completeness. The tissue defect formed after lesion excision is closed according to the reconstructive ladder.

7.2 Margin of clinically normal surrounding tissue

It is obvious that the extent of neoplastic infiltration affects the range of a peripheral and deep margin. On the other hand, the infiltration extent correlates with prognostic factors (Telfer et al., 2008) e.g. for primary morpheaform BCC resected with a 3-mm margin only 66% of radical excisions observed, with a 5-mm margin - 82% and with a 13-15-mm more than 95%. For that reason, the presence of prognostic factors should determine the extent of a margin. Nonetheless, a precise therapeutic algorithm has so far not been established (Telfer et al., 2008). The extent of suggested margins ranges from 2 to 15 mm (Table 4), is established empirically and what is the most important, it does not take prognostic factors into account.

As reports published so far are in the majority retrospective reviews of therapeutic outcomes for different margins, their conclusions should be treated more like advices rather than methodologically proven guidelines.

Although American recommendations of NCCN (National Comprehensive Cancer Network) recommend to remove low-risk BCCs with a 4-mm margin it has to be noted that, what is emphasised by the authors of these recommendations, this guideline was based on lower-level evidence (Clinical Practice Guidelines in Oncology, 2009). It is based on the prospective report by Wolf from 1987 (Table 4) where 117 primary lesions were resected with a 2-mm margin with subsequent histopathological evaluation according to Mohs. If excision was incomplete, the margin of resected tissues was expanded by 1 mm until the procedure was complete. When lesions were excised with 2-mm margins, completeness of 70% was achieved, with 3-mm margins excisions were complete in 85% of cases and when margins were 4 mm completeness was as high as 95%. Although these results are statistically significant, they are poorly reliable because the study did not take into account prognostic factors that have been identified until now. The study lacks in information regarding the site of a tumour, its histopathological subtype and regards only

Author	Suggested margin	Primary /recurrent	Site (%)	Size (mm)	Histological subtype (%)	Incomplete excision(%)	Recurrence (%)
Conway[59]	3-4 mm – intraperative frozen section control	114/0	medial/lateral canthus – 48,2 / 17,5 upper/lower lid – 33,4 / 0,9	mean 13,3 (2-32)	infiltrative – 21 others – 79	no data	0%
	4- 8 mm – conventional histopathological techniques	31/0	medial/lateral canthus – 35,5 / 22,6 upper/lower lid – 41,9 / 0	mean 12,9 (5-18)	infiltrative – 22,6 others – 77,4	no data	9,7
Beirne[60]	5-10 mm	169/0	no data	no data	no data	0 (10 mm margin)	no data
Bart[61]	3-5 mm	468/27	cheek – 18,1 lips – 1,1 forehead – 14,5 nose – 20,9 ear – 1,9 neck – 6,4 extremities- 7,5 trunk – 14,1 orbital region - 4,9 scalp – 4,1	0-5 – 22% 6-10 – 40,3% 11-15 – 20,7% 16-20 – 7,2% >20 – 9,8%	no data	6,8	no data
Emmett[62]	3 - 8 mm - nodular 3-10 mm - infiltrative, multifocal, poor-circumscribed >10mm - recurence	1411/258	head and neck – 75,5% trunk – 8,4% extremities - 16 %	no data	no data	12,7 (primary BCC) 0,7 (recurrent BCC)	no data
Epstein[63]	2mm - size < 10mm	131	b.d.	mean 8 (3-20)	nodular - 73 infiltrative – 6 superficial – 21	6 (1 mm margin) 2 (2 mm margin)	no data
Bisson[64]	3 mm	100	cheek – 19 nose – 25 forehead – 11 ear – 4 temple – 18 neck – 1 extremities – 10 trunk – 5 orbital region – 12 scalp – 2	mean 8,9 (1-30)	nodular – 68 micronodular- 6 superficial – 12 morpheaform -3 infiltrative - 4 others - 7	4	no data
Thomas[24]	4 mm – poor-circumscribed; 3mm -well-circumscriced	91	head and neck – 51	mean 12,1 (53% > 10 mm)	nodular -63 infiltrative – 10 superficial – 16 morpheaform – 2	4	no data
Hsuan[57]	2 mm	55	upper/lower lid – 56 / 11 medial/lateral canthus – 23,6 / 3,6 forehead – 0,5% cheek – 0,5 %	no data	no data	18	no data
Griffith[66]	3mm - well-circumscribed 10mm - poor-circumscribed and >10mm	634/49	cheek – 14,2 ear – 3,2 nose – 21,1 chin – 2,2 forehead - 21,0 neck – 4,9 extremities – 2,9 trunk – 5,5 orbital region – 9 scalp – 6,8	<5 – 38% 6-10 – 38,2% 11-20 – 17,5% 21-30 – 4,5% >30 – 1,8%	no data	no data	0,9
Breuninger[65]	7 mm	1757/259	forehead - 9,6 temple – 9,7 cheek – 10,2 neck – 2,6 nose – 17,1 scalp – 2,6 lower lid – 3,3 ear – 5,4 med./lateral canthus - 5,1 lips – 4,6	<10 – 48% 10-20 – 30% >20 – 9%	solidum -52 morpheaform - 13 superficial – 14 mixed – 20	46,7 (2 mm margin) 20,7 (4 mm margin) 14,7 (6-8 mm margin)	no data
Wolf[67]	4 mm - < 2 cm, well-circumscribed , non-aggressive growth pattern	177/0	no data	< 10 - 62% 10-20 – 29% >20 - 9%	no data	5 (4 mm margin) 15 (3 mm margin) 30 (2mm margin)	no data
Griffiths[68]	2-3 mm – well-circumscribed 5 mm - poor-circumscribed	1539	forehead - 10 temple – 14 cheek – 9 ear – 8 nose – 22 lips – 3 orbital region – 9 scalp – 5 neck – 5 trunk – 5 extremities– 10	no data	no data	8,4	
Collin[69]	3-5 mm	226/10	Lower/upper lid – 37,6 / 6,7 medial/ lateral canthus – 38,4 / 7,9	<5 – 25,2% 5-10 – 33,6% 10-20 -37,6% >25 – 3,6%	solidum - >50%	no data	2,3%

Table 4. Range of excision margin – analysis of selected studies.

well-demarcated lesions, and in 91% of cases the tumour diameter was below 2 cm, and the mean was 9 mm. Due to low reliability of studies published so far the need to perform prospective studies according to evidence based medicine (EBM) arises as it is necessary to determine unanimously the range of margins depending on prognostic factors. It is of special importance when BCCs are located in functionally and aesthetically important face areas such as nose (ala nasi, columella, naso-facial sulcus), eyelids, medial and lateral canthus, ear with preauricular and postauricular region, lips philtrum (Chicheł & Skowronek, 2005; Mohs & Parry, 2007). All anatomical regions mentioned above are associated with a high risk of recurrence (H -area– Figure 1), and the differences in suggested margin are extremely important although they are as small as several millimetres. The excision of a lesion with a larger margin may for example result in the removal of lacrimal ducts or cause ectropion. For that reason, during margin selection a surgeon resecting a lesion in these areas (a suggested margin for the face is from 2 to 10 mm) has to take into account such aspects as post-surgical function preservation, possibility of defect closure or, last but not least, achieving acceptable cosmetic results.

As it can be seen, due to varied and often not very reliable recommendations, the decision to choose an oncologically radical margin is extremely difficult and in most cases made based on operator's experience (his knowledge and skills.)

Prospective trials taking into account all factors affecting the range of a margin (including prognostic factors) would systematise the current state of knowledge and contribute to establishing consensus regarding the excision margins, what is indispensable in order to prepare a consistent algorithm for BCC treatment.

The deep margin range is less controversial. The majority of authors recommend to resect BCCs at the depth reaching the fat tissue (Telfer et al., 2008). In BCCs where the skin is directly above deep tissues (cartilages, bones) it is obligatory to perform imaging tests and if necessary, increase the depth of a margin (Australian Cancer Network Management of Non-Melanoma Skin Cancer Working Party, 2002).

7.3 Histopathological evaluation

In order to determine the location of a resected tumour with relation to the adjacent tissues, each specimen indicated for a histopathological examination should be equipped with a surgical marker (suture, cut, dye mark) and a precise diagram presenting its location with relation to the adjacent tissues. As a result, it will be possible to identify sites where excision was incomplete. Moreover, information regarding previous treatment and results of a biopsy are also necessary (Australian Cancer Network Management of Non-Melanoma Skin Cancer Working Party, 2002).

The aim of a histopathological examination is to determine a histological subtype of BCC and excision completeness.

From a histopathological point of view BCC is similar to the basement membrane cells but differs in that the nucleus/cytoplasm ratio is higher.

Moreover, BCC cells do not have intercellular bridges and mitotic figures (Bader, 2008).

According to the latest WHO classification there are several clinical-pathological types of BCC. It includes criteria of a clinical and histopathological picture of different subtypes of BCC (Kossard et al., 2006).

From a clinical point of view it is important to distinguish histopathological subtypes with a aggressive growth pattern, what is of importance when a surgical procedure is planned (Table 3.) In addition, infiltration along vessels and nerves is dangerous, and associated with a high risk of recurrence (Costantiono, 2006).

The literature also describes undifferentiated and differentiated BCC. Little or no differentiation is reffered to as a solid BCC and includes pigmented, superficial, morpheaform and infiltrative subtypes. Differentiated BCC is mainly nodular BCC which often differentiates into cutaneous appendages, including hair, sebaceous or tubular glands (Bader, 2008). For statistical purposes the classification including three types is often used: nodular (solid), fibrosing (desmoplastic) and metatypic (baso-spinocellular) (Bieniek et al., 2008). Based on precise histopathological evaluation it was determined that neoplastic infiltration is irregular and unpredictable; however, it is usually present to a limited extent (Burg et al. 1975).

The margin of clinically normal surrounding tissues viewed under a microscope is on average smaller by 24% from a macroscopic in vivo margin as a result of shrinking and fixing (Thomas et al., 2003).

Hendrix et al. proved that infiltration in the case of infiltrating BCC is on average 7.2 mm, whereas for nodular BCC it is 4.7 mm (primary /recurrent 5.6/10.4 vs 4.3/5.7 respectively) (Hendrix & Parlette, 1996). On the other hand, according to Salasche primary morpheaform BCC can infiltrate tissues even up to the width of 7 mm beyond macroscopic borders of a lesion (Salasche et al., 1981). Based on Burg's studies microscopic borders of primary BCC infiltration are estimated to be 3-6 mm, and 5-9 mm in the case of recurrent disease (Burg et al., 1975).

The most important factor determining the recurrence is to determine the extent of neoplastic infiltration and its relation to the edge of resection (Australian Cancer Network Management of Non-Melanoma Skin Cancer Working Party, 2002). It regards cases where tumor was identified at peripheral edge of resection and deep edge of resection what is associated with a more than a double risk of recurrence (17% peripheral vs 35% deep surgical edge in a 5-year follow-up period) (Liu et al., 1991).

In order to evaluate the risk of recurrence Pascal (Pascal et al., 1986) made the following classification:

- incomplete excision – a tumor is identified at a surgical edge. It is associated with a 33% risk of recurrence within 5 years follow-up.
- suboptimal excision - tumor is visible at the distance smaller than 0.5 mm from a surgical edge, what microscopically corresponds to one high-power field (400x.) In such cases there is a 12% risk of recurrence within 5 years follow-up.
- complete excision – tumor is visible at the distance larger than 0.5 mm, namely it is not present in one high-power field (400x) involving a surgical edge.

Although resecting a tumor in these cases is described as complete excision it is associated with a 1.2% risk of recurrence within 5 years follow-up.

It is mainly associated with the fact that histopathological techniques are not perfect. Conventional microscoping processing involves vertical sectioning at every 2-4 μm, perpendicular to the tumor surface (breadloaf sectioning -recommended for lesions <16 mm) (Rapini, 1990), when specimens from all four lesion quadrants are resected (cross sectioning – recommended >16 mm) (Rapini, 1990) or from its peripheral parts (peripheral sectioning) (Mohs & Parry, 2007) (Fig. 2: A, B, C.). Consequently, only representative vertical sections are evaluated and it is not possible to evaluate the whole tumor margin. It is claimed that using conventional methods it is possible to evaluate only from 0.01% to 44% of tumor margins (Kimyai-Asadi et al., 2005; Mohs & Parry, 2007).

The basic drawback of this method is an assumption that when a tissue margin in representative sections is considered as tumor-free, the whole lesion is considered to be excised completely. The method suggested by Mohs is significantly more precise than conventional techniques as it allows for collecting sections which are horizontal to the tumor surface, namely it is possible to evaluate the whole margin (Fig. 2:D.)

7.4 Incomplete excision

Incomplete excision of BCC is a situation when a tumor is identified at surgical edge or is at the distance of <0.5 mm from it (one high-power field at 400x magnification.) On average 4.7% - 7% (Griffiths, 1999; Kumar et al., 2000) of cases in the UK and 6.3% in Australia (Dieu & Macleod, 2002; Sussman & Liggins, 1996) are excised incompletely. These numbers prove that a problem is huge and although factors responsible for an increased risk of incomplete excision have already been identified until now it has not been possible to create a consistent algorithm of BCC management. The necessity to improve procedure completeness is undeniable; however, management following incomplete excision (follow-up, reexcision, radiation therapy) raises many controversies.

Followers of follow-up base their opinions on numerous studies proving that recurrent disease will occur only in 30-41% of cases (De Silva & Dellon, 1985; Park et al., 1994; Sussman & Liggins, 1996) out of all incompletely excised lesions, so as many as 2/3 of tumor tissue left in the skin will not recur.

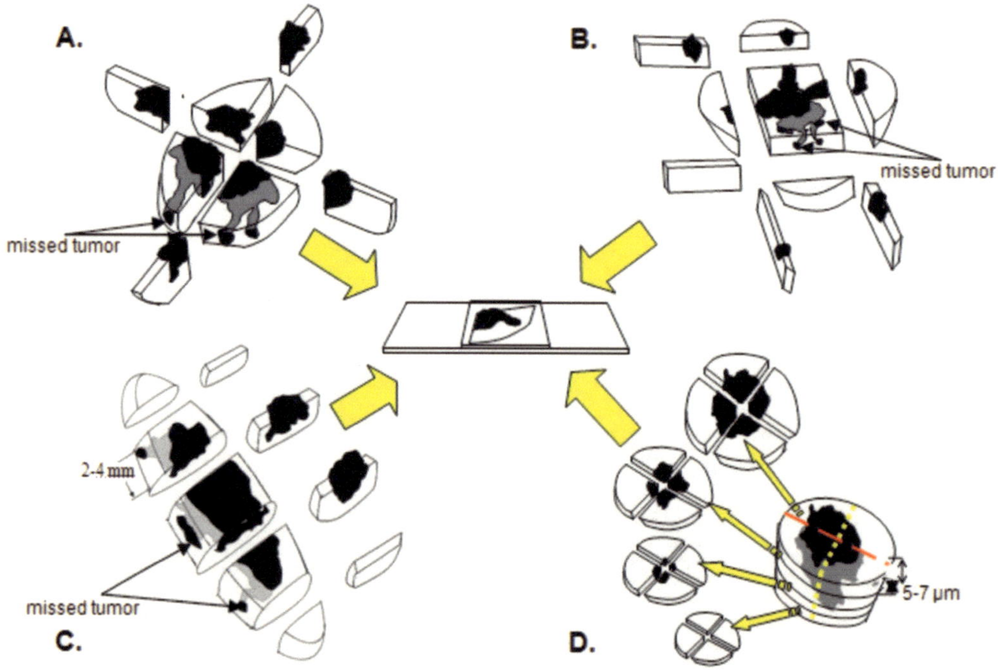

Fig. 2. Methods of microscopic processing: cross sectioning (A), peripheral sectioning (B), breadloaf sectioning (C), Mohs method (D).

In addition, prospective studies where incompletely excised BCCs were reexcised showed the presence of tumor tissue only in 45% (Wilson et al., 2004) and 54% (Griffiths, 1999) using conventional histopathological evaluation and 55% using the Mohs method (Bieley et al., 1992). It means that in almost half of cases the tumor tissue which was left regresses, possibly with the help of the immune system (Bieley et al., 1992).

Is a reexcision of an incompletely excised tumor justified?

Richmond et al. included in their study 92% patients who underwent reexcision of an incompletely excised tumors and 90% patients who were only observed (until recurrence occur, then it was excised immediately.) After a 10-year follow-up period recurrence occurred only in 9% of patients in the first group and in as many as 60% of patients in the other (Richmond & Davie, 1987).

Koplin recommends reexcision only in two cases: when a tumor is identified at surgical edge and when a tumor was excised suboptimally; however, only when expected life-time is long (Koplin & Zarem, 1980).

On the other hand, Robinson recommends only follow-up in the case of incomplete excision of an aggressive histopathological subtypes of BCC located on the nose, cheeks, around the lips, in men >65 years and in the case when a flap or split-thickness skin graft was used to cover a defect. His stand is based on the observation that in cases mentioned above significantly longer time is required for recurrence development (>5 years) than in other cases of BCC excised incompletely (Robinson & Fischer, 1996).

Similar controversies are associated with the use of radiation therapy following incomplete BCC excision. In a 10-year follow-up Liu compared the number of recurrence in the group of patients after immediate post-operative radiation therapy with the group of observed patients. Although in the group of patients subject to post-operative radiation therapy the recurrence rate was significantly lower the evaluation of all treatment aspects (costs analysis, complications) indicated that it is only recommended in cases after recurrence and when deep and lateral margins are involved. In the remaining cases the authors recommend careful observation stating a high presence of patients on follow-up examinations and significantly lower treatment costs as arguments for it (Liu et al., 1991).

On the other hand Wilson et al. recommend radiation therapy or reexcision of a tumor following its incomplete excision when a local flap or full-thickness skin graft was applied and when a deep margin in the H zone was involved. In all such cases recurrence would be difficult to detect and treat. In addition, Wilson does not recommend radiation therapy in young patients, especially in the forehead and scalp due to the risk of neoplastic transformation in scarred lesions in a long-term follow-up. In such cases, as well as in the cases of histologically aggressive BCC reexcision is recommended (Wilson et al., 2004).

Some authors have even more restrictive views on radiation therapy and they recommend it only in small lesions in patients who do not agree surgical treatment or in whom it is not possible to perform a surgery due to their physical condition (Australian Cancer Network Management of Non-Melanoma Skin Cancer Working Party, 2002).

7.5 Recurrence

Recurrence is defined as a new focus of tumor in a scar or in its vicinity formed after excision of a primary tumor occurring within 5 years since the excision and with the same histological type as the primary tumor. The incidence rate after surgical treatment of BCC in a 5-year follow-up is estimated to be 5% for primary and about 13% for recurrence BCC (Hauben et al., 1982). The factors increasing the risk of recurrence have been discussed in the Part II. Recurrence is the most frequent, namely as many as 82% of cases occur in the first five years, and about 30% of cases are present in the first year of observation, 50% in the second and 66% in the third year. The remaining 18% of cases occur in the period from 5 to 10 years since tumor excision (Marcil & Stern, 2000). The recommended follow-up for one patient in order to observe recurrence is 5 years (every 3 months during the first year, then every 6 months) (Liu et al., 1991) although the latest guidelines of the American NCCN recommend follow-up every 6-12 months for the whole lifetime (Clinical Practice Guidelines in Oncology, 2009). During follow-up control it is necessary to educate a patient with the possibilities of active prophylaxis against BCC, especially regarding sun protection. Moreover, it is also necessary to inform a patient about the need of skin self-examination. It is of special importance not only because of recurrence monitoring but also due to the risk of development of another BCC which is ten times higher in patients with a previous BCC than in the general population (Marcil & Stern, 2000). This risk is also significantly higher in elderly patients, in patients with multiple BCCs and with the lesion diameter > 1cm (Van Iersen, 2005).

In some countries general practitioners manage follow-up control after BCC excision (Park et al., 1994).

Clinical symptoms that should raise suspicion of recurrence:

- scarring with non-healing or recurrent ulceration,
- a scar that is becoming red, desquamating and looks like ichtyosis,
- an expanding scar with telangiectasia inside the scar
- a nodule appearing within a scar
- tissue destruction

Recurrence following non-surgical treatment (radiation therapy, cryotherapy, curettage) is associated with a higher risk of another recurrence or even with the possibility of metastases (Smith & Grande, 1991). Skin lesions due to such treatment (atrophy, hypopigmentation, scarring) make it difficult to assess the extent of recurrence precisely. In addition, recurrence following treating BCC with cryotherapy may be difficult to evaluate due to scarring associated with treatment and the fact that infiltration spreads deeply beneath normally looking skin (Australian Cancer Network Management of Non-Melanoma Skin Cancer Working Party, 2002). Moreover, recurrence diagnostics in skin creases such as the nasolabial sulcus may also be a huge problem. Due to diagnostic difficulties in all cases when recurrence is suspected it is necessary to perform a biopsy to confirm diagnosis.

Recurrence treatment is significantly more difficult than treatment of a primary lesion, and the success rate is considerably lower (Rowe et al., 1989a). The risk of another recurrence is by 50% higher that in the case of a primary lesion (Silverman et al., 1992). Furthermore, it is thought that some incompletely excised lesions recur in a more aggressive growth pattern (a more aggressive histological subtype), especially in the central face (Boulinguez et al., 2004).

Surgical methods are recommended to treat recurrence. Wide BCC excision with a scar and a margin ranging from 5 to 10 mm or Mohs micrographic surgery which is significantly more successful are performed.

7.6 Mohs micrographic surgery (excision controlled histopathologically)

The history how this method came into existence and evolved is tightly associated with its creator. In 1930s Frederic E. Mohs, who was a medicine student at those times, studied the effects of different substances on cancer cells in rats. When he injected 20% zinc chloride solution inside a tumour he accidentally observed tissue necrosis and at the same time in situ tissue fixation. As a result of in vivo tissue fixation with zinc chloride he was able to cut specimens horizontally (parallel to the skin.) As a result he was able not only to assess a tumor histopathologically, but also to assess its whole margin, what formed the base to excision of tumors under microscopic control. After a short period of laboratory tests Mohs replaced 20% zinc chloride solution with the zinc paste applied 24h before tumor excision and started clinical trials on the use of his method in the treatment of skin tumors. As early as in 1941 Mohs presented his first clinical trials in "Archives of surgery" and named his method chemosurgery (Mohs, 1941) (chemo - as tissue fixation is a result of a chemical reaction between tissues and zinc chloride) (Diagram 3).

It involves curettage of a tumour then applying a thick layer of the zinc paste under occlusive dressing which increases paste penetration and protects the surrounding skin. In the case of tumors with large hyperkeratosis before applying the zinc paste dichloroacetic acid with the keratolytic effects can be used and as a result, after the keratotic layer has been exfoliated, penetration of the zinc paste is greater. Tissues prepared in this way become necrotic after 6-24 hours what creates appropriate conditions for a surgical procedure (no pain, small bleeding at the operation site.) During the first stage a surgeon uses methylene blue, sutures or incisions to mark landmarks that will allow further identification of tumor areas that have been excised incompletely. Then the whole tumor with a 3-mm margin of clinically normal surrounding tissues is excised at the angle of 45°, what makes it possible to "tease up" a epidermal edge and facilitates histopathological evaluation, especially of superficial skin layers. The incision is continued at the angle of 45° around the tumor, and the deep surgical edge is parallel to the skin. After haemostasis a diagram presenting a defect formed after tumor excision and its relation to previously marked landmarks is prepared.

In the next stage, a histopathologist divides a lesion according to landmarks marked by an operator (usually into 4 quadrants), turns it deep surface up and marks edges of all quadrants formed after the division with two different dyes. Consequently, further identification of specimen areas excised incompletely is made easier. After marking quadrant edges the specimen is sectioned parallel to the skin and as a result 5-7 µm sections are obtained, therefore it is possible to assess the whole lesion margin. When a tumor fragment is found in the close vicinity of a surgical edge (suboptimal excision) or when a tumor is identified at surgical edge (incomplete excision) a histopathologist marks an area of incomplete excision in the diagram. Based on this diagram a surgeon locates the area with tumor cells that has been left, and then the whole process of fixation, excision and histopathological evaluation is repeated until complete excision is obtained.

In some cases when lesions were excised incompletely the whole process was repeated several times, what due to long time of tissue fixation with the zinc paste (6-24h) took even several days (high costs of treatment and hospitalisation.) Moreover, application of the zinc paste was painful for patients and induced tissue necrosis and ulceration in the lesion vicinity.

Therefore after tumor excision it was necessary to wait until necrosis areas became defined, and only then it was possible to close formed defect. All these features resulted in the fact that despite high efficacy this method did not gain much popularity. However, Mohs, who believed in the success of his method, focused more on its promotion than improvement. And in 1953 when he was doing a film demonstrating his technique an accident decided about a breakthrough discovery for yet another time. Mohs during resecting BCC of the lower eyelid omitted the stage of tissue fixation with the zinc paste in order to accelerate the whole process for the purposes of the film. Instead he excised BCC under local anaesthesia, then froze it and using cryotome obtained horizontal specimens of 5-7 µm. After their standard staining with haematoxylin-eosin he stated than the quality of specimens obtained in this way is the same when compared to the original method, and the duration of the procedure, costs and lack of ulceration and pain are significantly lower. Moreover, primary defect closure was possible what decided about the success of this method to a large extent. With time the fresh-tissue technique replaced the fixed-tissue technique that was originally developed by Mohs. The original name of the whole procedure (chemosurgery) was replaced by Mohs Micrographic Surgery (MMS) due to unfavourable associations and in order to confer its meaning, namely mapping out of the specific location of tumor extension by the use of microscopic evaluation.

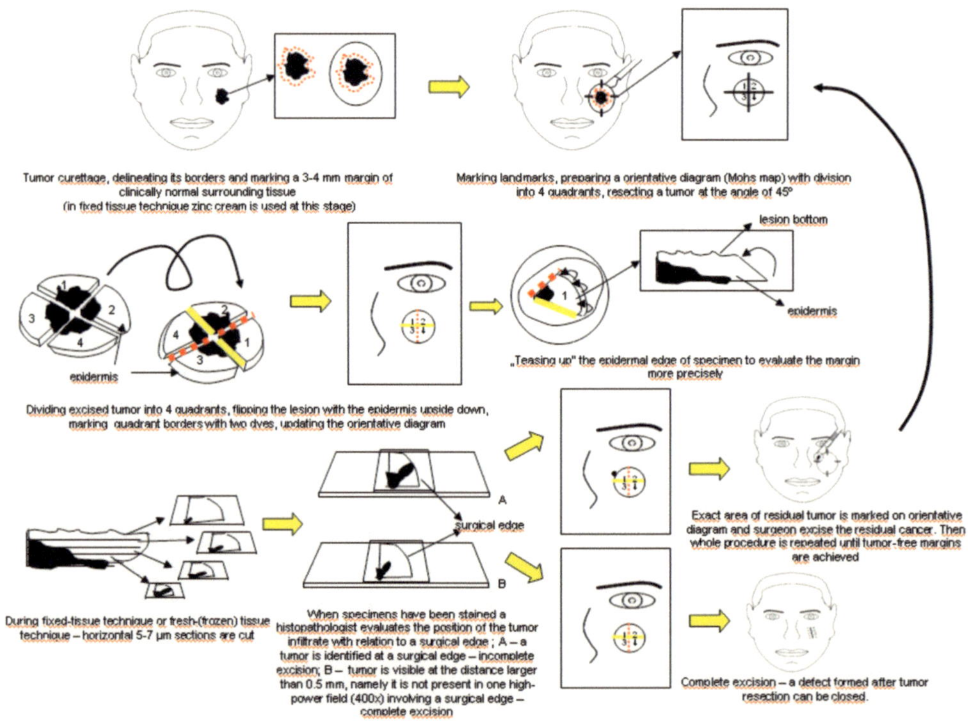

Diagram 3. Mohs micrographic surgery

Currently the fixed-tissue technique is used only in selected cases, mainly in order to eliminate excessive bleeding during lesion excision in areas which are well supplied with blood (e.g. penis.) The fresh-tissue technique has considerably more indications in BCC treatment (Table 5.)

A review of studies published since the mid-1940s confirms the high efficacy of this method reaching even 99% in a 5-year follow-up for primary (Rowe et al., 1989b) and 94.4 % for recurrent BCC (Rowe et al., 1989a). In prospective trials conducted in Australia in 819 patients with periocular BCC no recurrence were observed in 100% patients with primary and in 92.2% with recurrent BCC (Malhotra et al., 2004) in a 5-year follow-up, and in another study with 3370 patients with BCC on the head and neck no recurrence were observed in 98.8% patients with primary BCC and in 96% with recurrent BCC in a 5-year follow-up (Leibovitch et al., 2005).

Apart from its high efficacy other advantages of this method include the minimum amount of excised tissues and the possibility of primary defect closure knowing that a lesion was excised completely. Despite many advantages Mohs Micrographic Surgery has been fully approved only in the USA, where it is used in about 30% of cases (Gaston et al., 1999).

Indications for Mohs Micrographic Surgery:
• location: H area (Part II), especially in the areas where it is necessary to excise a lesion in a saving manner (tip and ala of the nose, lips, eyelids, ear, hands, feet, genitalia)
• size: lesion with the diameter > 2 cm
• histopathological subtype: BCC with an aggressive growth pattern (tab.4), perineural, perivascular or deep tissues involvement
• recurrent BCC
• BCC in patients with immunosuppression
• BCC in patients with a history of previous radiation therapy
• long-lasting BCC (neglected)
• Gorlin syndrome

Table 5. Indications for Mohs Micrographic Surgery (at least one of the mentioned above) (Mohs & Parry, 2007).

Also in the USA was formed the American College of Mohs Micrographic Surgery and Cutaneus Oncology that currently has more than 800 physicians of different specialities who are qualified to use this method when they have completed a 1-2 year training course. In other countries Mohs micrographic surgery is used more rarely, mainly due to high costs (equipment, service, qualified staff) (Cook & Zitelli, 1998) and more work contribution (Hsuan et al., 2004) (time of one procedure is 3h on average) compared to traditional surgical lesion excision. Moreover, contrary to a classic surgical procedure this method is laborious, time-consuming and exhausting for a patient.

Some researchers defend high costs of treatment using this method by the fact that it is possible to obtain better results, consequently, it is more effective in terms of treatment costs than classic surgery (Hsuan et al., 2004). However, Smeets in a prospective trial comparing this method with surgical excision of a lesion with a 3-mm margin of clinically normal surrounding tissue following 30 months of follow-up did not find statistically significant differences in the treatment efficacy between these two method (Smeets et al., 2004).

8. Conclusion

BCC is one of the most common human malignancies. Epidemiology and the increasing rate of incidence prove that BCC is and will be in the future a significant clinical problem. Studies published recently complete our knowledge on its pathogenesis and present new diagnostic and therapeutic methods. The majority of new therapeutic methods may be used only in highly selected cases.

The only universal method that can be used to treat all cases of BCC is surgical excision with a margin of clinically normal surrounding tissues. However, despite numerous advantages of this method and its versatility it has been impossible to determine until now what margin of clinically normal surrounding tissue should be applied when BCC is excised. It is of special importance when lesions in functionally and aesthetically important face areas are excised. In such cases margin differences as low as 1 mm may affect completeness of excision, its functional results, the method of reconstruction and its aesthetic results as well.

For that reason, the authors think that prospective studies in accordance with EBM are necessary in order to determine unanimously the range of margins depending on the prognostic factors mentioned above.

The results of such studies could allow for the unanimous determination of the excision margins and preparing a consistent and common algorithm of BCC treatment.

9. References

"11th ROC: Ultraviolet Radiation Related Exposures." 27 January 2005. U.S. Department of Health & Human Services. 15 April 2008.

American Cancer Society. Cancer Facts & Figures 2008. Atlanta: *American Cancer Society;* 2008.

American Cancer Society: http:www.cancer.org (2006).

American Joint Committee on Cancer, *AJCC Cancer Staging Manual,* 6th ed. New York: Springer-Verlag 2002.

Argenziano G, Zalaudek I, Corona R et al. Vascular structures in skin tumors: a dermoscopy study. *Arch. Dermatol.* 2004; 140(12): 1485-1489

Aston S.J., Beasley R.W., Thorne C.H. Grabb *and Smith's Plastic Surgery,* 5th Edition, Philadelphia, Lippincott-Raven; 1997

Australian Cancer Network Management of Non-Melanoma Skin Cancer Working Party. Non-melanoma skin cancer: *Guidelines for treatment and management in Australia;* 24 October 2002

Avril MF, Auperin A, Margulis A et al. Basal cell carcinoma of the face: surgery or radiotherapy? Results of a randomized study. *Br J Cancer* 1997; 76:100–6.

Bader RS, Basal Cell Carcinoma: Differential Diagnoses & Workup (2008): http://emedicine.medscape.com/article/276624-diagnosis

Bart RS, Schrager D, Kopf AW, Bromberg J, Dubin N. Scalpel excision of basal cell carcinomas. *Arch Dermatol* 1978(114),V,739-742

Bath-Hextall F, Perkins W, Bong J, Williams H. Interventions for basal cell carcinoma of the skin. *Cochrane Database Syst Rev* 2007; 1:CD003412.

Beirne GA, Beirne CG. Observations on the critical margin for the complete excision of carcinoma of the skin. *Arch Dermatol* 1959;80:344-5

Bers MH, Berkow R, *The Merck Manual of Diagnosis and Therapy.* 2001;Section 10,Chapter 126:1004-1010.

Bickers DR, Lim HW, Margolis D et al. The burden of skin diseases: 2004. *J Am Acad Dermatol* 2006; 55: 490-500.

Bieley HC, Kirsner RS, Reyes BA, Garland LD. The use of Mohs micrographic surgery for determination of residual tumor in incompletely excised basal cell carcinoma. *J Am Acad Dermatol* 1992; 26:754–6.

Bieniek A, Cisło M, Jankowska-Konsur A. Nowotwory skóry. Klinika, patologia, leczenie, *Galaktyka* 2008

Bisson MA, Dunkin CSJ, Suvarna SK, Griffiths RW. Do plastic surgeons resect basal cell carcinomas too widely? A prospective study comparing surgical and histological margins. *Br J Plast Surg* 2002;55:293-7

Boeta-Angeles L, Bennet RG: Features associated with recurrence. Cutaneus Oncology. Malden: *Blackwell Science*; 1998. p. 998

Boukamp P. Non-melanoma skin cancer: what drives tumor development and progression? *Carcinogenesis* 2005; 26: 1657-1667.

Boulinguez S, Grison-Tabone C, Lamant L et al. Histological evolution of recurrent basal cell carcinoma and therapeutic implications for incompletely excised lesions. *Br J Dermatol* 2004; 151:623–6.

Bouwes Bavinck JN, Hardie DR, Green A, Cutmore S, MacNaught A, O'Sullivan B, et al. The risk of skin cancer in renal transplant recipients in Queensland, Australia. A follow-up study. *Transplantation* 1996; 61:715–721.

Braun RP, Klumb F, Girard C et al. Three-dimensional reconstruction of basal cell carcinomas. *Dermatol Surg* 2005; 31:562–6.

Breuninger H, Schippert W, Black B, Rassner G. The margin of safety and depth of excision in surgical treatment of a basalioma. Use of 3-dimensional histologic study of 2016 tumors. *Hautarzt* 1989;40:693-700

Brodowski R, Lewandowski B. Rak skóry twarzy. Przegląd piśmiennictwa. *Przegląd Medyczny Uniwersytetu Rzeszowskiego* 2004;2-3:224-230.

Burg G, Hirsch RD, Konz B, Braun-Falco O. Histographic surgery: accuracy of visual assessment of the margins of basal-cell epithelioma. *J Dermatol Surg* 1975; 1:21–24.

Chicheł A, Skowronek J. Współczesne leczenie raka skóry - dermatologia, chirurgia czy radioterapia? *Współczesna Onkologia*; 2005;9;10; 429-435.

Chiller K, Passaro D, McCalmont T, Vin-Christian K. Efficacy of curettage before excision in clearing surgical margins of nonmelanoma skin cancer. *Arch Dermatol* 2000; 136:1327–32.

Clark C, Bryden A, Dawe R et al. Topical 5-aminolaevulinic acid photodynamic therapy for cutaneous lesions: outcome and comparison of light sources. *Photodermatol Photoimmunol Photomed* 2003; 19:134–41.

Clinical Practice Guidelines in Oncology: Basal Cell and Squamous Cell Skin Cancers V.I.2009: www.nccn.org

Cole P, Rodu B: Declining cancer mortality in the United States. *Cancer* 1996;78:2045

Collin JRO. Basal cell carcinoma in the eyelid region. *Br J Ophtalmol* 1976; 60:806-809

Conway RM, Themel S, Holbach LM. Surgery for primary basal cell carcinoma including the eyelid margins with intraoperative frozen section control: comperative interventional study with a minimum clinical follow up of 5 years. *Br J Ophtalmol* 2004;88:236-8

Cook J, Zitelli JA. Mohs micrographic surgery: a cost analysis. *J Am Acad Dermatol* 1998; 39:698–703.

Costantino D, Lowe L, Brown DL. Basosquamous carcinoma - an under-recognized, high-risk cutaneous neoplasm: case study and review of the literature. *J Plast Reconstr Aesthet Surg* 2006; 59:424–8

Cullen FJ, Kennedy DA, Hoehn JE. Management of basal cell carcinoma: current concepts. *Adv Plast Surg* 1993; 10:187

De Silva SP, Dellon AL. Recurrence rate of positive margin basal cell carcinoma: results of a five-year prospective study. *J Surg Oncol* 1985; 28:72–4.

DeVita VT Jr, Hellman S, Rosenberg SA. Cancer*: Principles and Practice of Oncology.* 6th Edition, Lippincot 2001: Chapter 41.

Dieu T, Macleod AM. Incomplete excision of basal cell carcinomas: a retrospective audit. *Aust NZ J Surg* 2002; 72:219–21.

Domarus H, Stevens P. J. Metastatic basal cell carcinoma. Report of five cases and review of 170 cases in the literature. *J.Am.Acad.Dermatol.* 1984;10:1043-60.

Dubin N, Kopf AW: Multivariate risk score for recurrence of cutaneous basal cell carcinomas. *Arch Dermatol* 1983;119 (5): 373-7.

Emmett AJJ, Broadbent GG. Basal cell carcinoma in Queensland. *Aust NZ J Surg* 1981;51:576-90

Epstein E. How accurate is the visual assessment of basal carcinoma margins? *Br J Dermatol* 1973;89:37-43

Farley RL, Manolidis S, Ratner D. Aggressive basal cell carcinoma with invasion of the parotid gland, facial nerve, and temporal bone. *Dermatol Surg* 2006; 32:307–15.

Franchimont C. Episodic progression and regression of basal cell carcinomas. *Br J Dermatol* 1982;106:305–10.

Gailani MR, Leffell DJ, Ziegler A et al. Relationship between sunlight exposure and a key genetic alteration in basal cell carcinoma. *J Natl Cancer Inst* 1996; 88:349–54.

Galletly NP, McGinty J, Dunsby C, Teixeira F, Requejo-Isidro J. Munro I, Elson DS., Neil MAA, Chu AC. French PMW, Stamp GW. Fluorescence Lifetime Imaging Distinguishes Basal Cell Carcinoma From Surrounding Uninvolved Skin; *Br J Dermatol.* 2008;159(1):152-161.

Gaston DA, Naugle C, Clark DP. Mohs micrographic surgery referral patterns: the University of Missouri experience. *Dermatol Surg* 1999;25:862-6

Gilbody JS, Aitken J, Green A. What causes basal cell carcinoma to be the commonest cancer? *Aust J Public Health* 1994; 18:218–21.

Giuffrida TJ, Jimenez G, Nouri K. Histologic cure of basal cell carcinoma treated with cryosurgery. *J Am Acad Dermatol* 2003; 49:483–6.

Global Cancer Statistics Globocan 2002: http://www-dep.iarc.fr/

Gloster Jr HM, Neal K, Skin cancer in skin of color, *J. Am. Acad. Dermatol.* 2006; 55: 741–760.

Godar DE, Urbach F, Gasparro FP, van der Leun JC. UV Doses of Young Adults. *Photochemistry and Photobiology* 2003; 77(4): 453-457.

Goldberg LH, Hsu SH, Alcalay J. Effectiveness of isotretinoin in preventing the appearance of basal cell carcinomas in basal cell nevus syndrome. *J Am Acad Dermatol* 1989; 21:144–145.

Goldsmith LA. Skin effects of fair pollution. *Otolaryn. Head and Neck Surg* 1996; 114:217.

Gorlin RJ. Nevoid basal cell carcinoma syndrome. *Dermatol Clin* 1995; 13:113–125

Graham G. Statistical data on malignant tumors in cryosurgery: 1982. *J Dermatol Surg Oncol* 1983; 9:238–9.

Griffith BH, McKinney P. An appraisal of the treatment of basal cell carcinoma of the skin. *Plast Rec Surg* 1973;51:563-571

Griffiths RW, Suvarna SK, Stone J. Basal cell carcinoma histological clearance margins: an analysis of 1539 conventionally excised tumours. Wider still and deeper? *J of Plast Rec and Aest Surgery* 2007,60:41-47

Griffiths RW, Suvarna SK, Stone J. Do basal cell carcinomas recur after complete conventional surgical excision? *Br J Plast Surg* 2005; 58:795–805.

Griffiths RW. Audit of histologically incompletely excised basal cell carcinomas: recommendations for management by re-excision. *Br J Plast Surg* 1999; 52:24–8.

Gupta AK, Cardella CJ, Haberman HF, Cutaneus malignant neoplasms In patients with renal transplants. *Arch Dermat.* 1986;122;1288-1293

Hauben DJ, Zirkin H, Mahler D, Sacks M: The biologic behaviour of basal cell carcinoma: analysis of recurrence in excised basal cell carcinoma. Part II. *Plast Reconstr Surg* 1982;69:110-116

Hendrix JD, Harry L, Parlette HL. Micronodular basal cell carcinoma. A deceptive histologic subtype with frequent clinically undetected tumor extension. *Arch. Dermatol.*1996;132:295.

Hendrix JD, Parlette HL, Duplicitous growth of infiltrative basal cell carcinoma. Analysis of clinically undetected tumor extent in a paired case-control study. *Dermatol Surg* 1996;22:535-539

Hsuan JD, Harrad RA, Potts MJ, Collins C. Small margin excision of periocular basal cell carcinoma: 5 year results. Br *J Ophthalmol* 2004; 88:358–60.

Ionesco DN, Arida M, Jukic DM. Metastatic Basal Cell Carcinoma. Four Case Reports, Review of Literature, and Immunohistochemucal Evaluation. *Arch Pathol Lab Med* 2006;130(1): 45-51.

Jabłońska S, Chorzelski T. *Choroby skóry. Dla studentów medycyny i lekarzy.* Wyd. V PZWL; 2002. p. 387-394.

Jeacock DA. *Dietary fats and antioxidants and BCC incidence.* 1998; Uni Qld. MSc.

Jemal A, Murray T, Samuels A, et al.: Cancer statistics, 2003, *CA Cancer J Clin* 2003; 53:5.

Jensen P, Hansen S, Moller B, Leivestad T, Pfeffer P, Geiran O, Fauchald P, Simonsen S, Skin cancer in kidney and heart transplant recipients and different long-term immunosuppressive therapy regimens, J. *Am. Acad. Dermatol.* 1999;40: 177–186.

Johnson TM, Tromovitch TA, Swanson NA. Combined curettage and excision: a treatment method for primary basal cell carcinoma. *J Am Acad Dermatol* 1991; 24:613–17.

Karagas MR, Stannard VA, Mott LA, Slattery MJ, Spencer SK, and Weinstock MA. Use of Tanning Devices and Risk of Basal Cell and Squamous Cell Skin Cancers. *J. Natl. Cancer Inst.* 2002; 94: 224.

Kimyai-Asadi A, Goldberg LH, Jih MH. Accuracy of serial transverse cross-sections in detecting residual basal cell carcinoma at the surgical margins of an elliptical excision specimen. *J Am Acad Dermatol 2005;* 53:469–74.

Koplin L, Zarem HA. Recurrent basal cell carcinoma: a review concerning the incidence, behavior, and management of recurrent basal cell carcinoma, with emphasis on the incompletely excised lesion. *Plast Reconstr Surg* 1980; 65:656–64.

Kordek R, Jassem J, Krzakowski M, Jeziorski A, *Onkologia. Podręcznik dla studentów i lekarzy.* Wyd. II: Via Medica; 2004. p. 191-196

Kossard S, Epstein EH Jr, Cerio R, Yu LL, Weedon D. Basal cell carcinoma. In: LeBoit P, Burg G, Weedon D, Sarasin A. The WHO classification of tumours. Pathology and genetics of skin tumours. *IARC Press*, Lyon 2006:13-19

Kossard S, Epstein EH Jr, Cerio R, Yu LL, Weedon D. Basal cell carcinoma. In: LeBoit P, Burg G, Weedon D, Sarasin A. The WHO classification of tumours. Pathology and genetics of skin tumours. *IARC Press*, Lyon 2006:13-19

Krajowy Rejestr Onkologiczny: http://epid.coi.waw.pl/krn/

Kricker A, English DR, Randell PL, Heenan PJ, Clay CD, Delaney TA, et al. Skin cancer in Geraldton, Western Australia: a survey of incidence and prevalence. *Med J Aust* 1990; 152:399–407.

Kumar P, Orton CI, McWilliam LJ, Watson S. Incidence of incomplete excision in surgically treated basal cell carcinoma: a retrospective clinical audit. *Br J Plast Surg* 2000; 35:563–6.

Kwan W, Wilson D, Moravan V. Radiotherapy for locally advanced basal cell and squamous cell carcinomas of the skin. *Int J Radiat Oncol Biol Phys* 2004; 60:406–11.

Leibovitch I, Huilgol SC, Selva D et al. Basal cell carcinoma treated with Mohs surgery in Australia II. Outcome at 5-year follow-up. *J Am Acad Dermatol* 2005;53:452-7

Leibovitch I, McNab A, Sullivan T et al. Orbital invasion by periocular basal cell carcinoma. *Ophthalmology* 2005; 112:717–23.

Liu FF, Maki E, Warde P, Payne D, Fitzpatrick P. A management approach to incompletely excised basal cell carcinomas of skin. *Int J Radiat Oncol Biol Phys* 1991; 20:423–428.

Lo JS, Snow SN, Reizner GT et al. Metastatic basal cell carcinoma: report of twelve cases with a review of the literature. *J Am Acad Dermatol* 1991; 24:715–19.

Maeda H, Akaike T. Nitric oxide and oxygen radicals in infection, inflammation, and cancer, *Biochemistry* (Mosc) 1998; 63:854-865.

Malhotra R, Huilgol SC, Huynh NT, Selva D. The Australian Mohs database, part II: periocular basal cell carcinoma outcome at 5-year follow-up. *Ophthalmology* 2004;111:631-6

Manusow D., Weinerman B.H., Subsequent neoplasia in chronic lymphocytic leukemia. *JAMA* 1975; 232: 267–269.

Marcil I, Stern RS. Risk of developing a subsequent nonmelanoma skin cancer in patients with a history of nonmelanoma skin cancer: a critical review of the literature and meta-analysis. *Arch Dermatol* 2000; 136:1524–30.

Marks R, Gebauer K, Shumack S et al. Imiquimod 5% cream in the treatment of superficial basal cell carcinoma: results of a multicenter 6-week dose–response trial. *J Am Acad Dermatol* 2001; 44:807–13.

Marks R, Jolley D, Lectsas S, Foley P. The role of childhood exposure to sunlight in the development of solar keratoses and non-melanocytic skin cancer. *Med. J. Aust.* 152 (1990):62-66.

Marks R, Staples M, Giles GG, Trends in non-melanocytic skin cancer treated in Australia: the second national sutvey. *Int J Cancer.* 1993;53:585-590.

Marks R. The epidemiology of non-melanoma skin cancer: who, why and what can we do about it. *J. Dermatol.*1995;22:853.

McCarthy EM, Ethridge KP, Wagner RF, Beach holiday sunburn: the sunscreen paradox and gender differences, *Cutis* 1999; 64:37–42.

McCormack CJ, Kelly JW, Dorevitch AP. Differences in age and body site distribution of the histological subtypes of basal cell carcinoma. A possible indicator of differing causes. *Arch Dermatol* 1997; 133:593–596.

Meads SB, Greenway HT. Basal cell carcinoma associated with orbital invasion: clinical features and treatment options. *Dermatol Surg* 2006; 32:442–6.

Menzies SW, Westerhoff K, Rabinovitz H, Kopf AW, McCarthy WH, Katz B. Surface microscopy of pigmented basal cell carcinoma. *Arch. Dermatol.* 2000; 136(8): 1012-1016

Miller DL, Weinstock MA. Nonmelanoma skin cancer in the United States: incidence. *J Am Acad Dermatol* 1994; 30:774–8.

Mogensen M, Jemec GB. Diagnosis of nonmelanoma skin cancer/keratinocyte carcinoma: a review of diagnostic accuracy of nonmelanoma skin cancer diagnostic tests and technologies. *Dermatol. Surg.* 2007;33(10): 1158-1174.

Mohs FE: Chemosurgery: A microscopically controlled method of cancer excision. *Arch Surg* 1941;42:279-295

Mohs Mooney M, Parry E. Mohs Micrographic Surgery(2007): www.emedicine.com/derm/topic542.htm

Morawiec Z., Rykała J., Kołacińska A., Antoszewski B., Kruk-Jeromin J., Czy metoda fotodynamiczna będzie diagnostyką przyszłości? *Acta Clinica et Morphologica* 2004; 7(1):10-14

NCNN Clinical Practice Guidelines in Oncology: Basal Cell and Squamous Cell Skin Cancers V.I.2009: www.nccn.org

Nelson BR, Railan D, Cohen Scott Moh's micrographic surgery for nonmelanoma skin cancers. *Clin in Plast Surg* 1997;24(4): 705-718

Nordin P, Stenquist B. Five-year results of curettage-cryosurgery for 100 consecutive auricular non-melanoma skin cancers. *J Laryngol Otol* 2002; 116:893–8.

Nouri K, Chang A, Trent JT, Jimenez GP. Ultrapulse CO_2 used for the successful treatment of basal cell carcinomas found in patients with basal cell nevus syndrome. *Dermatol Surg* 2002; 28:287–90.

Olmedo JM, Warschaw KE, Schmitt JM, Swanson DL. Optical coherence tomography for the characterization of basal cell carcinoma in vivo: a pilot study. *J. Am. Acad. Dermatol.* 2006; 3: 408-412

Park AJ, Strick M, Watson JD. Basal cell carcinomas: do they need to be followed up? *J R Coll Surg Edinb* 1994; 39:109–11.

Parkin DM, Pisani P, Ferley J: Global cancer statistics. *CA Cancer J Clin* 1999; 49:33.

Parrish JA. Ultraviolet radiation affects the immune system, *Pediatrics* 1983;71: 129–133.

Pascal RR, Hobby LW, Lattes R, Crikelair GF, Prognosis of "incompletely" versus "completely excised" basal cell carcinoma. *Plast Rec Surg* 1968;41;328-332

Petit JY, Avril MF, Margulis A et al. Evaluation of cosmetic results of a randomized trial comparing surgery and radiotherapy in the treatment of basal cell carcinoma of the face. *Plast Reconstr Surg* 2000; 105:2544–51.

Pietrzykowska-Chorążak A.: Odczyny skórne na promieniowanie UV w zależności od wieku. *Przegl. Dermatolog.* 1978;61:3.

Presser SE, Taylor JR. Clinical diagnostic accuracy of basal cell carcinoma. *J Am Acad Dermatol* 1987; 16:988–990.

Preston DS, Stern RS. Nonmelanoma cancers of the skin. *N Engl J Med* 1992;327:1649–62.

Raasch BA, Buettner PG. Multiple nonmelanoma skin cancer in an exposed Australian population. *International journal of Dermatology* 2002;41(10):652–8.

Randle HW. Basal cell carcinoma: identification and treatment of the highrisk patient. *Dermatol Surg*. 1996;22:255–261.
Rapini RP, Comparison of methods for checking surgical margins. *J Am Acad Dermatol* 1990;23:288-94
Reymann F. 15 years' experience with treatment of basal cell carcinomas of the skin with curettage. *Acta Derm Venereol* (Stockh) 1985; 120 (Suppl.):56–9.
Rhodes LE, de Rie M, Enstrom Y, Groves R, Morken T, Goulden V, et al.Photodynamic therapy using topical methyl aminolevulinate vs surgery for nodular basal cell carcinoma. *Arch Dermatol* 2004;140:17–13.
Rhodes LE, de Rie MA, Leifsdottir R et al. Five year follow-up of a randomized, prospective trial of methyl aminolevulinate photodynamic therapy vs surgery for nodular basal cell carcinoma. *Arch Dermatol* 2007; 143:1131–6.
Richmond JD, Davie RM. The significance of incomplete excision in patients with basal cell carcinoma. *Br J Plast Surg* 1987; 40:63–67.
Robinson JK, Fisher SG: Recurrent basal cell carcinoma: A management dilemma? *Aust NZ J Surg* 1996, 66;276-278
Robinson JK. Sun Exposure, Sun Protection, and Vitamin D. *JAMA* 2005; 294: 1541-43.
Rowe DE, Carroll RJ, Day CL Jr et al. Long-term recurrence rates in previously untreated (primary) basal cell carcinoma: implications for patient follow-up. *J Dermatol Surg Oncol* 1989; 15:315–28.
Rowe DE, Carroll RJ, Day CL. Mohs surgery is the treatment of choice for recurrent (previously treated) basal cell carcinoma. *J Dermatol Surg Oncol* 1989; 15:424–31.
Safai B, Good RA. Basal cell carcinoma with metastasis: review of literature. *Arch Pathol Lab Med*. 1977;101:327–331.
Salasche SJ, Amonette RA. Morpheaform basal-cell epitheliomas. A study of subclinical extensions in a series of 51 cases. *J Dermatol Surg Oncol* 1981; 7:387–394.
Schreiber MM. Moon TE, Fox SH, Davidson J. The risk of developing subsequent nonmelanoma skin cancers. *J Am Acad Dermatol* 1990;23:1114–18.
Sieroń A, Gibiński P, Woźnica T. Spektrometryczny system wczesnego wykrywania i diagnostyki nowotworów. *Acta Bio-Optica et Informatica Medica* 2007; 13(4):
Silverman MK, Kopf AW, Bart RS, Grin CM, Levenstein MS. Recurrence rates of treated basal cell carcinomas. Part 3: Surgical excision. *J Dermatol Surg Oncol* 1992; 18:471–476.
Silverman MK, Kopf AW, Grin CM et al. Recurrence rates of treated basal cell carcinomas. Part 2: curettage-electrodesiccation. *J Dermatol Surg Oncol* 1991; 17:720–6.
Smeets NWJ, Krekels GAM, Ostertag JU, Essers BAB, Dirksen CD, Nieman FHM, et al.Surgical excision vsMohs' micrographic surgery for basal-cell carcinoma of the face: randomised controlled trial. *Lancet* 2004;364:1766–72.
Smith SP, Grande DJ. Basal cell carcinoma recurring after radiotherapy: A unique difficult treatment subclass of recurrent basal cell carcinoma. *J Dermatol Surg Oncol* 1991; 17:26
Snow SN, Sahl, W, Lo, J S, Mohs FE, Warner T, Dekkinga ,JA. et al. Metastatic basal cell carcinoma. Report of five cases. *Cancer*. 1994;73:328-35.
Soler AM, Warloe T, Berner A, Giercksky KE. A follow-up study of recurrence and cosmesis in completely responding superficial and nodular basal cell carcinomas treated

with methyl 5-aminolaevulinate-based photodynamic therapy alone and with prior curettage. *Br J Dermatol* 2001; 145:467–71.

Spiller WF, Spiller RF. Treatment of basal cell epithelioma by curettage and electrodesiccation. *J Am Acad Dermatol* 1984; 11:808–14.

Sussman LA, Liggins DF. Incompletely excised basal cell carcinoma: a management dilemma? *Aust NZ J Surg* 1996; 66:276–8.

Swanson N.A., Mohs surgery: Technique, indications, applications, and the future. *Arch. Dermatol* 1983;119:761-773.

Swindle L, Freeman M, Jones B, Thomas S. Fluorescence confocal microscopy of normal human skin and skin lesions in vivo. *Skin Res Technol* 2003b; 9:167.

Swindle LD, Thomas SG, Freeman M, Delaney PM. View of normal human skin in vivo as observed using fluorescent fiber-optic confocal microscopic imaging. *J Invest Dermatol* 2003a; 121:706–12.

Szepietowski J, Sworszt-Pączek W, Wąsik F, Cisło M, Bliżanowska A. Mnogie raki kolczystokomórkowe u chorego z łuszczycą. *Przegl. Dermatol* 1996;83:127.

Taylor CR et al. "Photoaging/Photodamage and Photoprotection" *J. Am Acad Dermatol* 1990: 22.

Telfer NR; Colver GB; Morton CA; Guidelines for the Management of Basal Cell Carcinoma. *Br J Dermatol.* 2008;158(7): 35-48

The Burden of Skin Cancer. National Center for Chronic Disease Prevention and Health Promotion. 13 May 2008.

The skin Cancer Foundation: Skin Cancer Facts 2008: www.skincancer.org

Thissen MRTM, Nieman FHM, Ideler AHLB. Cosmetic results of cryosurgery versus surgical excision for primary uncomplicated basal cell carcinomas of the head and neck. *Dermatological Surgery* 2000; 26:759–64.

Thomas DJ, King AR, Peat BG. Excision margins for nonmelanotic skin cancer. *Plast Reconstr Surg* 2003;112:57-63

Ulrich M., Astner S., Stockfleth E., Röwert-Huber J. Noninvasive Diagnosis of Non-melanoma Skin Cancer: Focus on Reflectance Confocal Microscopy, *Expert Rev Dermatol.* 2008;3(5):557-567.

Van Iersel CA, van de Velden HV, Kusters CD et al. Prognostic factors for a subsequent basal cell carcinoma: implications for follow up. *Br J Dermatol* 2005; 153:1078–80.

Viac J, Chardonnet Y., Euvrard S, Chignol MC, Thivolet J. Langerhans cells, inflammation markers and human papillomavirus infections in benign and malignant epithelial tumors from transplant recipients, *J. Dermatol.* 1992; 19: 67–77.

Vogt M, Ermert H. High Resolution Ultrasound In: Bioengineering of the Skin. Skin, Skin imaging and Analysis; second edition, KP Wilhelm, P Elsner, E Berardesca, H Maibach (eds.). *Informa Healthcare USA Inc*, NY, USA, 2007; 17–29.

Wade T., Ackerman A.B.: The many faces of basal-cell carcinoma. *J. Dermatol. Surg. Oncol.* 1978;4:23.

Wagner RF, Casciato DA: Skin cancers. In: Casciato DA, Lowitz BB, eds.: *Manual of Clinical Oncology*. 4th ed. Philadelphia: Lippincott; 2000. p. 336-373.

Walker P, Hill D. Surgical treatment of basal cell carcinomas using standard postoperative histological assessment. *Australas J Dermatol* 2006; 47:1–12.

Weedon D, Wall D. Metastatic basal cell carcinoma. *Med J Aust.* 1975;2: 177–179.

Wei Q, Matanoski GM, Farmer ER, Strickland P, Grossman L. Vitamin supplementation and reduced risk of basal cell carcinoma. *J Clin Epidemiol* 1994; 47:829–836.

Weinstock MA, Bogaars HA, Ashley M, Litle V, Bilodeau E, Kimmel S. Nonmelanoma skin cancer mortality: a population-based study. *Arch Dermatol.* 1991; 127:1194–1197.

Welzel J, Bruhns m, Wolff H. Optical coherence tomography in contact dermatitis and psoriasis. *Arch Dermatol Res* 2003; 295:50–5.

Welzel J, Lankenau E, Birngruber R et al. Optical coherence tomography of the human skin. *J Am Acad Dermatol* 1997; 37: 958–63.

Williams LS, Mancuso AA, Mendenhall WM. Perineural spread of cutaneous squamous and basal cell carcinoma: CT and MR detection and its impact on patient management and prognosis. *Int J Radiat Oncol Biol Phys* 2001; 49:1061–9.

Wilson AW, Howsam G, Santhanam V et al. Surgical management of incompletely excised basal cell carcinomas of the head and neck. *Br J Oral Maxillofac Surg* 2004; 42:311–14.

Włodarkiwicz A, Muraszko-Kuźma M. Czynniki zwiększonego ryzyka wznowy w raku podstawnokomórkowym skóry. *Przegl. Dermatol.* 1998,85,405.

Wolf DJ, Zitelli JA, Surgical margins for basal cell carcinoma. *Arch Dermatol* 1987;123:340-4

Wronkowski Z, Dąbska M, Kułakowski A. *Rak skóry.* PZWL, Warszawa 1978.

Wu JK, Oh C, Strutton G, Siller G. An open-label, pilot study examining the efficacy of curettage followed by imiquimod 5% cream for the treatment of primary nodular basal cell carcinoma. *Australas J Dermatol* 2006; 47:46–8.

Zak-Prelich M, Narbutt J, Sysa-Jedrzejowska A. Environmental risk factors predisposing to the development of basal cell carcinoma. *Dermatol Surg* 2004; 30:248–52.

3

Implant Retained Auricular Prostheses

Metin Sencimen[1] and Aydin Gulses[2]
[1]*Gulhane Military Medical Academy, Department of Oral and Maxillofacial Surgery*
[2]*2ndArmy Corps, Commando Troop No 5. Dental Service, Gokceada Canakkale*
Turkey

1. Introduction

Reconstruction of a facial defect is a complex modality either surgically or prosthetically, depending on the site, size, etiology, severity, age, and the patient's expectation. The loss of an auricle, in the presence of an auditory canal, affects hearing, because the auricle gathers sound and directs it into the canal. The auricle acts as a resonator to slightly amplify lower frequency sounds and helps to localize sounds, especially in conjunction with the other ear. (Wright et al., 2008 Karakoca et al., 2010, Toljanic et al., 2005)

Recently developed surgical reconstruction techniques, including microsurgical tissue transfer and autogenous or alloplastic grafts, have been used for the reconstruction of auricular defects. More than 40 different cartilaginous, osseous, and alloplastic frame materials for auricular reconstruction have been described since 1891. Reconstructive techniques for auricular defects include second intention healing simple linear closures, skin grafts if the perichondrium and soft tissue are intact, local rotation flaps, two-lobed advancement flaps from the post-auricular sulcus, and post-auricular interpolation flaps for larger defects of the ear ear rim(Vergilis-Kalner et al, 2010, Goldberg et al, 1996). Away from the helical rim, donor skin from the posterior surface of the ear is easily obtainable and the defect can be closed with a vertically oriented side-to-side closure. Other reconstruction options for an auricular defect, adjacent to and on the helical rim, include the helical rim advancement flap, helical advancement flap, wedge excision, or a post-auricular interpolation flap from the scalp (Justiniano & Eisen, 2009, Vergilis-Kalner et al, 2010). Most of the local options involve extensive undermining, often into the hair-bearing portions of the scalp (Cordeiro et al, 2007, Vergilis-Kalner et al, 2010) [3]. Closing the ear defects still represents a reconstructive challenge because of the lack of available freely mobile skin anteriorly, superiorly, and inferiorly to the defect. (Vergilis-Kalner et al, 2010) According to Vergilis-Kalner et al., the choice of the bilobed flap circumvents this challenge by using skin from the posterior surface of the ear and, as necessary, from the post-auricular groove. In addition, bilobe flap is a one-stage repair in which donor tissue is transferred from the area of excess, such as from the post-auricular sulcus, lower pole of the posterior ear, or superior neck adjacent to the posterior ear, rotated anteriorly, folded forward, and fitted into the defect over the exposed cartilage. (Vergilis-Kalner et al, 2010) Vergilis Kalner et al suggested that, the bilobed flap is a useful technique for transferring local tissue while simultaneously minimizing donor-site deformity and described two cases in which a bilobed flap was used to rotate skin from the post-auricular surface to reconstruct full thickness skin defects involving the helical rim and posterior ear, with excellent cosmetic resultsCombined with coverage of the framework by a temporoparietal fascia flap and autologous skin grafts, this surgical approach of auricular reconstruction is reported not only to yield reliable results but also to be associated with a low complication rate. However, an auricular prosthesis is the efficient alternative, when aesthetic and functional demands cannot be surgically fulfilled. Complete rehabilitation of patients with auricular defect is achieved using a multidisciplinary team approach, involving surgical and prosthetic personnel. Treatment requires cooperation between those treating the disease and those responsible for the emotional wellbeing of the patient. Retention and stability of prostheses improve the patient's confidence and sense of security.

However, especially in pediatric patients, the impact of surgical invasion and donor-site morbidity can be severe, and the collectable volume of autologous cartilage is limited. Therefore, Yanaga et al (Yanaga et al ,2009) proposed regenerative surgery for microtia using cultured ear chondrocytes. Through the development of a multilayer chondrocyte culture system and two-stage implantation technique, the authors successfully generated human ears. In culture, the chondrocytes are expanded to a sufficiently large volume, produce rich chondroid matrix, and form immature cartilaginous tissues. First, the cultured chondrocytes are injection-implanted into the lower abdomen of the patient, where the cells grow into a large, newly generated cartilage with neoperichondrium in 6 months. Following this, the cartilage is harvested surgically, sculptured into an ear framework, and implanted subcutaneously into the position of the new ear. The cultured chondrocytes formed a mature cartilage block with sufficient elasticity for use as an auricular cartilage. The formed block had the same histologic origin as elastic cartilage. The ear framework was implanted into the auricular defect area, and an auricle with a smooth curvature and shape was subsequently configured. In the 2 to 5 years of postoperative follow up, the neocartilage maintained good shape, without absorption. The authors have suggested that, the benefits of the technique are minimal surgical invasion, lower donor-site morbidity, lessened chance of immunologic rejection, and implantation stability. (Yanaga et al, 2009)

The use of medical-grade skin adhesives, solvents, eyeglasses, the use of hard and soft tissue undercuts, and other modalities became traditional means of retaining facial prostheses. However these techniques were often wrought with difficulties associated with retention, stability, adverse tissue reactions, discoloration and prosthesis deterioration, inconvenience of use or application, poor hygiene, discomfort, and lack of acceptance. The use of osseointegrated implants in craniofacial reconstruction has minimized some of these disadvantages and has provided patients with predictable cosmetics, improved retention, and stability of the episthesis. (Wright et al., 2008 Karakoca et al., 2010, Toljanic et al., 2005, Karayazgan Saracoglu et al., 2010, Tolman& Taylor, 1996)

Nowadays, methods of retention varied within each prosthesis type. Retention methods for auricular prostheses are bars, adhesives, magnets, and mechanical devices. Since the early 1970s, the use of osseointegrated implants to retain facial prostheses has become an integral part of treatment planning for facial reconstruction. Implant retention is currently considered the standard of care in many situations because of the advantages it offers over conventional retention methods such as the use of adhesives. (Arcuri & Rubinstein, 1998, Karakoca et al., 2010, Toljanic et al., 2005, Karayazgan Saracoglu et al., 2010, Tolman& Taylor, 1996, Gumieiro et al, 2009, Niparko et al., 1993)

This chapter reviews the history, planning, surgical technique and complications of osseointegrated implants in auricular reconstruction and briefly discusses the surgical and non surgical treatment alternatives of auricular defects. In adition, a simple surgical technique was described herein.

2. Implant retained auricular prosthesis

2.1 Historical perspective

Since the introduction of endosseous implants for use with bone conduction hearing aids in 1970s, the use of osseointegrated implants to retain facial prostheses has acquired an important role in the prosthetic rehabilitation of patients with craniofacial defects and became an integral part of treatment planning for facial reconstruction. (Granström, 2007, Brånemark & Albrektsson, 1982, Scolozzi & Jaques, 2004)

Implant retention is currently considered as the gold standard in prosthetic reconstruction of these structures. The success of bone-anchored auricular prostheses could base upon the patients' acceptance, contribution to quality of life and use of the prostheses as replacement prosthesis for either a developmental defect or acquired defect. (Karayazgan Saracoglu et al., 2010, Karakoca et al., 2010)

The use of cranial implants has also provided an alternative approach towards rehabilitating patients with severe auricular defects since 1977 (Niparko et al., 1993) and has become a viable option that can offers several advantages over traditional reconstructive techniques. (Miles et al, 2006) It has been suggested that, auricular implants enhance retention and stability of prostheses, improving the patient's confidence and sense of security.(Karakoca et al., 2010) In addition, attachment systems aid in the proper positioning of prostheses, facilitating insertion by the individuals with auricular defects. The etiology of the loss of an auricle can be either acquired or congenital. Among acquired cases, gun shot injuries, traffic accidents etc, burns, ablative cancer surgeries are the reasons. (Karakoca et al., 2010, Toljanic et al., 2005, Karayazgan Saracoglu et al., 2010, Tolman& Taylor, 1996) (Table 1)

Defect etiology
Gunshot injuries
Traffic accidents
Dog bite
Burns
Ablative cancer surgeries
Congenital

Table 1. The etiology of the auricular defects

Another advantage of the implant retained auricular prostheses is that the skin and mucosa are less subject to mechanical and chemical irritation from mechanical retention or adhesives. (Karakoca et al., 2010) Cosmetically, a fine feathered margin in implant-retained prostheses allows the creation and maintenance of more esthetic results and patient satisfaction. The elimination of the marginal degradation due to daily application and removal of adhesives improves extension in functional life of the prostheses. (Arcuri &

Rubinstein, 1998, Karakoca et al., 2010, Toljanic et al., 2005, Karayazgan Saracoglu et al., 2010, Tolman& Taylor, 1996)

The use of osseointegrated implants in extraoral prosthetic rehabilitation has resulted in several studies which are primarily focused on implant osseointegration success and soft tissue complication rates. (Karakoca et al., 2010, Tolman& Taylor, 1996, Karayazgan Saracoglu et al., 2010)

Extraoral prostheses are usually made of silicone elastomers, acrylic resin, or of both of these. According to the literature survey of Karakoca et al, the use of silicones have been used for over 50 years in the field of craniofacial prosthetics, with desirable material properties including flexibility, biocompatibility, ability to accept intrinsic and extrinsic colorants, translucency, chemical and physical inertness, moldability, and ease of cleaning. (Arcuri & Rubinstein, 1998, Karakoca et al., 2010, Toljanic et al., 2005, Karayazgan Saracoglu et al., 2010, Tolman& Taylor, 1996, Gumieiro et al, 2009, Niparko et al., 1993, Scolozzi & Jaques, 2004, Miles et al, 2006, Granström, 2007, Brånemark & Albrektsson, 1982, Wazen et al., 1999, Kamish et al 2008) (Fig 1)

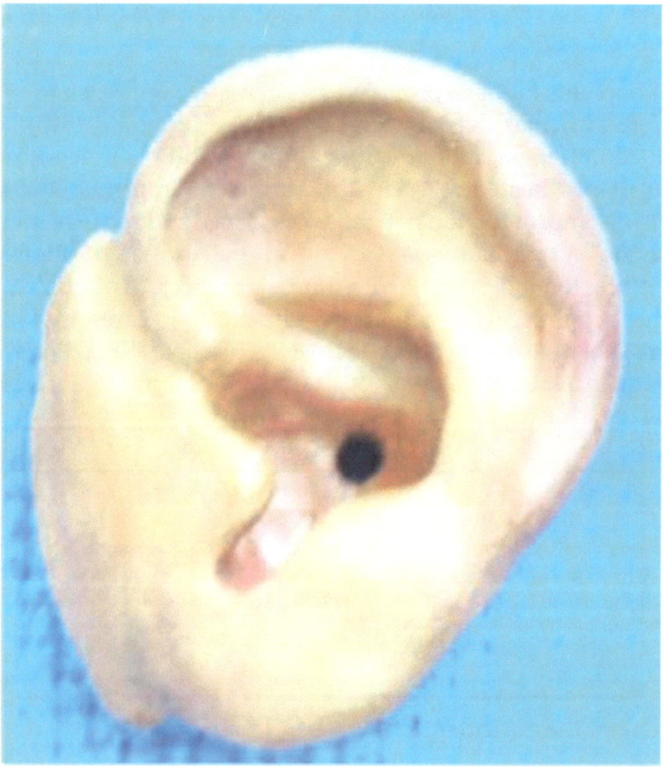

Fig. 1. An auricular episthesis made of silicone.

Gumieiro et al have reviewed the literature and stated the indications for implant retained auricular prosthesis in adult and paediatric patients. According to their results, among pediatric patients, autogenous reconstruction is the procedure of choice. (Gumieiro et al, 2009)

Adult patients	*Paediatric patients*
• The presence of an acquired total or subtotal auricular defect, most often traumatic or ablative in origin • When plastic surgery is impossible or when the final cosmetic result is unsatisfactory	• Failed autogenous reconstruction • Severe soft-tissue/skeletal hypoplasia • A low or unfavorable hairline
• Lack of adequate tissue for reconstruction	• Severe congenital or acquired microtia
• Absence of the lower half of the ear	
• Failed attempts at reconstruction • Major cancer excision • Poor operative risks • Selection of the technique by the patient	

Table 2. Indications for implant retained auricular prosthesis in adult and paediatric patients. (Adopted from Gumieiro et al., 2009)

2.2 Retentive system

Although the concept of osseointegration is the same whether implants are placed intraorally or extraorally, craniofacial implants should have modified design features to match the anatomical and biomechanical differences in the facial area. (Kamish et al 2008) Compared with the maxilla and the mandible, in spite of having limited thickness, facial bones are dense. The load and frequency of loading forces on craniofacial implants are limited when compared to implants placed intraorally. In the literature, some researchers have recommended that 2 implants are enough for auricular function, because the episthesis is not heavy. (Wazen et al., 1999) (Fig 2)

According to the literature survey, three or four implants were also preferred, when the CT scans were examined and the temporal bone quality seemed to be appropriate for osteointegration. (Brånemark et al., 1985) (Fig 2)

The choices of retentive mechanisms to be applied on the implants depend on the patient, the number of the implants and the flexibility of the episthesis. The conventional retention techniques involve magnetic or clip retention provided by golden bars (Fig 4) and ball clip (Fig 5) or magnet retentive cap systems (Fig 6).

For the use of a golden bar, at least two bone-fitting implants and a moderately hand-skilled patient are needed.(Sencimen et al., 2008) Magnets can be used with at least 3 bone-connected implants.(Fig. 7) In cases with three implants, a cantilever extension of the bars could be planned. (Fig 8) If four bone connected implants were used, there is no need for a cantilever extension of the bars.(Fig 9) Episthesis connected on bars between four implants by ball shaped caps are also used. (Fig10)

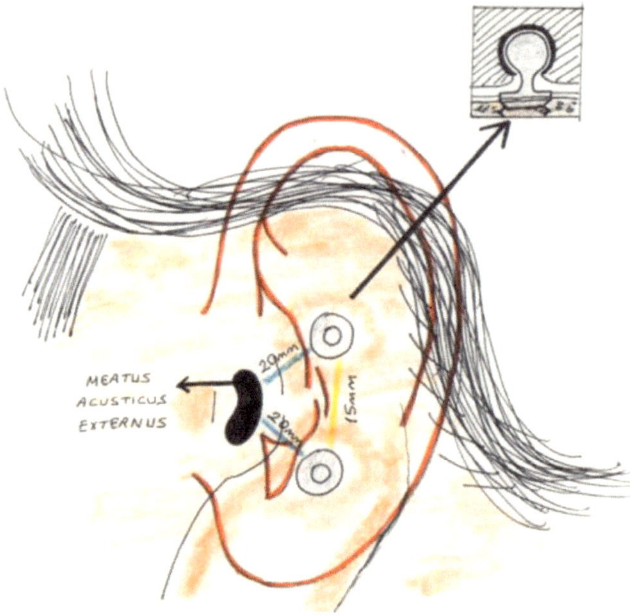

Fig. 2. Auricular prosthesis retained on ball shaped retentive caps of two implants

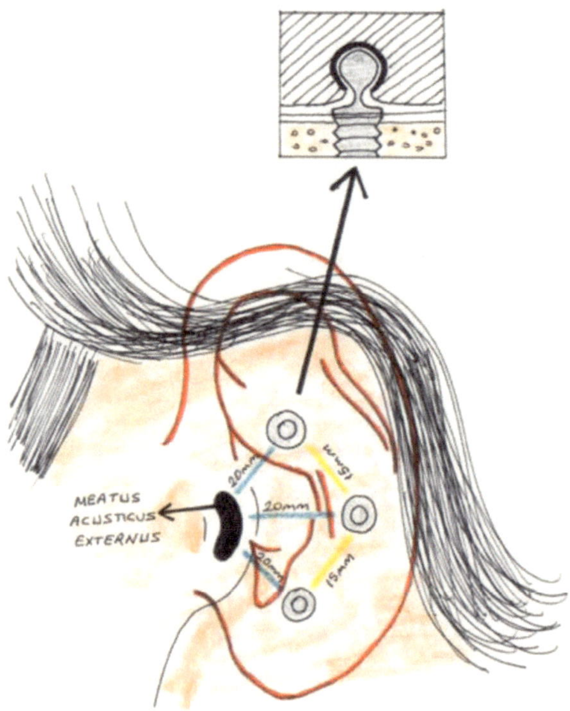

Fig. 3. Auricular prosthesis retained on ball shaped retentive caps of three implants

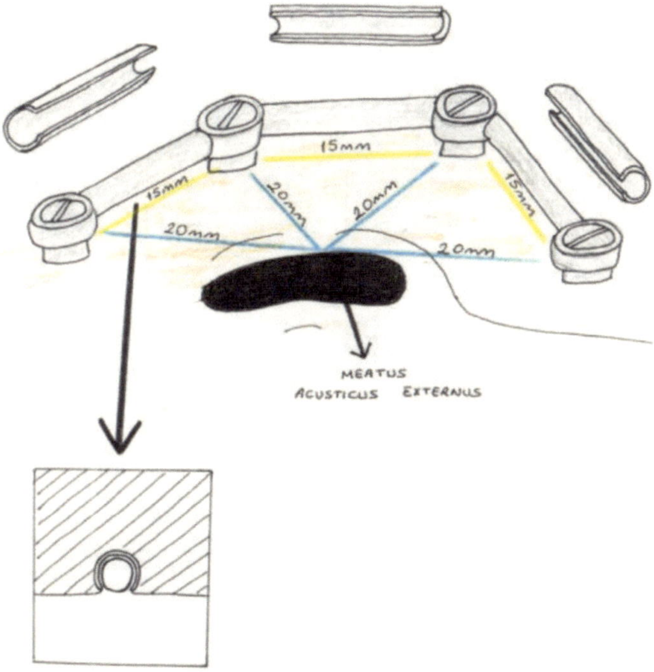

Fig. 4. Retention provided by golden bars

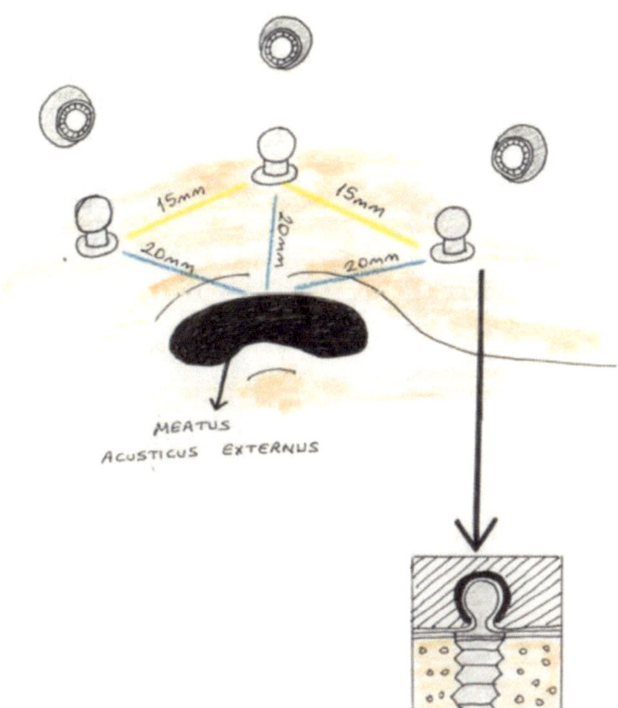

Fig. 5. Retention provided by ball clips

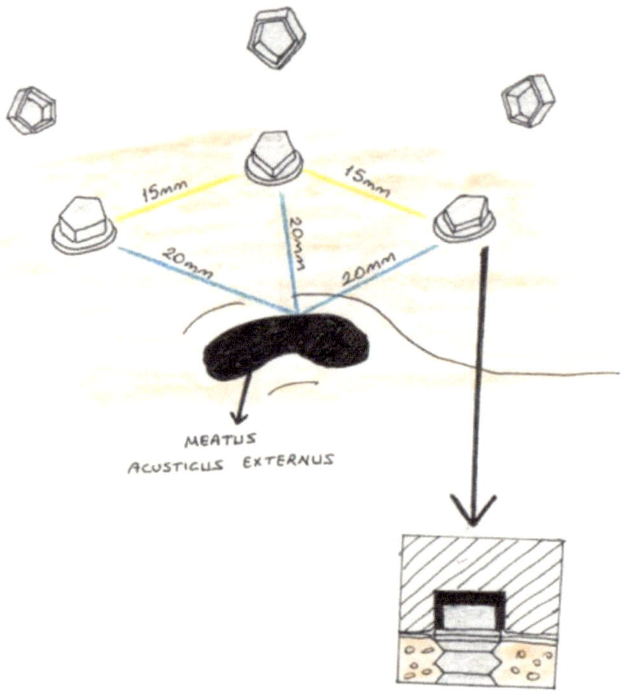

Fig. 6. Retention provided by magnet retentive caps

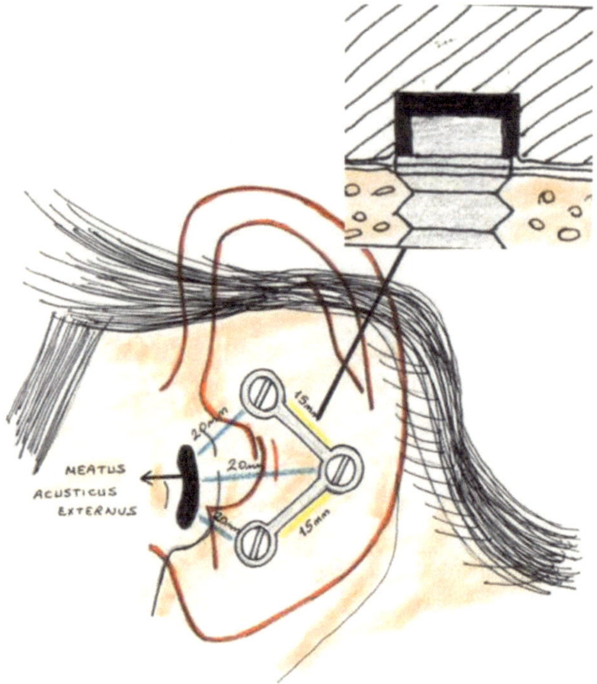

Fig. 7. Bars connected to magnets used with 3 bone-connected implants

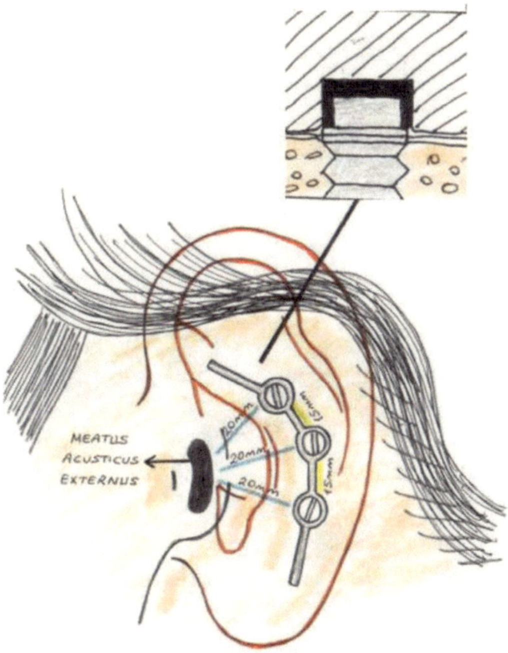

Fig. 8. In cases with three implants, a cantilever extension of the bars could be planned.

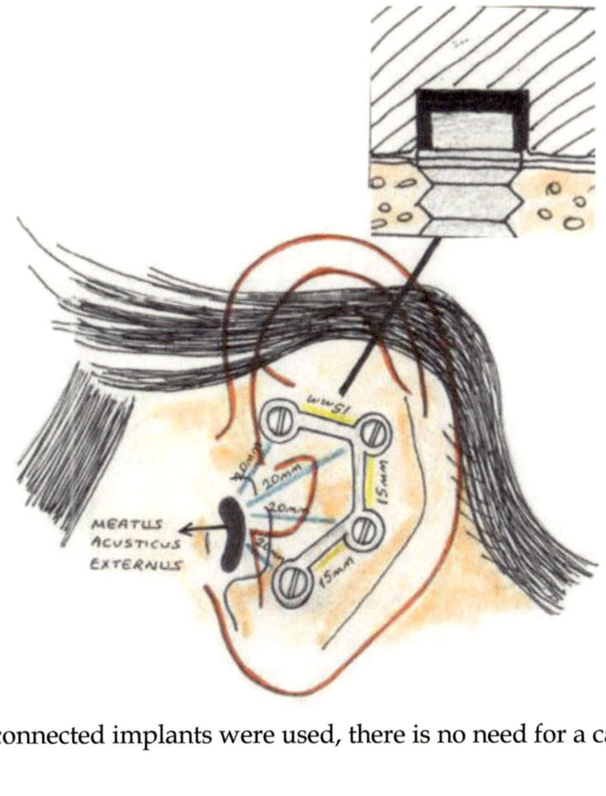

Fig. 9. If four bone connected implants were used, there is no need for a cantilever extension of the bars.

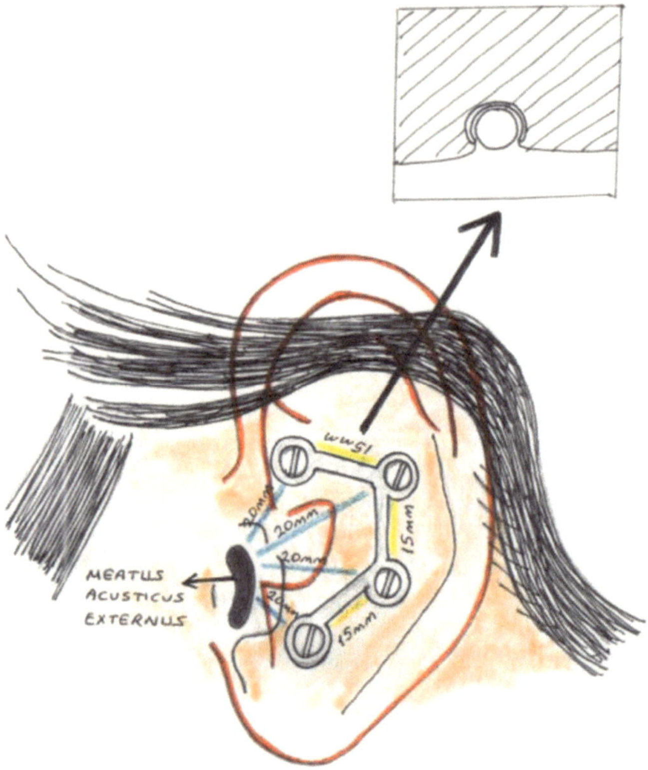

Fig. 10. Episthesis connected on bars between four osseointegrated implants by ball shaped caps are also used.

Khamis et al described a new technique with modified abutments in implant-retained auricular prostheses, using a single- stage surgical procedure. (Kamish et al 2008) They have screwed the modified O-ring abutments directly onto the implants at the time of surgery. Plastic washers were attached to the O-ring heads of the exposed abutments to avoid skin overgrowth to allow a single-stage surgical procedure. After a osseointegration period of 4 months, a silicone prosthetic ear was fabricated and retained using clips over the O-ring abutments.

According to Wright et al, several factors could affect the choice of bars and clips versus magnets.(Wright et al., 2008) To distribute functional loads and reduce bending moments by avoiding the use of cantilevers or to distribute the loads if magnets were used, three implants in a nonlinear alignment are recommended. When magnets are used for retention, three implants placed in a tripod fashion could provide the best stabilization. When bar and clip systems are planned, two implants often sufficed. (Wright et al., 2008)

Magnets offered the advantages of easier fabrication, shortened appointments, and access for peri-abutment hygiene procedures. Magnets also could maintain a longer, more predictable level of retention than clips, which tended to loosen in a shorter period of time. However, bar and clip systems were advantageous biomechanically in that they effectively splinted the implant sites together, and these systems could offer stronger immediate retention. (Sencimen et al., 2008, Wright et al., 2008)

2.3 Planning

The diagnostic step is an important point that must be clearly defined in construction of an auricular prosthesis. CT of the temporal bone and clinical photographs of the patient should be obtained preoperatively to plan the placement and appropriate size of the implants and to evaluate the thickness and spaces of mastoid cortical bone in order to preserve the duramater. (Ciocca et al., 2009) (Fig 11) However, CT scans could reveal errors in the planning of the implant position. Usually, measurements do not consider the difficulty transferring the diagnostic CT data to the surgical template. (Ciocca et al., 2009)

The position of landmarks registered during CT and the duplication of the diagnostic template as a surgical one might introduce error during implant insertion into the recipient site of the bone. (Ciocca et al., 2009) Therefore, a virtual elaboration for maxillofacial implant positioning could be used to define the correct implant site in relation to the available bone. (Sencimen et al., 2008, Ciocca et al., 2009)

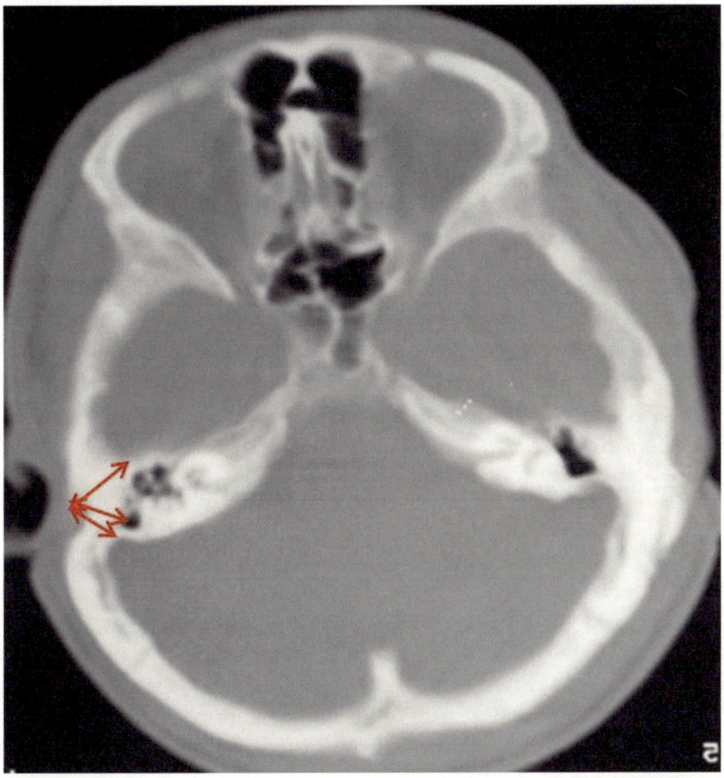

Fig. 11. The axial CT scan of the cranium. The arrows show the distances from the masoid region to the adjacent anatomical structures such as external auditory canal, duramater and the orbita.

A new approach to the diagnosis of bone available for craniofacial implant positioning based on Computer-aided design and manufacturing (CAD-CAM) system was described by Ciocca et al. (Ciocca et al., 2009) A mirrored volume of the healthy ear was rapidly prototyped for a clinical trial in an appropriate position relative to the patient's face. Three ideal positions for the implant were chosen in the inner of the volume of the mirrored ear. The same positions were transferred to a diagnostic template that was rapidly prototyped with a positioning arm extending to the zygomatic arch, and two craniofacial implants were correctly positioned in the temporal bone. Ciocca et al have stated that this protocol allows the correct diagnosis of the available bone and perfect transfer in the surgical environment. In addition, the use of CAD–CAM technology allowed visualization in a virtual environment that was previously elab orated on film, and allowed to prototype the final volume of the prosthesis and its consequent surgical template with a 3D printer. This feature assured perfect transfer of the projected and CT-registered implant positions to the surgical template. (Ciocca et al., 2009)

In cases with aetiology of cancer, the surgeon should be aware of the risk of osseointegration failures and such patients who have undergone irradiation should be treated with caution, because differences in volume and density could result in irradiation having a more destructive effect on the vascularity of this site, thereby compromising the potential for osseointegration. (Gumieiro et al, 2009)Basically, the adverse biological changes that occur when osseous tissues are exposed to ionizing radiation results from alterations in the cellular components of bone, involving significant reductions in the numbers of viable osteoblasts and osteocytes, as well as the development of areas of fatty degeneration within the bone marrow spaces. In addition, regional ischemia could also be seen as results of the blood vessels undergo progressive endarteritis, hyalinization and fibrosis. As a conclusion, radiotherapy is not a contraindication for the use of osseointegrated implants in the maxillofacial region, but the loss of implants is higher in irradiated sites than in non-irradiated sites. (Gumieiro et al, 2009)

2.4 Surgical technique

It has been suggested that the mastoid region as a recipient site could offer the best results in implant retained auricular epistheses. Wright et al have stated that, the mastoid region in nonirradiated patients has provided a high degree of predictable individual implant survival. (Wright et al., 2008)

The implants should be placed at least 20 mm away from the external acustic meatus and 15 mm from each other. (Sencimen et al., 2008) (Fig 12) In addition, in cases with two implants, 9 and 11 o'clock positions are recommended. (Nishimura et al., 1995) (Fig 13) After marking the implant sites with surgical pen, a curved incision is used in the skin over the mastoid process approximately 30 mm posterior to the opening of the expected position of the external auditory canal.(Fig 14) Skin and subcutaneous tissue are reflected until the periost was seen. Then the periost is incised and bone surface is exposed. The implants placed are inserted at the sites that were marked with surgical pen parallel to each other under minimum trauma to prevent heat injury to the surrounding bone and to ensure a stable osseointegration. (Sencimen et al., 2008)

It has been known that implant surgery may be performed in single or two stages. However, because the operation area is covered with a previous scar tissue formation, the two-stage procedure is not recommended so as not to compromise the vascular supply of the area. (Sencimen et al., 2008) Using single-stage procedure, recovery screws are placed and the skin incision closed with wire sutures, with ointment-soaked gauze used to protect the skin. The sutures are removed 1 week after the surgery, and the patient is asked to apply antibacterial ointment once or twice a week for the first 3 months. (Sencimen et al., 2008)

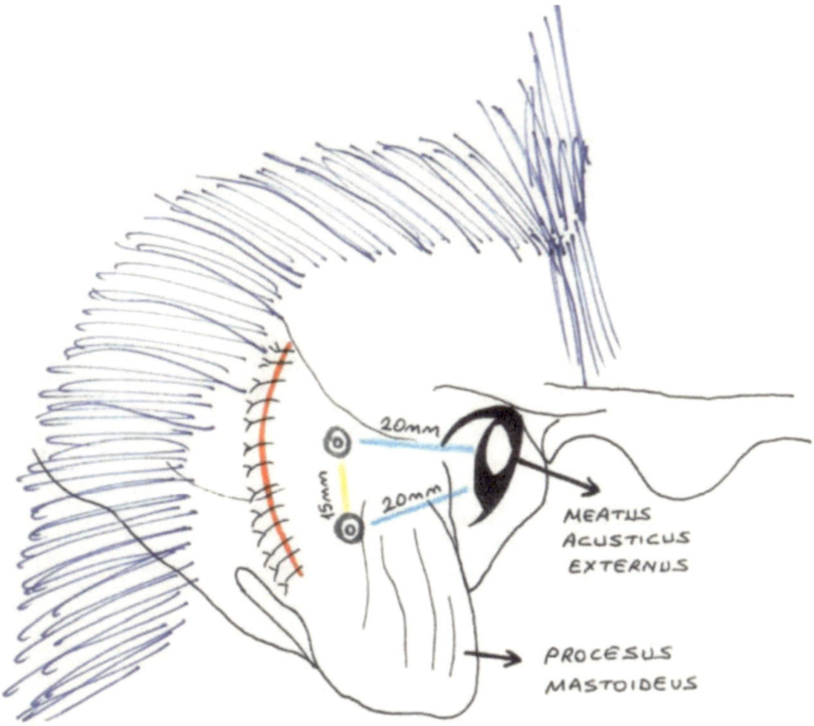

Fig. 12. The implants should be placed at least 20 mm away from the external acustic meatus and 15 mm from each other.

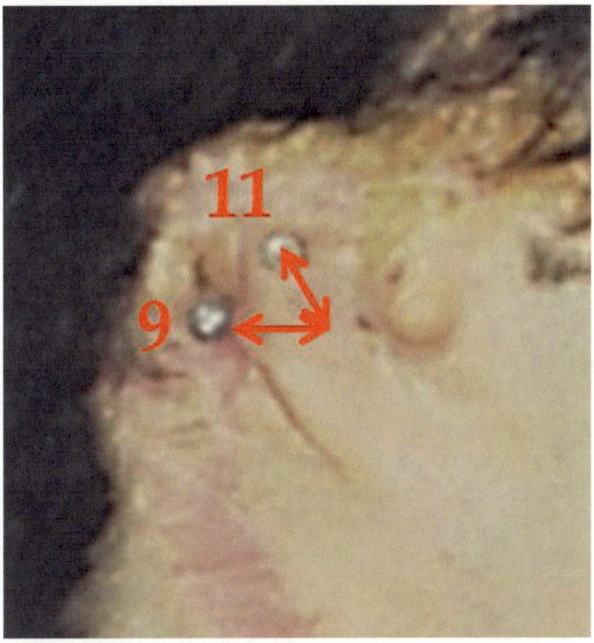

Fig. 13. In cases with two implants, 9 and 11 o'clock positions are used.

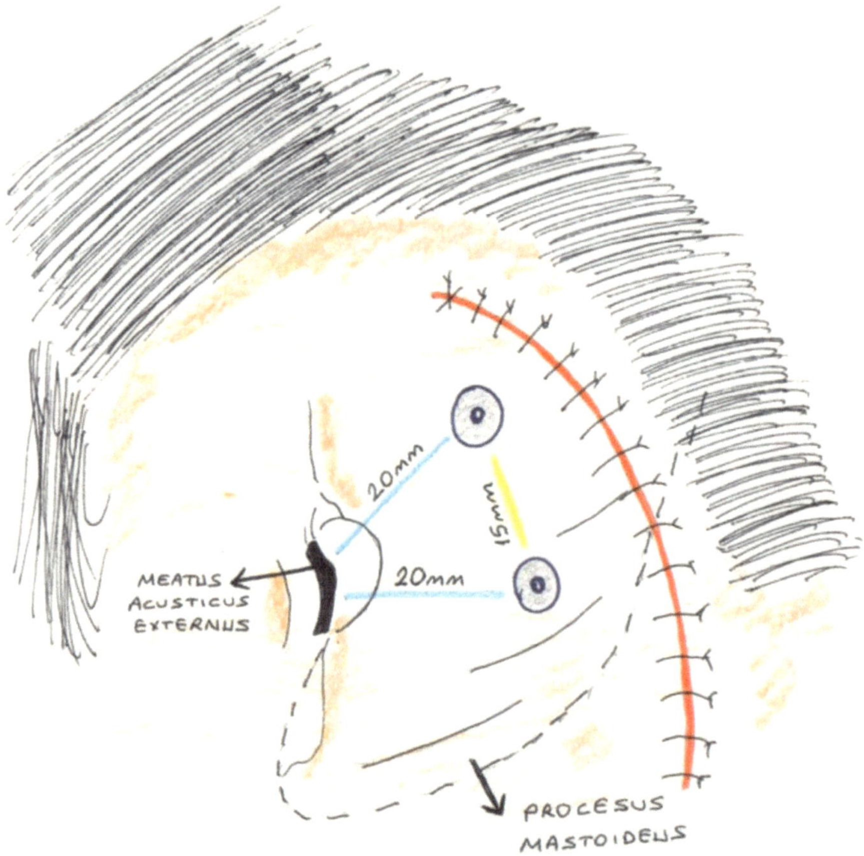

Fig. 14. A curved incision is used in the skin over the mastoid process approximately 30 mm posterior to the opening of the expected position of the external auditory canal. Please note the safety distances between the implants and the external auditory canal.

2.5 Prosthetic procedure

At the end of the recommended period of 4 months for osteointegration, the recovery screws are removed and titanium bone graft retentive anchors or bars are placed. The wax model of the missing ear is prepared according to a cast model of the opposite ear which is obtained with an optosil-xantopren impression paste. The ear episthesis is completed with flexible acrylic recine. (Tjellström et al., 1985, Sencimen et al., 2008) The gold matrixes are placed parallel on retentive anchors or bars. To provide symmetry with the opposite ear, the episthesis is placed by hand, according to the position of the external auditory canal, the retentive mechanism and the relation with the hairy skin. (Figure 15) At the same time, the connection between gold matrix and episthesis should be secured by self-curing acryl. After setting the self-curing acryl, gold matrixes and episthesis are separated from the retentive anchors. A tunnel should be prepared not to hinder the hearing of the patient. (Adell et al., 1981, Lemon et al., 1996)

The patient is advised to take his episthesis off during bathing and sleeping. The use of saline cleaning solution and ointment once or twice a week is recommended.

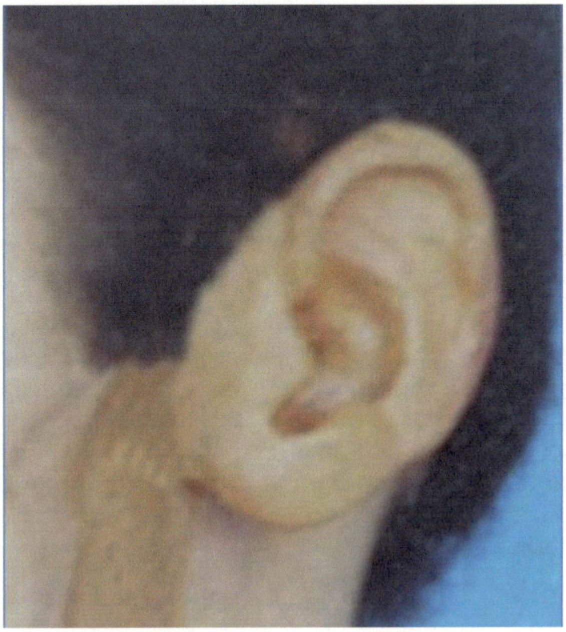

Fig. 14. Application of the auricular prosthesis

2.6 Complications

Complications related to auricular prosthesis are the loosening of abutment, broken bar or extensions, loosening of prosthetic bar screws, broken or lost clips, loss of clip retention, loss of magnet retention, fractured acrylic resin substructure, loss of bonding between substructure and silicone, deposits on tissue surface of the prosthesis, and tear or rupture of the prosthesis. (Karakoca et al, 2010)

Loosening of bar screws is another relatively frequent complication noted in auricular prosthesis; therefore, the screws should be placed with proper torque control, ensuring complete seating of the driver into the screw head.

The most frequent complications are mechanical failures of the substructure and retentive attachments, including acrylic resin substructure fracture, clip fracture, and loss of atta chment between the silicone and substructure. Loss of clip retention was a frequent complication in bar-retained auricular prostheses. Clips were activated using the activator device of the attachment system. (Karakoca et al, 2010)

Clip activation was also dependent on the patient's request for activation, along with the objective evaluation of the prosthodontists. Karakoca et al have suggested that, loss of retention might be attributed to the demand of patients who actively sought optimal stability for their prostheses and adequate clip activation is required. (Karakoca et al, 2010)

It has been suggested that, maxillofacial elastomers perform well initially, but deterioration associated with either degradation of mechanical properties or changes in appearance commonly occurs. This deterioration limits the service life of extraoral prostheses, and refabrication of these prostheses is time consuming, labor intensive, and costly.

According to the literature survey of Gumieiro et al, auricular osseointegrated implants have presented survival rates varying according to the length of follow-up, ranging from 92% after 8 years to 100% with shorter follow-up. (Gumieiro et al, 2009) However, there have been limited clinical studies on the life span of extraoral prostheses. (Aydin et al., 2008, Jebreil, 1980) Two studies reported on the life span of adhesive retained prostheses.(Jani & Schaaf, 1978, Jebreil, 1980) Jani and Schaaf indicated that 36% of prostheses were refabricated within 6 months, 33.6% within 7 to 12 months, 17.6% within 13 to 18 months, 8% within 19 to 24 months, and 4.8% were refabricated after 24 months.(Jani & Schaaf, 1978) Jebreil reported that adhesive-retained orbital prostheses were refabricated after 6-9 months. (Jebreil, 1980)

Wright et al have reported on the survival rate of 16 patients treated with extraoral implants in the auricular region and encountered no surgical complication, implant failures, or prosthetic failures; however, the follow-up visits were scheduled at 1 week, 6 months, and 1year. Hooper et al reported a 14-month mean life span for implant-retained extraoral prostheses. A study performed by Aydin et al. demonstrated a 17-month mean survival time for implant-retained auricular prostheses. (Aydin et al, 2008) In a recent study performed by Visser et al, it was indicated that a new prosthesis had to be made every 1.5 to 2 years. (Visser et al, 2008, Karakoca et al, 2010)

Karakoca et al performed a study to estimate the survival rates of implant-retained extraoral prostheses and to analyze the frequency of prosthetic complications. (Karakoca et al, 2010) They have evaluated 32 auricular, 25 orbital, and 13 nasal prostheses. According to the results of the same study, mean survival was 14.5 months for the patients' first prostheses. The survival times for the first implant-retained auricular prostheses were 14.1 months. In addition, the survival times for the second implant-retained auricular prostheses were estimated as 14.4 months. The summary of the patient data of the studies peformed by Karakoca et al and Karayazgan Saracoglu et al were shown in Table 4. (Karayazgan Saracoglu et al., 2010, Karakoca et al, 2010)

Number of patients	*Gender*	*Age (Range and mean)*	*Observation period (Range and mean)*	*Retention*
32*	20 male 12 female	9-72 (31.5)	12-46 (27.7) (months)	31 bar clips 1 magnet
14**	10 male 4 female	7-70 (37.63)	Not declared	Not declared

Table 4. Summary of the data of the review performed by Karakoca et al. (* Adopted from Karakoca et al., 2010, ** Adopted from Karayazgan Saracoglu et al, 2010)

Frequency distribution of complications of auricular prosthesis of the study performed by Karakoca et al were shown in Table 5 and survival rates of the study performed by Karakoca et al were shown in Table 6.

The frequency of adverse skin reactions around the soft tissues of the percutaneous implant is generally very low and the main symptomatic reactions may consist of slight redness, reddened and moistened peri-implant tissues, granulation tissue associated with the implants or infection of the peri-implant soft tissues. (Tjellström et al, 1985, Nishimura et al., 1995) Gumieiro et al have stated that good patient hygiene compliance combined with thin and immobile peri-implant soft tissues have been found to result in minimal soft tissue complications. (Gumieiro et al, 2009)

Complication	Once	Twice	Thrice	Total
Bar fracture	6.5%	-	-	6.5%
Clip activation	22.6%	41.9%	6.5%	7%
Clip replacement	9.7%	-	-	9.7%
Loosening bar screws	29.0%	3.3%	-	32.3%
Loosening abutment	40.6%	6.3%	-	46.9%
Substructure fracture	15.6%	6.3%	-	21.9%
Loss of attachment between silicone and substructure	25%	6.3%	-	31.1%
Tear of prosthesis	9.4%-	-	-	9.4%

Table 5. Frequency distribution of complications of auricular prosthesis (Adopted from Karakoca et al., 2010)

Estimated mean survival time of the first auricular prosthesis	Estimated mean survival time of the second auricular prosthesis
14.1 month±(0.75)	**14.4 month± (0.67)**

Table 6. Mean survival rate for the first and second auricular prostheses (Adopted from Karakoca et al., 2010)

According to Gumieiro et al, the surgical techniques required for prosthetic reconstruction are less demanding than those for autogenous reconstruction are, construction of prostheses is a time-consuming task requiring experience and expertise.Compared with the autogenous reconstruction, despite the technical challenge of autogenous reconstruction, prosthetic reconstruction requires lifelong attention and may be associated with late complications and necessitates dependence on the health services. (Gumieiro et al, 2009)

Karayazgan-Saracoglu et al reviewed the survival rates and soft tissue responses of extraoral implants and observed the mean loss period throughout the 159 extraoral implants as 12.64 weeks. (Karayazgan Saracoglu et al., 2010) In total, 52 patients were examined, including 16 with auricular defects. (Karayazgan Saracoglu et al., 2010) According to their results, craniofacial implants in the auricular region are more reliable in the long term when compared with those in the other areas. In addition, soft tissue complications are fewer in the auricular area. In most of the studies focusing on the peri-implant soft tissue condition, the criteria proposed by Holgers et al. is used. (Holgers et al, 1989) According to this classification, the peri-implant soft tissue condition is recorded by a 5- point scale (Likert scale) as grade 0 (no irritation), grade 1 (slight redness), grade 2 (red and slightly moist tissue), grade 3 (granulation and red and moist tissue), and grade 4 (infection). The peri-implant soft tissue response on auricular implants evaluated by Karayazgan-Saracoglu et al was shown on Table 7. (Karayazgan Saracoglu et al., 2010)

Implant loss associated with auricular episthesis were also reported in the literature. Karayazgan-Saracoglu et al evaluated the implant loss based on the variables such as

Grade	Frequency
0	61%
I	13%
II	21%
III	4%
IV	1%

Table 7. The peri-implant soft tissue response on auricular implants evaluated by Karayazgan-Saracoglu et al., 2010

diabetes, alcohol consumption, tobacco use, and alcohol and tobacco use and radiotherapy history. (Karayazgan Saracoglu et al., 2010) According to their results, the relationship of implant loss with diabetes and alcohol use was found statistically significant. Relationships between implant loss and radiotherapy history and smoking with and without alcohol use were not found as statistically significant. In addition, it has been suggested that smoking has a relationship with implant loss might be expected to be significant with a further wider sample studies. (Karayazgan Saracoglu et al., 2010)

3. Conclusion

In 1979, Branemark proposed craniofacial implants that have been used worldwide in facial prosthesis. Nowadays, the extraoral use of osseointegrated implants for the retention of auricular prosthesis has been used for better support, stability, retention and cosmetics. The surgical technique for osseointegrated implant retained auricular prostheses s seems to be simple and is associated with a low failure and perioperative complication rates. The major advantages of this technique are that it puts less strain on the patient and provides superior cosmetic results, compared with traditional surgical reconstructive techniques. The main disadvantage of the implant retained auricular prosthesis is the need for a lifelong daily skin care.

Osseointegrated titanium implants may provide patients with a safe and reliable method for anchoring auricular prostheses that enables restoration of their normal appearance and offer an improvement in their quality of life. The use of osseointegrated prostheses should be considered to be a simple and viable alternative to surgical reconstruction and as a gold standard in the management of individuals with massive auricular defects.

Other than the clinical experiences, treatment outcomes of implant retained auricular prostheses should be evaluated for predicting the long-term success.

4. Acknowledgement

None declared.

5. References

Adell, R.; Lekholm, U.; Rockler, B.& Brånemark, P.I.(1981) A 15-year study of osseointegrated implants in the treatment of the edentulous jaw. Int J Oral Surg. Vol. 10, No. 6, (Dec 1981), pp.387-416, ISSN: 0300-9785

Arcuri, M.R.& Rubenstein, J.T.(1998) Facial implants. Dent Clin North Am. Vol. 42, No.1, (Jan 1998), pp. 161-175, ISSN: 1558-0512

Aydin, C.; Karakoca, S.; Yilmaz, H.& Yilmaz, C.(2008) Implant-retained auricular prostheses: an assessment of implant success and prosthetic complications. Int J Prosthodont. Vol. 21, No. 3, (May-Jun 2008), pp.241-244, ISSN: 1942-4426

Brånemark, P.I., & Albrektsson, T.(1982)Titanium implants permanently penetrating human skin. Scand J Plast Reconstr Surg, Vol. 16, No. 1, (June 2008), pp. 17-21, ISSN: 0036-5556

Brånemark,, P.I.; Zarb, G.A.,;& Albrentsson, T. (1985) Tissue-iintegrated pros theses osseointegration in clinical dentistry. Chicago, London, Berlin, Sao Paulo, Tokyo, Quintessence Publishing, 1985, ISBN: 10: 0867151293

Ciocca, L.; Mingucci, R.; Bacci, G.& Scotti, R.(2009) CAD-CAM construction of an auricular template for craniofacial implant positioning: a novel approach to diagnosis. Eur J Radiol. Vol 71, No. 2, (Aug 2009), pp. :253-256, ISSN: 1872-7727

Cordeiro, C.N.; McCarthy, C.M.; Mastorakos, D.P.& Cordeiro, P.G.(2007) Repair of postauricular defects using cervical donor skin: a novel use of the bilobed flap. Ann Plast Surg, Vol. 59, No. 4, (Oct 2007), pp. 451-452, ISSN: 1536-3708

Goldberg, L.H.; Mauldin, D.V.& Humphreys, T.R. (1996) The postauricular cutaneous advancement flap for repairing ear rim defects. Dermatol Surg Vol 22, No. 1, (Jan 1996), pp. 28-31. ISSN:1087-2108

Granström, G.(2007) Craniofacial osseointegration. Oral Dis. Vol. 13, No. 3.,(May 2007), pp. 261-269, ISSN: 1601-0825

Gumieiro, E.H.; Dib, L.L.; Jahn, R.S.; Santos Junior, J.F.; Nannmark, U.; Granström, G.& Abrahão, M.(2009) Bone-anchored titanium implants for auricular rehabilitation: case report and review of literature. Sao Paulo Med J. Vol. 127, No. 3, (2009), pp. 160-165, ISSN: 1806-9460

Holgers, K.M.; Bjursten, L.M.; Thomsen, P.; Ericson, L.E.& Tjellström, A.(1989) Experience with percutaneous titanium implants in the head and neck: a clinical and histological study. J Invest Surg. Vol. 2, No. 1, (1989), pp.7-16, ISSN: 1521-0553a

Hooper, S.M.; Westcott, T.; Evans, P.L.; Bocca, A.P.& Jagger, D.C.(2005)Implant-supported facial prostheses provided by a maxillofacial unit in a U.K. regional hospital: longevity and patient opinions. J Prosthodont. Vol. 14, No. 1,(Mar 2005), pp.32-38, ISSN: 1532-849X

Jani, R.M.& Schaaf, N.G.(1978) An evaluation of facial prostheses. J Prosthet Dent. Vol. 39, No. 5, (May 1978), pp.546-550, ISSN: 1097-6841

Jebreil, K.(1980) Accetability of orbital prostheses. J Prosthet Dent. Vol. 43, No. 1, (Jan 1980), pp.82-85, ISSN: 1097-6841

Justiniano, H. & Eisen, D,B.(2009) Pearls for perfecting the mastoid interpolation flap. Dermatology Online Journal, Vol.15, No. 6, (June 2009),pp. 2. ISSN:1087-2108

Karakoca, S.; Aydin, C.; Yilmaz, H.& Bal, B.T. (2010) Retrospective study of treatment outcomes with implant-retained extraoral prostheses: survival rates and prosthetic complications. J Prosthet Dent. Vol. 103, No. 2, (Feb 2010), pp. 118-126, ISSN: 1097-6841

Karayazgan-Saracoglu, B.; Zulfikar, H.; Atay, A.& Gunay, Y.(2010) Treatment outcome of extraoral implants in the craniofacial region. J Craniofac Surg. Vol. 21, No. 3, (May 2010), pp.751-758.

Khamis, M.M.; Medra, A.& Gauld, J.(2008) Clinical evaluation of a newly designed single-stage craniofacial implant: a pilot study. J Prosthet Dent. Vol. 100, No. 5, (Nov 2008), pp. 375-383, ISSN: 1097-6841

Lemon, J.C.; Chambers, M.S.; Wesley, P.J.& Martin, J.W.(1996) Technique for fabricating a mirror-image prosthetic ear. J Prosthet Dent.Vol. 75, No. 3, (Mar 1996), pp.292-293, ISSN: 1097-6841

Miles, B.A.; Sinn, D.P.& Gion, G.G.(2006) Experience with cranial implant-based prosthetic reconstruction. J Craniofac Surg. Vol. 17, No. 5, (Sep 2006), pp. 889-897, ISSN: 1536-3732

Niparko, J.K.; Langman, A.W.; Cutler, D.S.& Carroll, W.R.(1993), Tissue-integrated prostheses in the rehabilitation of auricular defects: results with percutaneous mastoid implants. Am J Otol.Vol. 14, No. 4, (Jul 1993), pp. 343-348, ISSN: 0192-9763

Nishimura, R.D.; Roumanas, E.; Sugai, T.& Moy, P.K.(1995) Auricular prostheses and osseointegrated implants: UCLA experience. J Prosthet Dent. Vol. 73, No. 6, (Jun 1995), pp. 553-558, ISSN: 1097-6841

Scolozzi,P.& Jaques, B. (2004)Treatment of midfacial defects using prostheses supported by ITI dental implants. Plast Reconstr Surg. Vol. 114, No.6, (Nov 2004), pp. 1395-404, ISSN: 1529-4242

Sencimen, M.; Bal, H.E.; Demiroğullari, M.; Kocaoglu, M.& Dogan, N.(2008) Auricular episthesis retained by an attachment system (2 case reports). Oral Surg Oral Med Oral Pathol Oral Radiol Endod. Vol. 105, No. 2, (Feb 2008),pp. e28-34, ISSN: 1528-395X

Tjellström, A.; Yontchev, E.; Lindström, J.& Brånemark, P.I.(1985) Five years' experience with bone-anchored auricular prostheses. Otolaryngol Head Neck Surg. Vol. 93, No. 3, (Jun 1985), pp.366-372, ISSN: 1097-6817

Toljanic, J.A.; Eckert, S.E.; Roumanas, E.; Beumer, J.; Huryn, J.M.; Zlotolow, I.M.; Reisberg, D.J.; Habakuk, S.W.; Wright, R.F.; Rubenstein, J.E.; Schneid, T.R.; Mullasseril, P.; Garcia, L.T.; Bedard, J.F.& Choi, Y.G. (2005) Osseointegrated craniofacial implants in the rehabilitation of orbital defects: an update of a retrospective experience in the United States. J Prosthet Dent. Vol. 94, No. 2, (Aug 2005), pp. 177-182, ISSN: 1097-6841

Tolman, D.E.& Taylor, P.F. Bone-anchored craniofacial prosthesis study: irradiated patients. Int J Oral Maxillofac Implants. Vol. 11, No. 5, (Sep-Oct 1996), pp. 612-619, ISSN: 1942-4434

Tolman, D.E.& Taylor, P.F. Bone-anchored craniofacial prosthesis study. Int J Oral Maxillofac Implants.Vol. 11, No. 2, (Mar-Apr 1996), pp. 159-168. ISSN: 1942-4434

Vergilis-Kalner, I.J.& Goldberg, L.H. (2010) Bilobed flap for reconstruction of defects of the helical rim and posterior ear.Dermatol Online J.Vol.10, No. 15, (Oct 2010), pp. 9, ISSN:1087-2108

Visser, A.; Raghoebar, G.M.; van Oort, R.P.& Vissink, A.(2008) Fate of implant-retained craniofacial prostheses: life span and aftercare. Int J Oral Maxillofac Implants. Vol. 23, No. 1,(Jan-Feb 2008),pp.89-98, ISSN: 1942-4434

Wazen, J.J.; Wright, R.; Hatfield, R.B.& Asher, E.S.(1999) Auricular rehabilitation with bone-anchored titanium implants. Laryngoscope.Vol. 109, No. 4, (Apr 1999), pp. 523-527,ISSN: 1531-4995

Wright, R.F.; Zemnick, C.; Wazen, J.J. & Asher, E. (2008) Osseointegrated implants and auricular defects: a case series study. J Prosthodont., Vol. 17, No. 6, (August 2008), pp. 468-475. ISSN: 1532-849X

Yanaga, H.; Imai, K.; Fujimoto, T.& Yanaga, K. (2009) Generating ears from cultured autologous auricular chondrocytes by using two-stage implantation in treatment of microtia. Plast Reconstr Surg. Vol.124, No. 3, (Sep 2009), pp.817-825, ISSN:0032-105

Part 2

Breast

4

Contralateral Breast Augmentation in Heterologous Breast Reconstruction

Paolo Persichetti, Barbara Cagli, Stefania Tenna, Luca Piombino,
Annalisa Cogliandro, Antonio Iodice and Achille Aveta
Campus Bio-Medico University
Plastic Surgery Department, Rome
Italy

1. Introduction

Breast cancer is the most frequent, after skin cancer, in women in industrialized countries, and is the leading cause of cancer morbidity and mortality. The latest epidemiological data in USA, updated in 2010, reported 207,090 new cases of breast cancer with a death toll of 39,840. (National Cancer Institute US). This disease is highly debilitating, even in the treatable forms, due to the emotional and psychological implications that come with it: even though it's not an organ essential to life, the breast is, in all cultures of the world, the deepest and purest expression of femininity, a pivotal aesthetic element, symbol of sexual and psychological identity and seduction. At the time of diagnosis the woman faces, on one hand a real threat to her survival and safety, and on the other the fear of witnessing her body image being irreversibly altered. Therefore in recent years, the need to provide the possibility for a breast reconstruction treatment after total mastectomy, in addition to specific treatment procedures for such tumors, has become increasingly pressing. The objective of post-cancer breast reconstruction is to restore the importance of the breast and maintain a good quality of life with no effect on the prognosis or the monitoring for tumor recurrence. Numerous studies confirm that breast reconstruction not only restores the body image, but it improves vitality, femininity and sexuality and has a positive effect on the sense of well being and quality of life of the patient. Modern breast reconstruction has seen many technical advances, which has provided valuable tools to the plastic surgeon for such procedures, including: improved models of silicone and saline breast implants, tissue expanders and the identification of several muscle-skin flaps that can provide well-vascularized tissue for breast reconstruction, as well as the tendency to perform modified total mastectomy as opposed to total mastectomy. Each surgical technique can be used both, for the delayed reconstruction (secondary), and for the immediate reconstruction, one that is performed at the same time as the mastectomy.

Nowadays acellular dermal matrices (ADMs) are being used for increasingly wider applications in breast reconstruction, both in primary and revision implant-based reconstructive procedures. ADM is helpful in subpectoral implant-based reconstruction, where it can be used as an interposition substrate between the released origin of the pectoralis major muscle and the inframammary fold (IMF).

Breast reconstruction with implants is the most frequently used technique after mastectomy. About 70% of breast reconstructions are performed using heterologous techniques that include the use of tissue expanders or breast implants.

Breast implants, in fact, allow the achievement of a good symmetry, in selected patients, with relative simplicity, and virtually no tissue transfer and scarring at the donor site. This supporting evidence makes breast reconstruction with implants seem to be the better accepted choice than flap reconstruction.

Patients who require radiation therapy for management of their breast cancer pose a unique set of challenges to the reconstructive surgeon. For the patient who has already received radiotherapy or will receive it after reconstructive surgery, implant-based procedures are often problematic. Tissue expansion is difficult in the previously irradiated tissues, and the risk of infection and the risk of subsequent extrusion of an implant are increased, but considering that some patients are not ideal candidates for flap based procedures it is crucial to individualize a specific surgical planning/timing.

For the last 20 years, the quality of breast implants has continued to evolve with the intent to improve the aesthetic results of this type of surgical procedure. The implant's shapes, surfaces, contents and materials typically used have been repeatedly modified to produce more reliable and resistant implants, with increased similarity to the natural breast, while maintaining a high degree of patient and surgeon satisfaction alike. However, in the case of unilateral breast reconstruction, the long term stability cannot account for variations which the contralateral breast may physiologically undergo. The achievement and preservation of symmetry is therefore the most important challenge for the surgeon especially in the case of unilateral reconstructions with heterologous materials. The achieve symmetry on the healthy breast the use of well known techniques such as breast reduction (procedure most frequently used), breast augmentation and ultimately mastopexy may be warranted. Whatever the technique used, good cosmetic result will depend on the stability over time, thus the choice of the procedure must take into account both functional and aesthetic results by allowing for possible minor corrections in the future. However, this data is poorly documented in the literature. There are only a few articles where the long-term aspect of breast reconstruction is analyzed and the most important series reveal that, despite a high percentage of good results during the first two years after surgery (approximately 84%), about 30% of surgeries worsen in a linear fashion over time and only 54% of patients retain a good result after five years. The deterioration of the aesthetic result is due to the appearance of breast asymmetry that worsens over time, due mainly to changes in the contralateral breast, weight fluctuations, the appearance of ptosis, and the aging of the patient. In the case of heterologous reconstruction, the breasts age differently (the implant on one side and autologous tissue on the other) and the development of tissue atrophy around the implant with the gradual appearance of folds and an increasingly spherical look of the reconstructed breast further contribute to the deterioration of the aesthetics results. If the use of a heterologous reconstruction technique has been selected, it becomes necessary to try to minimize the long-term issues associated with the implant.

In agreement with the data reported in the literature on long-term satisfaction of patients, our institute chooses implants for heterologous breast reconstruction when possible.

2. Heterologous breast reconstruction

2.1 History of implants and heterologous breast reconstruction

The first attempt at breast reconstruction with a material that did not present any rejection problems dates back to 1895 with Czerny, who used autologous adipose tissue. In 1899, Gersuny described a technique for breast augmentation achieved by percutaneous injection of paraffin wax. In 1930, Shwarzman implanted glass beads under the skin and in 1950 Polystan was introduced, a spongy material derived from polyethylene rarely recommended because it was invaded by connective tissue after the insertion. The research to use inert substances arrived to 1951 with Wallace and Pangmann who introduced the use di Ivalon, a sponge made of polyvinyl alcohol and formaldehyde. This substance was introduced under the breast tissue in a polyurethane casing. The implant was molded according to the patient's needs, soaked for 24 hours, sterilized and implanted. In 1960 the ethron was introduced, a polymethane derivative, which was used with some success because it induced low peripheral fibrosis and did not cause calcification.Since then many substances and methods have been tested, but the era of the current breast implants began only in 1963 when Cronin implanted prosthesis made of solid silicone casing with a smooth surface, filled with gel of the same polymer. On the back side, the mammary prosthesis were provided with dacron disks in order to adhere to tissues better. The casing did not stick to tissues and did not lead to phlogistic reactions. Since the introduction of Cronin's breast implants in 1963, the implants have always been composed in a similar manner. Over the years the manufacturers of breast implants have been trying to improve the quality by changing the thickness of the outer silicone casing, adding texture to the surface and introducing new filling substances as saline, hydrogel, soybean oil and silicone gel. In 1970, Ashley presented a model of breast implant made of a thin and soft silicone casing filled with low viscosity silicone gel, fully surrounded externally by a one-millimeter thick layer of polyurethane microfibers. In early 1989, textured surface implants have been introduced for clinical use; such implants would theoretically have the advantage of limiting the percentage of incidence of periprosthetic capsule retraction, thanks to their rough surface.

3. Classification and current status of breast implants

The heterologous reconstruction is based on the installation of prosthetic devices, whose morphological and structural features are constantly evolving. However, it's been shown in numerous studies that these materials do not increase the risk of developing cancer or autoimmune diseases.

Currently there are three types of commercially available implants: provisional tissue expanders, permanent tissue expanders and definitive implants. The definitive implants available on the market offer a wide variety in regards to the type of surface, the filling, the shape and the size that the consumer may choose. They are made of a silicone elastomer casing filled with silicone gel or saline.

The surface can be of three kinds: smooth, textured and polyurethane (Image 1,2,3). The smooth surface implants are now used very rarely. The polyurethane surface made it possible to reduce the phenomenon of capsular contracture by covering elastomers with an irregular surface and as a result it inspired further research for alternative solutions that will minimize capsular contracture even more. The texturized implants are the outcome of this research; in fact, their rough surface limits the periprosthetic capsular contracture even more so than the polyurethane surface. In recent years, the shape of the implants was of great importance to the business aspect of plastic surgery. Primarily, there are two shapes that are available: round and anatomic.

The round implants were the first available and today are the most frequently used. They are available with any type of surface, filling and profile, pre-filled, inflatable, with single and double chamber.

The anatomic implants were designed to give the breast a more natural look. The upper pole is flattened and slopes down to a fuller lower pole, where generally the maximum implant projection is situated. The anatomical implants, especially those filled with cohesive silicone

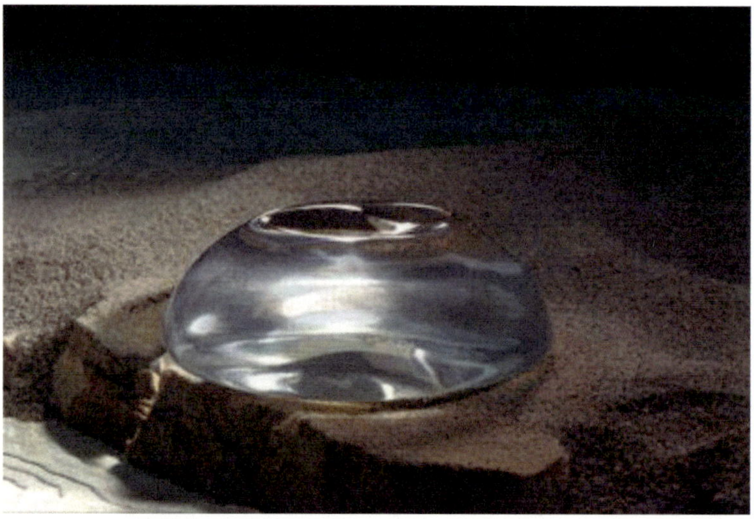

Image 1. Smooth surface implants filled with silicon gel.

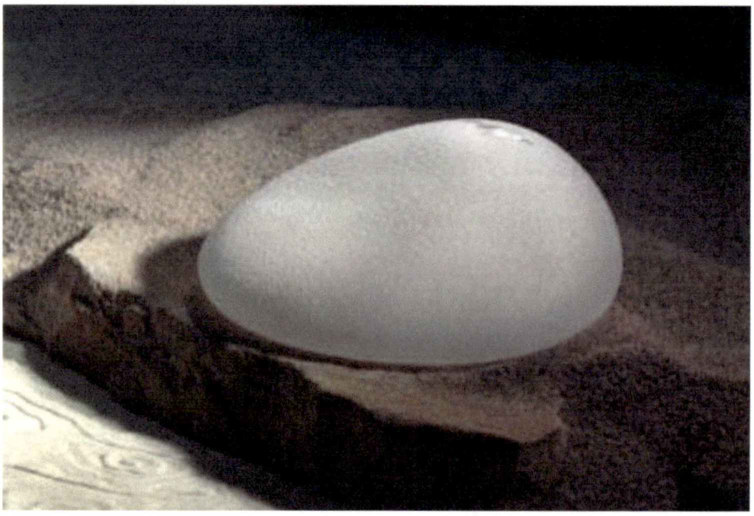

Image 2. Textured surface implants saline filled with saline solution.

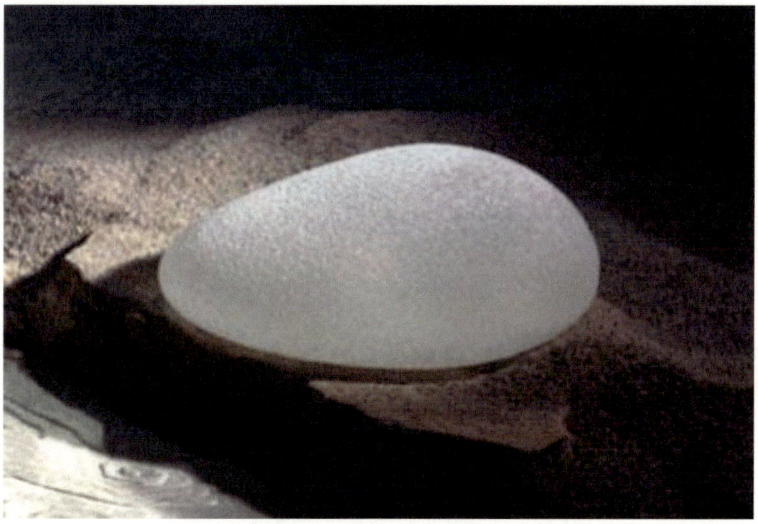

Image 3. Textured surface implants saline filled with silicon gel.

gel, maintain their shape both in ortho and clinostatism and guarantee a more predictable result. The possibility to choose the implant height according to chest proportions and the absence of collapse effect, assure a stable upper pole. With regard to the size, the implants may vary according to three basic parameters: height (Height: full, moderate, low), projection (Variable projection: full, moderate, low), and base diameter. They should be evaluated according to the patient's body habitus and preferences.

The most used implants are:

- double-lumen implants with silicone gel-filled core and outer chamber with saline content.
- double-lumen implants with saline-filled inner chamber and outer chamber made of silicone gel.
- double-lumen implants with chambers filled with silicone gel in different density.
- single-lumen implants containing uniform or differentiated density silicone gel.
- single-lumen implants containing oil of various types (so far not sufficiently tested and safe).
- single-lumen implants containing saline solution.

The provisional tissue expanders are implants whose purpose is to stretch the breast tissue and to reconstruct the mammary relief by creating the necessary space to accommodate a definitive implant. This process, known as tissue expansion, is carried out by progressive fillings of saline through a valve that allows the expander to inflate until the desired volume is reached. The expander is then left inside the breast for a period of approximately 4 to 6 months, the time required for the breast tissue to adequately expand in order to accommodate the definitive implant at a later date. The valve of the expander can be integrated into the implant itself or placed at a distance, or rather be connected through a small silicone tube. The embedded valve reduces the risk of expander depletion. However, this implies that the progressive saline fillings are performed with the needle piercing the tissues (skin, subcutaneous tissue and muscle). Also, the tissue expanders can vary according to some parameters: shape (round, oval to drop, crescent), base, height and projection (classically with a greater projection and wider bending to the inferior pole) (Image 4). The permanent tissue expanders, or Becker's expansion implants, are devices that have the dual function of tissue expanders and long term breast implants, and are designed to be left inside the breast permanently at the end of the expansion. The goal is to avoid a second surgery for the placement of the definitive implant and to maintain the possibility of volume manipulation through a remote valve usually located in the axillary region. There are several models differing by shape, dimension and volume. The disadvantage; however, is a higher rate of implant depletion compared to provisional tissue expanders.

3.1 Status of breast implants filled with silicone gel

On April 10, 1991, the FDA (Food and Drug Administration) asked manufacturers to have silicone gel breast implants to undergo a pre-market test for safety and effectiveness. Unfortunately, they were not able to provide this information to the FDA. Without sufficient data on the safety and effectiveness, the FDA determined that these implants could not be approved. Therefore, the silicone implants were withdrawn from the market. However, these implants were still available through the following studies approved by the FDA:

- an additional study.
- A study investigating patterns in installments (IDE).

In April 1992, after a careful consideration of the public's needs of the alternatives to silicone implants and of their risks, the FDA concluded that the implants should continue to be available for women who require breast reconstruction or revision of an existing implant. Consequently, the additional study was developed to make the implants available for reconstruction and revisions and to collect short-term data on complications. Women who wanted silicone implants to increase the volume, for aesthetic reasons, could not be included in the additional studies. According to the protocol of the additional study, every woman would be followed for a minimum of 5 years.

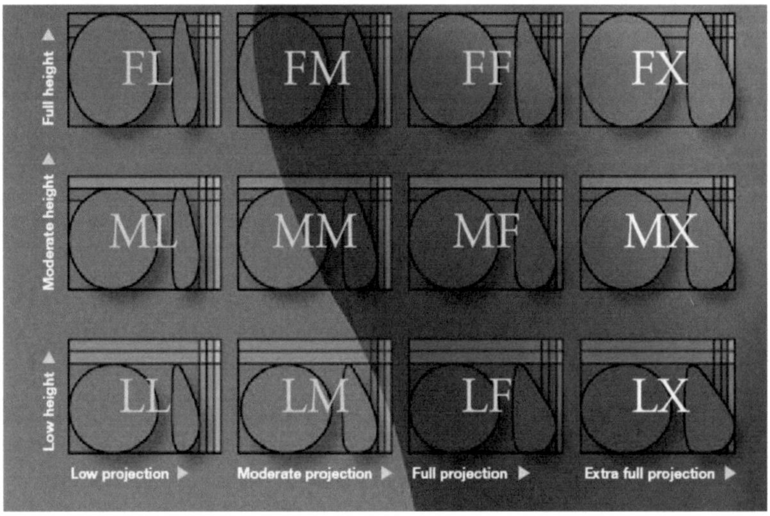

Image 4. Different profile of silicone implants.

The IDE study is a clinical study, reviewed and approved by the FDA in order to ascertain the significance of the data and check for any risks or complications associated with the use of silicone gel implants. Generally, IDE study data is used as the basis for a future application on the market. The women participating in an IDE study can receive their implants for the uses described by the study protocol. A detailed informed consent is mandatory for IDE study. In addition, an IRB (Institutional Review Board), composed of scientists and health professionals, must supervise the study.

On November 17th, 2006, the FDA approved the distribution in the U.S. market of silicone breast implants manufactured by companies Mentor Corp. and Allergan Corp. In addition to having allowed the distribution of silicone breast implants of only two manufacturers (Mentor ed Allergan) that provided complete documentation for the approval, the FDA has limited the use of silicone implants to women aged 22 years and older when the surgery is performed for cosmetic reasons. There is no age limit, however, for the use of silicone implants in breast reconstruction.

3.2 Study of saline solution Implants

The manufacturers of saline implants have had notification from the FDA in January 1993 that the agency would require data on the safety and efficacy of their products. While the manufacturers were carrying out the required studies, the saline implants remained on the market. On May 10, 2000 the FDA approved the pre-market testing of Mentor and McGhan. Currently, saline implants of all other manufacturers are considered experimental.

4. Surgical technique

In the first breast reconstruction surgeries with heterologous material, implants were placed beneath the skin layer, but since the overlying skin appeared visibly irregular with this technique and the use of saline implants, surgeons progressively moved to the placement of implants under the musculofascial layer, between the pectoralis major and the pectoralis minor muscle, in continuity with the serratus anterior, providing better protection for the implant as well as a better aesthetic result. Breast reconstruction with heterologous material includes three different procedures using different prosthetic devices:

- expander-implant technique.
- insertion of immediate definitive implant.
- insertion of permanent expander implant.

4.1 Expander-implant technique

It's the most common technique used today for the immediate reconstruction, but it can also be used for delayed reconstruction. The first surgical stage involves the construction of a lodge under the muscle-fascial layer between the Pectoralis Major muscle and the Pectoralis Minor muscle which is in continuity with the Serratus Anterior muscle and the cephalic portion of the Rectus Abdominis muscle fascia with the disconnection of the Pectoralis Major muscle from distal costal and mid-distal sternal plane. Then, the placement of the expansion implant is performed, pre-injected with saline solution (about 20% of the total volume), and two suction drainages are placed in the axillary region and in the muscular lodge. The expansion, carried out through a valve within the implant (sometimes remote), may begin nearly two weeks after surgery and continue for about 6-8 weeks to reach the desired volume and shape. Chemotherapy does not impair the expansion which can be performed in parallel to chemotherapy (except in cases of severe neutropenia in which it is preferable to suspend the expansion). Once the desired volume is reached, the surgeon then proceeds with the removal of the expansion implant and the insertion of the definitive implant (the second stage of breast reconstruction). However, this procedure must await the end of the chemotherapy treatment and must be preceded by careful assessment of the patient's general state of health. To insert the definitive implant, subject to scarstomy of the previous surgery (gesture oncologically important since surgical scars are a frequent site for local recurrence), a sub-muscular access is performed until the expander is located and removed. This is followed by capsulotomy or radial incisions for tissue relaxation, the creation of a breast neo-fold through prefascial upper abdominal dissection, the anchoring flap with underdermal points on the groove to the V and VI rib periosteum, the placement of suction drainage and of the definitive implant, previously soaked in saline. Accesses are sewed and elasto-compressive dressing is applied. Such reconstruction can be performed regardless of contralateral breasts volume or ptosis status.

The advantages of this technique are as follows:

- technique versatility;
- reconstruction adaptability to ancillary treatments;
- short duration of the first surgical stage (average time 35 minutes);
- immediate reconstruction contextual to mastectomy;
- same access path as used during the demolitive stage;
- possible even if the skin of the mastectomy flap is insufficient;
- achievement of a good level of symmetry of folds, volume and shape;
- adequate expansion of skin and muscles;
- scars confined to the breast area;
- lack of "sacrifice" of working muscles;
- absence of aftereffects on gait and posture as a consequence of the reconstruction method;
- neo-breast skin and sensitivity with typical characteristics of mammary region;
- low immediate and delayed surgical morbidity;

The disadvantages are:

- two surgical stages;
- outpatient procedures necessary for the expansion;
- final outcome can be obtained only after some time;
- three surgical stages to complete the reconstruction (following reconstruction of nipple-areola complex, when requested);
- presence of foreign body (implant);
- possible alterations of the implant due to time and interaction with biological tissues;
- need to use "standard" implants, not always adaptable to shapes and dimensions of biological tissues;
- need to adapt the contralateral breast to the reconstructed one;
- the method is not recommended if residual tissues present precarious conditions (in post-actinic or surgical cases);

Complications associated with the use of breast implants may occur either in the immediate post-operative period or at a later date. They include exposure, extrusion or infection of the implant, asymmetry, displacement or implant rupture and capsular contracture.

4.2 Immediate definitive implant

Patients with contralateral breast of medium or small volume, in the absence of ptosis or mild ptosis, can be treated with the placement of immediate permanent implants. The advantage of such technique is that the entire reconstruction can be performed in a single surgical stage, but several factors have to be considered for this procedure. To start with, this technique cannot be executed if the mastectomy skin flap turns out to be inadequate for the purpose of the mammary relief reconstruction. In addition, frequently the intra-operative result does not match with the surgical outcome later and additional surgeries are commonly needed to achieve satisfactory cosmetic, clinical and morphological outcomes. Therefore, it is extremely difficult to achieve symmetry in shape, volume and the submammary fold in a single surgical stage.

4.3 Permanent expander implants

The use of permanent expansion implants follows the same instructions with respect to immediate definitive implants (small or medium-volume breasts without ptosis or mild ptosis) with the only difference in the possibility of intra- and postoperative volume adjustments. Similarly to the definitive implant, their placement is limited by the precarious conditions of the mastectomy flap and by the difficulty in reaching symmetry in shape, volume and the submammary fold in a single surgery. Besides the obviously higher cost, the disadvantages are the presence of the remote valve which eventually requires an additional surgical procedure for its removal and the fact that the models on the market, compared to implants, are not always adaptable to the shapes and dimensions of the biological tissues.

5. The contralateral breast

Symmetry is one of the main purposes of breast reconstruction, with the need to perform a surgical procedure on the healthy contralateral breast in most cases. Obtaining symmetry represents a great challenge for plastic surgeons, especially in case of unilateral heterologous reconstruction rather than unilateral autologous reconstruction. In addition, surgical techniques should allow an adequate oncological follow-up. The choice of the surgical procedure depends on the oncological stage of the patient, the characteristics of the contralateral breast, the type of mastectomy, the surgeon and patient's preferences. As a matter of fact the evaluation of the contralateral breast during pre-operative planning is essential to achieve an aesthetically pleasing result. The patient should be adequately informed about the whole reconstructive procedure, especially about the need for further surgery and other possible adjustments. The timing for symmetrization procedures is highly controversial. Some surgeons argue that it's easier to re-shape the contralateral breast during the first stage of the reconstruction rather than during a secondary procedure: in these cases the contralateral breast may be a model for the reconstruction rather than a corollary and the symmetrization procedure may be an opportunity to explore the contralateral gland, since the risk of occult cancer. Others prefer to perform the symmetrization surgery after the adjuvant therapy on account of the possibility to further reshape the reconstructed breast. In case of heterologous reconstruction the choice of the surgical technique for symmetrization depends on volume, shape and position of the healthy breasts and must necessarily refer to the reconstructed breast and to the type of prosthesis chosen after the expander. Depending on the above mentioned parameters, it's possible to perform breast reduction and/or mastopexy, or breast augmentation.

5.1 Breast reduction and mastopexy

Breast reduction is performed on the large healthy breast, to adapt it to the reconstructed breast. Several authors recommend the use of a less traumatic as possible technique for the breast parenchyma to facilitate the oncological monitoring of breast cancer. The most common techniques rely on a superior or an inferior pedicle and do not generally require significant mobilization of tissue or glandular flaps. Anyway, the excised tissue is sent for histologic examination due to the risk of developing contralateral breast cancer. The patterns of skin resection vary depending on the size and shape of the breast (inverted-T, J or vertical scar). The "Round block" technique is quite frequently used because it decreases the projection of the breast, allowing a better symmetry with the reconstructed breast over time. Breast mastopexy is preferred if adequate breast volume, with only skin excess and ptosis of the nipple areola complex exclusively, is present. Again, the pattern of resection must minimize scars.

5.2 Breast augmentation

Breast augmentation using implants is generally used to achieve symmetry in patients who underwent heterologous reconstruction, when the contralateral breast has small or medium volume (hypotrophic or normotrophic). The breast reconstructed with heterologous techniques looks less natural and it often presents a rounded appearance, especially in the upper pole; moreover, it doesn't vary in volume like the contralateral breast if the patient changes weight. Therefore, both breasts will have, over time, a different aging process with the onset of asymmetry and the need for surgical procedures to be performed. Consequently, the placement of a contralateral prosthesis can give better symmetry both immediately and over time. The symmetrization using breast implants is comparable to the traditional breast augmentation procedures, therefore the surgeon will have to realize an accureate pre-operative planning about the incision, the choice of the implant and its placement.

5.3 Choice of the implant

Generally, the implants commonly used in Italy and Europe consist of a hard silicone surface wall that encloses silicone gel. The surface can be textured, smooth or made of polyurethane. The shape of the prosthesis can vary essentially between round and anatomical. There are no general rules to make this choice, that is generally made according to the personal preference of the surgeon and the patient. One of the aims of this work is to try to obtain, retrospectively, a decision algorithm for the selection of the contralateral prosthesis in heterologous breast reconstruction.

5.4 Incision placement

Incision placement is a crucial choice, because it greatly affects the final result. Moreover, the placement of the scar is critical to achieve a good cosmetic result and for patients' satisfaction. The choice surely depends on the preference of the surgeon, agreed with the patient, but it must also consider certain anatomical features. The most frequently used incisions are the hemiperiareolar, inframammary fold and axillar. Hemiperiareolar incision: this is the most versatile approach. It provides a central access to all quadrants and it is compatible with all types of breast implants and plans for dissection. It is preferable when the inframammary fold should be lowered of several centimeters, and it is the best choice when a round block technique is simultaneously performed. It is also the most appropriate approach for the remodelling the gland, as in cases of tuberous breast. A little areolar diameter may limit the viability of this access; anyway, it must be considered that an areolar diameter of 2.5 cm can still provide an access at least 4 cm. Caution should be taken with the nipples that lacks net color contrast, because the scar would be very visible. There is also evidence that this incision may cause alterations in the sensitivity of the nipple and areola.

Incision in the inframammary sulcus: this is undoubtly the most simple approach in breast augmentation. It gives direct access to both the subglandular and submuscular plans, which can be reached without the need for a trans-glandular dissection. The scar can be hidden from the lower pole, but the quality of these scars is often worse than hemiperiareolar ones. The length of the incision can be considerable, allowing the placement of large implants. In patients with lower pole hypoplasia, after positioning the implant, the IMF may fall more than planned, thus resulting in an ugly scar in the lower pole of the breast. Incision in the armpit: This type of access is preferred when the patient does not want any scar on the breast. The scar is hidden well behind the anterior pillar of the axilla. The access to the surgical plans is more difficult than the two previously described approaches, but the use of an endoscope may facilitate the operation. However, the technique lacks precision in the dissection and placement of the implant, increasing the risk of asymmetry and malpositioning. Furthermore, it is impossible, if necessary, to manipulate the breast parenchyma to insert large silicone gel implants. Trans-umbilical incision: trans umbilical access is certainly the latest innovation in breast augmentation. Through an invisible incision inside the navel, a subcutaneous tunnel is created just above the fascia of the rectus muscles up to the breast. Although it has been described for positioning of the implant in both subglandular or submuscular pockets, the latter is very difficult. The risks and limitations are the same of the axillary approach as both the accesses are far from the mammary gland. In addition, it is impossible to insert a silicone-gel implant and it should be used with caution in patients with a very thin subcutaneous tissue.

5.5 Implant placement

The mainly used pockets created for implants placement breast augmentation are the retroglandular, partially submuscular, totally submuscular and dual-plane.

Subglandular: In the history of breast augmentation the subglandular pocket was the first to be described. It is generally viable with patients in whom there is enough tissue to cover the implant. In patients with poor adipo-glandular tissue the risk of implant visibility and palpability is very high. In addition the prosthesis becomes very visible in the upper quadrants of the breast, resulting in a typical deformation of the breast. Moreover, the subglandular pocket is associated with an increased risk of capsular contracture compared to submuscular or partially submuscular ones. In addition, the subglandular implant interferes with mammography more than the submuscular.

Submuscular: The totally submuscular pocket was developed in order to reduce the visibility and palpability of the implant and the incidence of capsular contracture. Unfortunately, with this technique the definition of the lower pole is poor, often worse than with other techniques. In addition, there is a higher incidence of upper dislocation of the implant.

Subpectoral: Generally the term subpectoral refers to a pocket partially under the pectoralis major muscle, with the lower portion of the implant located under the gland. This localization seems to be associated to a lower incidence of capsular contracture; it also facilitates mammography. This pocket should be used with caution in women with postpartum atrophy or glandular ptosis, because in these cases the risk of creating a double-bubble deformity is very high.

Dual-Plane: This technique has been developed as an evolution of the subpectoral pocket to minimize the risk of double bubble. The technique, recently described by Tebbets, achieves a good shape of the breast using both the submuscular and subglandular plans. The main difference with the subpectoral technique is the subglandular dissection, which may extend to the upper edge of the areola. In patients with poor breast tissue, dissection proceeds to the lower edge of the areola. In patients with more soft tissue coverage and ptosis, the dissection extends until the top edge of the areola.

6. Aim of the study

The aim of this retrospective study was to critically analyze the outcome of breast reconstruction after mastectomy using tissue expander followed by permanent implant placement and contralateral symmetrization trough augmentation mammaplasty with a follow up at least of three years.

The overall aesthetic results was analyzed on the base of grade of symmetry, shape, volume, implant position, patient and surgeon satisfactions, thus evaluated with objective method (physical examination with clinical measures) and with a subjective one trough a questionnaire administered to patients. Thus a flow chart was developed based on the volume, contour, and position of the natural and reconstructed breast and on the base of the data collected trough the study.

7. Materials and methods

A review of about 360 tissue/expander breast reconstructions performed at University Campus Bio-Medico of Rome from 2003 to 2009 was performed. Out of 360 288 reconstructions (80%) were eterologous with two stage technique. 35 patients operated with permanent implant placement and contralateral symmetrization trough augmentation mammaplasty were included in the present study.

The exclusion criteria were contralateral symmetrisation with reduction mammaplasty or mastopexy.

Preliminarily, patients were classified according age, tumour stage (Table 1), chemotherapy (after either quadrantectomy or mastectomy), radiation therapy timing of reconstruction (immediate vs delay), expander volume, definitive implant (in both sides), numbers of reoperation.

Grouping in stages

N°	stage0	stage1	stage 2A	stage 2B	stage 3A	stage 3 B
Pz	5	10	11	7	1	1

Table 1.

Tissue expander were choosen according to contralateral breast width, volume and shape and patients heigth. The follow up was completed in 17 patients (48%). The Authors evaluated in both breasts the following measures immediately after nipple areola reconstruction (time 0) and after at least 3 years (time 1):

- emiclavear –nipple distance
- sternal notch-nipple distance
- nipple –IMF distance
- breast width
- grade of contracture

Patient and surgeon satisfaction were assesed trough a questionnaire with numerical score form 1 to 5 (poor, fair, good, very good, excellent) regarding breasts appearance in terms of:

- Shape
- Volume
- Projection
- Inframmary fold
- Ptosis
- Countour of the device
- Grade of contracture
- Symmetry
- Overall aesthetic result

Accurate photographic documentation was thus evaluated by surgeons.

8. Results

Of the 35 patients the mean age of patients identified was 54 years ranging from 38 to 74 years.

Immediate reconstruction was performed in 25 patients (71%), delay reconstruction in 10 patients (29%). Volume range of tissue expander was from 300cc to 850 cc with median volume of 500 cc.

Volume range of anatomical implants of the reconstructed breast was from 210cc to 640 cc with median volume of 427 cc. In all reconstructed breasts the implant was anatomical shape, style 410. The implant style was 410 (Table 2), Low Height-Full Projection (LF) in 8 cases (23%), Low Height - Extra projection in 4 cases (11%), Medium height- Full Projection (MF) in 14 cases (40%), Medium height-Extra Projection in 8 cases (23%) and Full Height-Full Projection in 1 case (3%).

Height	Projection			
	L	M	F	X
F	0	0	0	1
M	0	0	14	8
L	0	0	8	4

Table 2.

For the contralateral symmetrization the implant volume range was from 90cc to 440 cc with median volume of 220cc. In 23 cases (83%) a round implant style 110 was used while in only 6 cases (17%) anatomical implant was preferred , style 410 LL in 1 case, style 410 ML in 1 case, style 410 FL in 1 case, style 410 MM in 1 case and style 410 MF in 2 cases (33%) as showed in Table 3.

Height	Projection			
	L	M	F	X
F	0	1	0	0
M	1	1	2	0
L	1	0	0	0

Table 3.

23 patients underwent adjuvant chemotherapy, 2 patients underwent both chemotherapy and radiotherapy. Thirteen patients underwent re operation: 7 capsulotomies for capsular contracture grade III of the reconstructed breast, 6 lipofilling for breast contour irregolarities. Follow up ranged from 1 to 5 years with median of 4 years. Seventeen patients patients after at least 3 years of follow-up were evaluated. A comparison between time 0 and time 1 of the reconstructed breast is shown on Table 4, of the contralateral breast is shown on Table 5.

Parameters	Medium value		Variation
	T0	T1	
distance midclavicular-nipple	19,8125	18,906	1 ↓
distance jugular-nipple	20,9375	19,94	1 ↓
distance nipple-furrow	7,7666	7,4063	0,5 ↓
mammary base	13,125	12,81	0,4 ↓

Table 4.

Parameters	Medium value		Variation
	T0	T1	(Δm)
distance midclavicular-nipple	19	20,58	1,58 ↑
distance jugular-nipple	21,53	22,02	0,5 ↑
distance nipple-furrow	8,12	8,11	↔
mammary base	14,03	13,61	0,4 ↓

Table 5.

Capsular contracture grades classified with modified Baker classification was higher on the reconstructed breast compared to the healthy one. (Table 6).

Breast	Medium value		Δ Avarage
	T0	T1	
Reconstructed	1,43	2,68	1,25
Controlateral	1,06	1,25	0,19

Table 6.

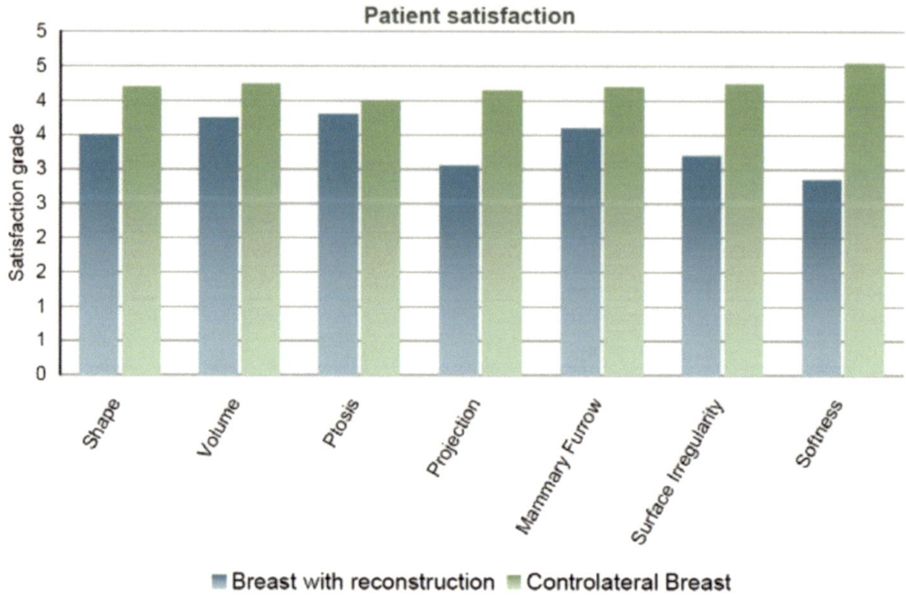

Image 5.

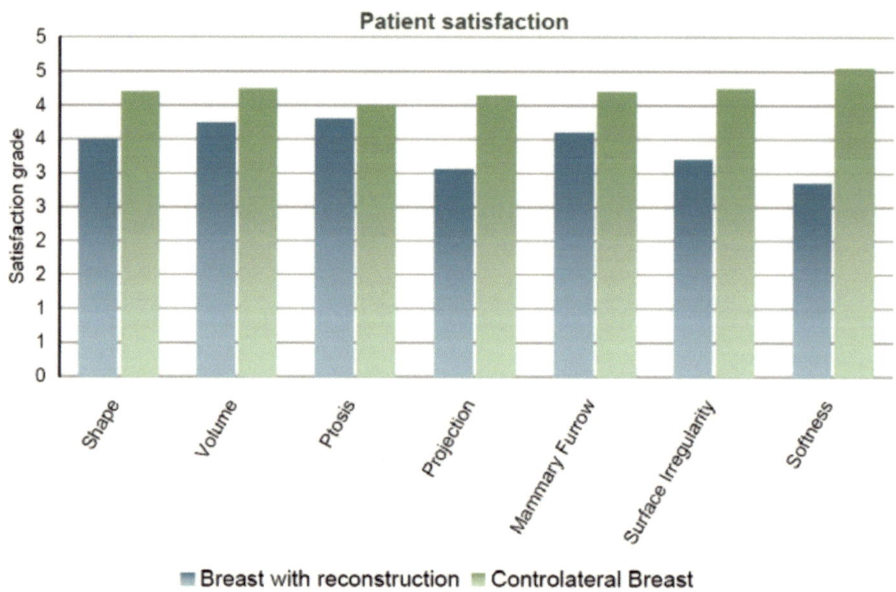

Image 6.

Patient and surgeon satisfaction were assesed trough a questionnaire with numerical score form 1 to 5 (poor, fair, good, very good, excellent). Patient satisfaction was scored and showed in Image 5 while surgeon satisfaction was scored in Image 6. For the contralateral breast the score ranged in all patients between good and excellent. Symmetry was scored good in majority of case, while global satisfaction was scored good for surgeon, very good for patients in most cases

On the base of our results we developed a flow chart to guide the surgeon to preoperatively choice the right implant on the base of the shape of contralateral breast:

- Normal shape, glandular hypomastia: round implant
- Normotrophic, ptotic breast: round implant
- Normal shape, hypertrofic breast: round implant
- Normotrofic breast wih hypoplasia of 1 or 2 quadrants: round implant
- Hypoplasic breast with mild deformity of 1 or 2 quadrants: anatomical or round implant
- Hypoplasic breast with severe deformity of 2 or more quadrants: anatomical implant

9. Discussion

In plastic surgery a good result is not influenced only by technical competence but also depends on other factors such as few surgical prestiges, short operating time, absence of pain, no touch up which of course highly increase patient's satisfaction. Patients undergoing breast reconstruction usually expected full recovery of the body image without further complications and they pay more attention to the oncological aspects than to the reconstructive ones, especially in immediate procedures. No interference with adjuvant therapies, very limited scars and perfect match with the contralateral breast are strongly considered in women's final evaluation. On the opposite, a technical opinion on the breast reconstruction mostly considers whether all anatomical features have been recovered and maintained for the longest. The goal is not "to fill the cup of a bra" but to "rebuild" an organ that has been mutilated. Shape, volume and projection of the breast are the main issues but many details need to be adequately restored such as fullness of the lower pole, definition of the inframammary fold (IMF) and nipple areola complex (NAC) position. In eterologous breast reconstruction the development of capsular contracture is probably the main cause for the loss of symmetry at 5 years follow up, which show a very high incidence in all studies (over 60 %) of revisions, so the challenge to maintain the result remains open. As other groups have already published our limited experience confirm some important considerations and suggest some refinements in implant based reconstruction that is still the major reconstructive procedure performed (80%, 288 out of 360 patients in our series). Simmetrization of controlateral breast is a key point. As Loske demonstrated and published, in fact, breast reduction, mastopexy and breast augmentation must be required to remodel the healthy breast (67%), and particularly contralateral breast augmentation seemed more used in implant based reconstruction (41%). Nahabedian et al. also introduced the necessity to revise surgical procedure along the years. In our experience simmetrization of controlateral breast has been done in almost 90% and breast augmentation revealed to be a precious tool to enhance long lasting symmetry in eterolougus reconstruction. Shape and position of the healthy breast unfortunately vary as time pass, breast reduction and mastopexy may age more rapidily while the presence of a submuscular implant improving upper pole fullness and volume symmetry may require minor revisions especially when a capsular contracture occurs on the reconstructed breast. The choice of which implant to use in these cases is crucial but represents just a step in the ongoing debate about round and anatomical in common cosmetic breast augmentation. Our review suggested that for normal shaped breast requiring just volume adjustment a round implant can be used, on the contrary in case of severe hypoplasia an anatomical implant is preferable. In our series 83% of patients had a round implant while the 17% need an anatomical one. Round implants have some advantages as they do not rotate, can be easily inserted even trough small incisions and can be used also in mild to moderate hypertrophy combining implant position with a minor breast reduction. On the other hand round implants improve just volume and uppur pole fullness but they do not correct asymmetry of breast diamters. According to our chart they must be chosen if the breast is normal shape or if the deficiency is limited to one quadrant. In case of more severe alterations involving 2 or more quadrants the anatomical implants are ideal. The vast sort of different width, height and projection, commonly available for anatomical implants, allowed an easy matching of the extra projected implant which is often chosen on the reconstructed side. Anyway, the long term analysis of 35 patients who have underwent breast augmentation on the contralateral side and completed the three years follow up, showed in the 49% the presence of asymmetry mainly due to capsular contracture. As well as in other studies also in our series most of the variations, such as implant dislocation, loss of lower pole projection and IMF definition occurred on the reconstructed breast. These modifications required in the 37% of cases a further surgical correction which has been achieved by means of lipostructure and lipofilling. Finally it is interesting to underline that patient's opinion, from the VAS questionnaire we have asked and registered, demonstrated a higher satisfaction when a contralateral implant is employed. This result was confirmed even in patients older than 65 years. The reason is probably a better symmetry with a upper pole fullness especially wearing the bra. All these patients, in fact, realized and described the development of modifications during the years but at the same time continued to positively judge the surgical procedure declaring an overall improvement of body image after the reconstruction with a full recovery of relationship and quality of life.

10. Conclusions

Heterologous breast reconstruction still represents a first option in a great majority of patients due to easy and rapid technique, no donor site morbidity and technological improvement in implant industry. Contralateral breast symmetrization should be performed during the second stage of breast reconstruction. Nevertheless long term follow up confirm after 3 years a progressive loss of symmetry that may require further corrections. Lipostructure may be also useful in order to harmonize the volume and shape of both breasts, to acquire a better shape of the reconstructed breast or to manage the implant based breast contracture. In conclusion we underline that breast symmetrization with augmentation mammaplasty enhances long term satisfaction of patients and it should be consider as an important tool also in case of older patients or in case of mild to moderate breast hypertrophy.

11. Clinic cases

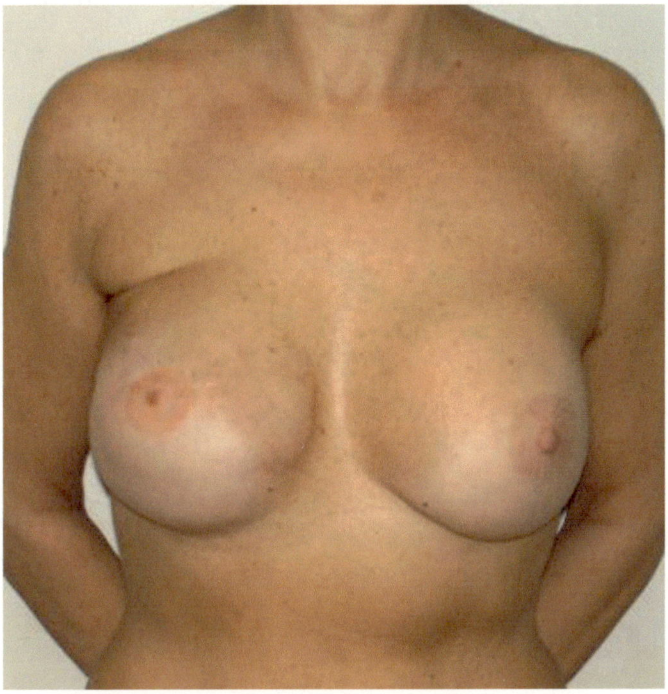

A

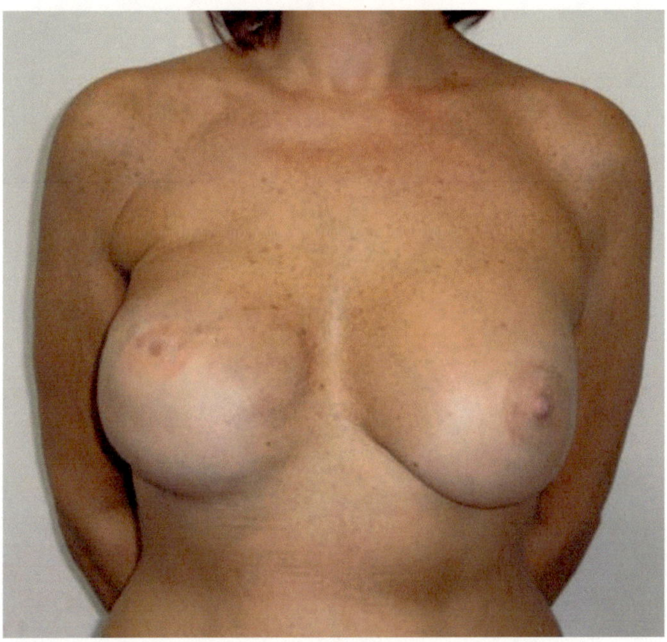

B

Fig. 1. Post-operation: (A) time T0; (B) time T1 follow-up 5 years

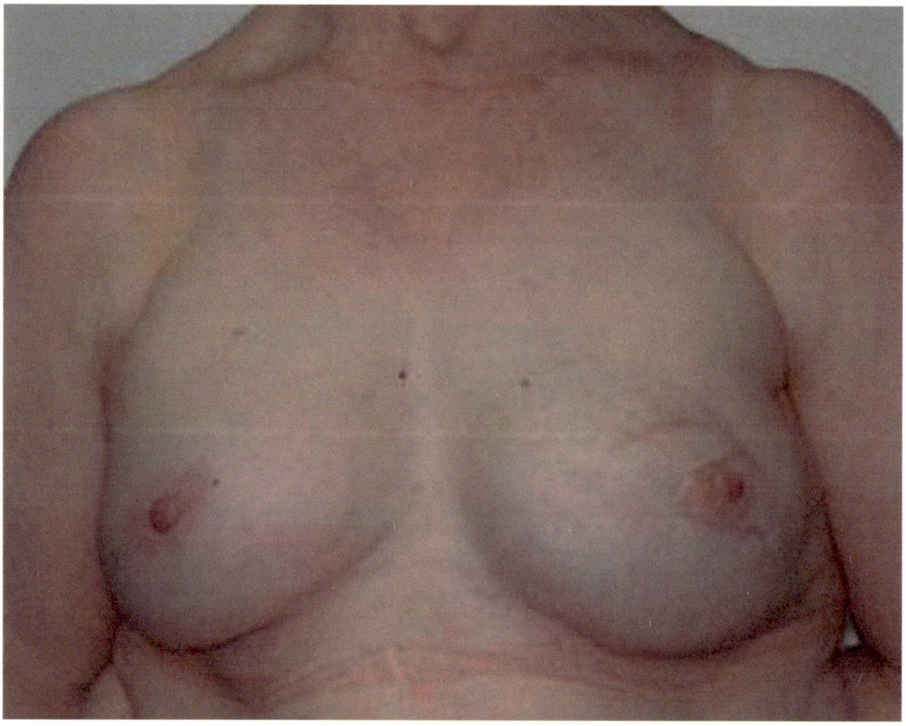

A

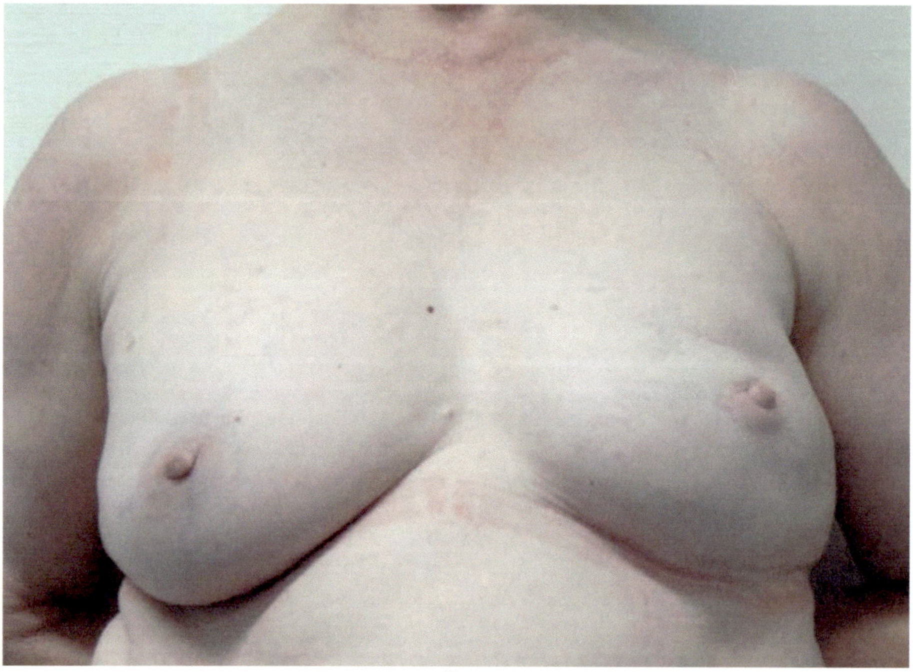

B

Fig. 2. Post-operation: (A) time T0; (B) time T1 follow-up 5 years

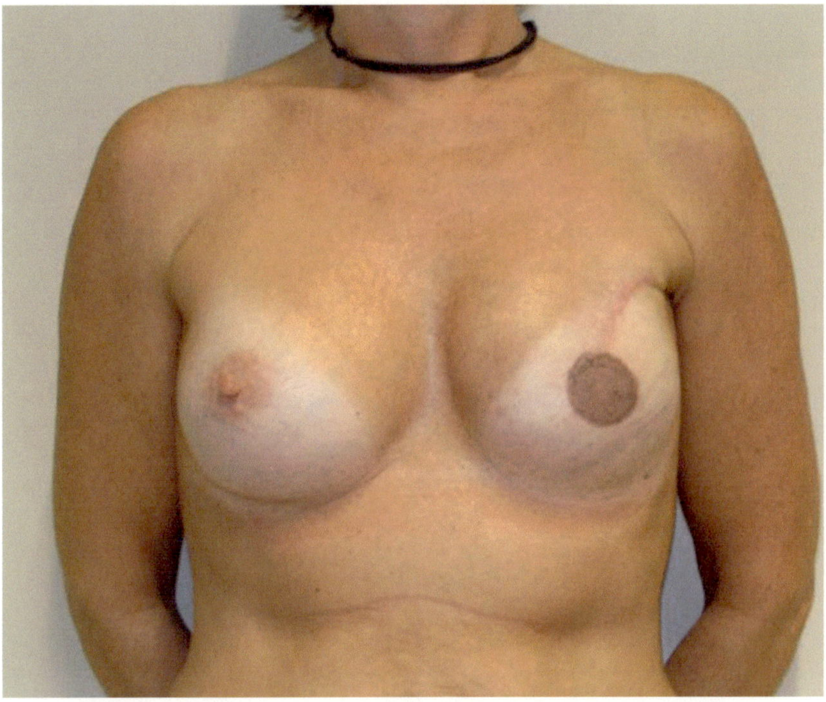

A

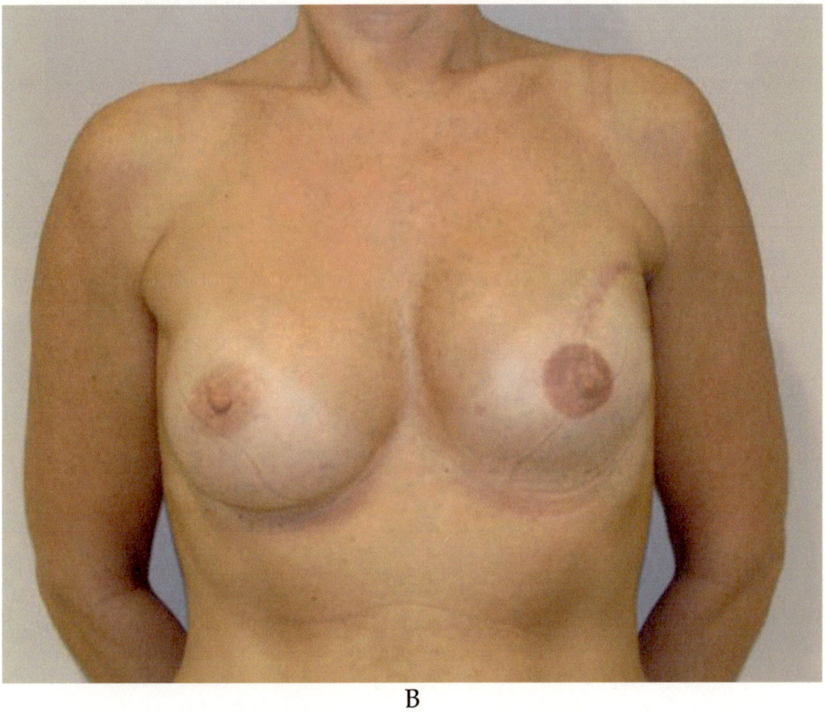

B

Fig. 3. Post-operation: (A) time T0; (B) time T1 follow-up 5 years

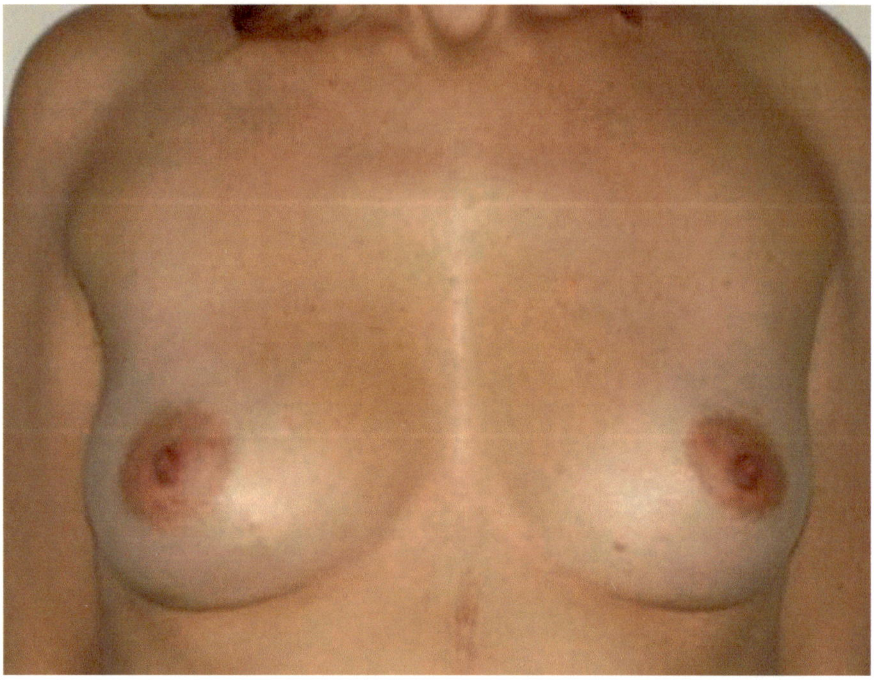

A

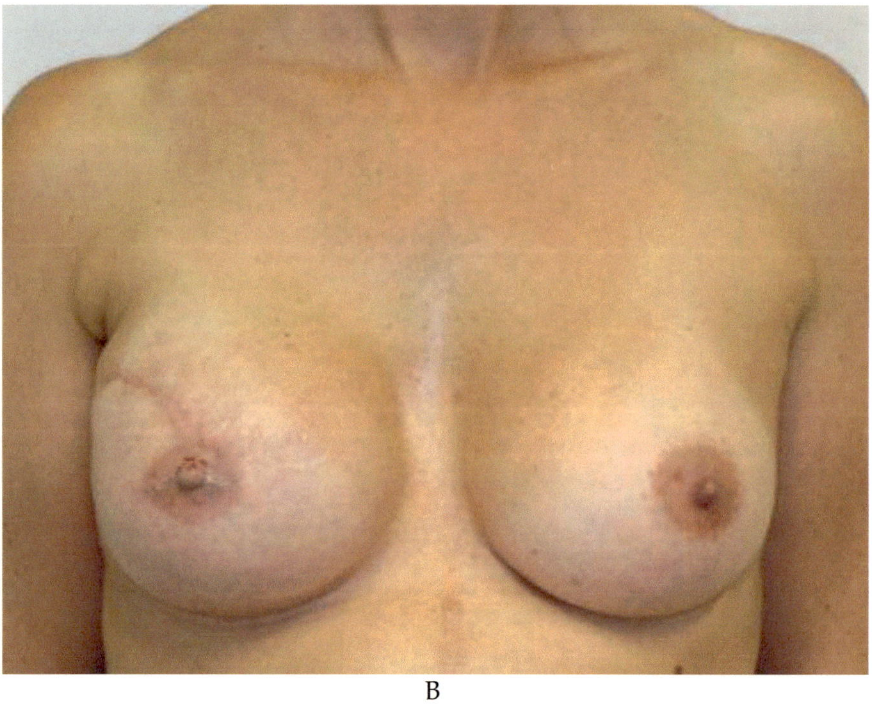

B

Fig. 4. (A) Pre-operation. (B)Post-operation:reconstruction right breast :anatomic implant H media /P extra; controlateral left breast : round implant P moderate

12. References

A.D. Fitoussi, B. Couturaud. Evaluation of asymmetric implants in breast augmentation surgery. Annales de chirurgie plastique esthétique 50 (2005) 517–523.

Albert Losken, M.D., Grant W. Carlson, M.D., John Bostwick, III, M.D.,† Glyn E. Jones, M.D., John H. Culbertson, M.D., and Mark Schoemann, B.A. Trends in Unilateral Breast Reconstruction and Management of the Contralateral Breast: The Emory Experience. Plastic and reconstructive surgery. July 2002; Vol. 110, No.

Asplund O, Korlof B. Late results following mastectomy for cancer and breast reconstruction. Scand J Plast Reconstr Surg 1984;18:221–5

Bogetti P, Boltri M, Balocco P, Spagnoli G. Augmentation mammaplasty with a new cohesive gel prosthesis. Aesthetic Plast Surg 2000;24(6):440–4

Bostwick J Iii. Breast reconstruction following mastectomy. CA Cancer J Clin 1995; 45: 289-304.[

Dean C, Chetty U, Forrest AP. Effects of immediate breast reconstruction on psychosocial morbidity after mastectomy. Lancet 1983;1:459-62.

Elder EE, Brandberg Y, Björklund T, et al. Quality of life and patient satisfaction in breast cancer patients after immediate breast reconstruction: a prospective study. Breast 2005;14:201-8.

Emily S. Hu e all. Plast Reconstr Surg.- July 2009-V. 124, Number 1.2

Emily S. Hu, Andrea L. Pusic, Jennifer F. Waljee, Latoya Kuhn, Sarah T. Hawley, Edwin Wilkins, Amy K. Alderman. Patient-Reported Aesthetic Satisfaction with Breast Reconstruction during the Long-Term Survivorship Period. Plastic and Reconstructive Surgery, July 2009-Volume 124, Number 1.

Garson S, Delay E, Sinna R, Carton S, Delaporte T, Chekaroua K. 3D evalution and breast plastic surgery: preliminary study. Ann Chir Plast Esthét 2005;50(4):296–308.

K.B.Clough, I.Sarfati, A. Fitoussi, P. Leblanc-Talent. Breast reconstruction: late cosmetic results of implant reconstruction. Annales de chirurgie plastique esthétique 50 (2005) 560–574.

Kroll SS, Baldwin B. A comparison of outcomes using three different methods of breast reconstruction. Plast Reconstr Surg 1992;90:455. [4(1)

Lagergren J, Jurell G, Sandelin K, et al. Technical aspects of immediate breast reconstruction with implants: Five year follow-up. Scand J Plast Reconstr Surg Hand Surg 2005;39:147–52

Leis HP Jr. Managing the remaining breast. Cancer. 1980 Aug 15;46(4 Suppl):1026-30.

Linell F, Ljungberg O, Andersson I. Breast carcinoma. Aspects of early stages, progression and related problems. Acta Pathol Microbiol Scand Suppl. 1980;(272):1-233.

Metcalfe KA, Semple JL, Narod SA. Satisfaction with breast reconstruction in women with bilateral prophylactic mastectomy: a descriptive study. Plast Reconstr Surg 2004;114:360-6.

Nahabedian MY. Managing the opposite breast: contralateral symmetry procedures. Cancer J 2008 Jul-Aug;14(4):258-63.

Niechajev I. Mammary augmentation by cohesive silicone gel implants with anatomic shape: technical considerations. Aesthetic Plast Surg 2001;25(6):397–403

Olle Asplund and Gunilla Svane. Adjustment of the contralateral breast following breast reconstruction. Scand J Plast Reconstr Surg 17: 225-232, 1983. (

P.Panettiere, L. Marchetti, D.Accorsi, G.A. Del Gaudio. Aesthetic Breast Reconstruction. Aesthetic plast. surgery. 26:429-435, 2002

Parker PA, Youssef A, Walker S, et al. Short-term and long-term psychosocial adjustment and quality of life in women undergoing different surgical procedures for breast cancer. Ann Surg Oncol 2007; 14:3078-89.

Peter G. Cordeiro, M.D. Breast Reconstruction after Surgery for Breast Cancer. N.Engl.J.Med. 359-15; October 9, 2008.

Petit, J. Y., Rietjens, M., Contesso, G., Bertin, F., and Gilles, R. Contralateral mastoplasty for breast reconstruction: A good opportunity for glandular exploration and occult carcinomas diagnosis. Ann. Surg. Oncol. 4: 511, 1997.

Ringberg A, Palmer B, Linell F. The contralateral breast at reconstructive surgery after breast cancer operation a histopathological study.. Breast Cancer Res Treat. 1982;2(2):151-61.

Roldán, J. A. Lozano, J. Oroz. An. Sist. Sanit. Navar. Treatment of the contralateral breast in breast reconstruction. Nipple- areola reconstruction. P.. 2005; 28 (Supl. 2): 81-90.

Rowland JH, Desmond KA, Meyerowitz, BE, Belin TR, Wyatt GE, Ganz PA. Role of breast reconstructive surgery in physical and emotional outcomes among breast cancer survivors. J Natl Cancer Inst 2000; 92:1422-9.

Sigurdson L, Lalonde DH. MOC-PSSM CME article: Breast reconstruction. Plast Reconstr Surg. 2008 Jan;121(1 Suppl):1-12

Tebbetts JB. Dual plane breast augmentation: optimizing implant-soft-tissue relationships in a wide range of breast types. Plast Reconstr Surg. 2006 Dec;118(7 Suppl):81S-98S; discussion 99S-102S.

Vandeweyer E, Hertens D, Nogaret JM, Deraemaecker R. Immediate breast reconstruction with saline-filled implants: no interference with the oncologic outcome? Plast Reconstr Surg 2001;107: 1409-12.

5

The Role of Free Fat Graft in Breast Reconstruction After Radiotherapy

Pietro Panettiere, Danilo Accorsi and Lucio Marchetti
Dipartimento di Scienze Chirurgiche Specialistiche ed Anestesiologiche, University of Bologna Italy

1. Introduction

Free fat grafts in plastic surgery and in regenerative medicine are extremely promising. Their use in breast reconstruction and in particular after radiotherapy is radically changing the approach to the problem.

2. Radiotherapy and tissue damage

Radiotherapy is a fundamental therapeutic resource in a large majority of neoplastic diseases. But adverse reactions and complications can severely damage the irradiated tissues. Adverse effects can be distinguished into early (within few weeks to 90 days from treatment) and late ones (months to years from exposure). Late adverse effects are primarily the result of radiation-dependent reduction of stem cells or progenitors (Brush, 2007; Rodemann & Blaese, 2007). Fibrosis, teleangiectasias and atrophy are the most common late effects for skin and subcutaneous tissues and those most frequently observed in irradiated breast cancer patients. The mean concentrations of collagen are two times higher in irradiated skin than in non-irradiated skin thus leading to fibrosis (Autio et al, 1998; Riekki et al, 2002). There seems to be a genetic predisposition for fibrosis and teleangiectasias as a response to radiotherapy. Fibrosis risk is also associated with an inflammatory response, whereas telangiectasia is linked to endothelial cell damage. Atrophy is related to an acute response, but no genetic predisposing factors have yet been identified. (Quarmby et al, 2003; Andreassen et al, 2005; Giotopoulos et al, 2007). The reconstructive properties of adipose tissue are also significantly altered (Poglio et al, 2009) as the stromal microenvironment is unable to self-repair the injury suffered. Depletion of the stromal compartment leads to a loss of the precursor reservoir, thus compromising its ability to maintain tissue homeostasis. In response to ionizing radiation, fibroblasts and macrophages remain in an activated state, continuously generating growth factors and free radicals (Barcellos-Hoff et al, 2005) which are the main reasons for fibrosis. Radiations also severely harm the homeostatic network connecting parenchymal, mesenchymal, and vascular cells within tissues and normal interactions between cells are therefore altered (Barcellos-Hoff et al, 2005; Bentzen, 2006). Late adverse effects of radiotherapy in breast reconstructions can consequently cause flap failure, implant exposure, and capsular contracture in prosthetic breast reconstructions. The final aesthetic results can also be compromised due to liponecrosis.

The Late Effects of Normal Tissue-Subjective Objective Management Analytical (LENT-SOMA) scale (Pavy et al, 1995) is considered the gold standard when evaluating radiation injury (Hoeller et al, 2003), as it provides both subjective and objective analyses and a detailed and specific description of the nature and severity of the injury.

3. Adipose-Derived Stem/Stromal Cells (ADSCs)

3.1 The features of the ADSCs

The ideal stem cell for use in tissue regeneration needs to be abundantly available, harvested with minimal morbidity, reliably differentiated down various pathways and able to be safely and efficaciously transplanted. Adult human adipose tissue contains a population of mesenchymal stem cells (MSC), named "adipose-derived stem cells" or "adipose-derived stromal cells" (ADSC), which seem to fulfil most, if not all, of these criteria. They are part of the stromal vascular fraction (SVF) that also contains a large amount of mature endothelial and hematopoietic cells. ADSCs can be harvested readily, safely, and in relative abundance by liposuction techniques. Their abundance in adipose tissue is 100 to 500 fold higher than that of MSCs in bone marrow. Their functional properties are: multipotency, functional cell support (stromagenesis), and modulation of immuno-inflammatory functions. Most of these effects are believed to be mediated via paracrine activity (Caplan & Dennis, 2006; Phinney & Prockop, 2007), so that the fat is considered as a true endocrine tissue (Casteilla et al, 2005; Gimble et al, 2007; Uccelli et al, 2008; Wang et al, 2008). The multipotency of ADSCs was first proved *in vitro* by Zuk (Zuk et al, 2002) and several works proved that they can differentiate into other mesenchymal tissue types, including adipocytes, chondrocytes (Erickson et al, 2002), myocytes and osteoblasts (Cowan et al, 2004) as well as they are claimed to differentiate also into nerves (Kang et al, 2003), cardiomyocytes, hepatocytes and pancreatic endocrine cells, even if their *in vivo* potential still remains unclear. Therefore, fat cells are supposed to effectively supply any tissue texture both in trauma reconstruction and for aesthetic needs (Wickham et al, 2003; Gimble & Guilak, 2003). Angiogenic properties were also observed, even more efficient than the bone marrow MSCs one (Y. Kim al, 2007), probably linked to the secretion of vascular endothelial growth factor (Cousin et al, 2003; Planat-Benard et al, 2004; Mazo et al, 2008; Ebrahimian et al, 2009) or other cytokines/chemokines (HGF, placental growth factor, FGF-2, TGF-β, and angiopoietin-1). This suggests that ADSCs may have a potential as cell sources for therapeutic angiogenesis (Murohara et al, 2009). Angiogenic activity was shown to increase in hypoxic conditions (Rehman et al, 2004; Weil et al, 2009), but aging could reduce angiogenic potentials (Efimenko et al, 2011). A very efficient immunosuppressive capability and modulation of inflammation both in vitro and in vivo were also shown (Puissant et al, 2005; Yañez et al, 2006; González et al, 2009; Constantin et al, 2009) as demonstrated in healing chronic wounds in Crohn's fistulae (Garcia-Olmo et al, 2008, 2009; Ebrahimian et al, 2009).

3.2 Adipose-tissue Derived Stem Cells (ADSCs) in irradiated tissues

An increasing number of studies addressed lipofilling in irradiated tissues (Rigotti et al, 2007; O. Amar et al, 2008; Phulpin et al, 2009; Faghahati et al, 2010). The rationale for the use of ADSCs in irradiated tissue repair stems from the consideration that late adverse effects of radiotherapy derive from the destruction or the loss of functionality of ADSCs and, in particular, the loss of self-repair properties, chronic inflammation and destruction of microcirculation. The fat grafts can replace atrophic functional niches (the complex made of cell, extracellular and biochemical elements whom the adipose cell interacts with) with physiologic ones, thus playing their normalizing role on the receiving tissue. The normalizing role of free fat grafts in tissue regeneration was pointed out by several clinical studies (Moseley et al, 2006; Rigotti et al, 2007; Locke & de Chalain, 2008; Panettiere et al, 2009; Sarfati et al, 2011). In a recent work (Panettiere, 2011), USG and MR of a free fat grafts reconstructed breast suggested that the proliferation and differentiation of the ADSCs allowed the formation of a perfectly normal structural tissue. Moreover, a quite high density of perivascular stem elements was found, demonstrating a persistent regenerative potential.

An important reduction of fibrosis was also observed (Rigotti et al, 2007; Panettiere et al, 2009, 2011). The immunoregulatory activity and the capacity to modulate inflammation displayed by ADSCs can at least partially explain such behaviour. Recent studies therefore started challenging the dogma of the relative contraindication of prosthetic reconstruction after radiotherapy (Percec, 2008; Panettiere et al, 2009; Salgarello et al, 2010).

3.3 Neoplastic degeneration of the ADSCs or activation of dormant neoplastic cells

The immunosuppressive effect associated with angiogenic properties of ADSCs, as well as their paracrine activity, raised questions about their interactions with cancer cells. A positive correlation between obesity and cancer is well-known (Roberts et al, 2010). Some authors observed that ADSCs can promote tumour growth (Zhang et al, 2009; Lin et al, 2010; Prantl et al, 2010; Zhao et al, 2010; Nomoto-Kojima et al, 2011; Zimmerlin et al, 2011). Tumour growth beyond the size of 1-2 mm is angiogenesis-dependent. Therefore, it was hypothesized that the angiogenic spike induced by MSCs or ADSCs could awake dormant cancer cells (Naumov et al, 2006; Vessella et al, 2007; Indraccolo et al, 2006; Favaro et al, 2008); but more recent studies (Donnenberg et al, 2010; Zimmerlin et al, 2011) concluded that ADSCs could trigger tumour growth from active cancer cells, but not from dormant ones. Moreover, ADSCs promoted tumour growth only when transplanted at the beginning of the neoplastic process. An unusual cell line was observed to emerge from a culture of human ADSCs. Though being proved to be unable to form tumours, they presented alarming similarities with human angiosarcoma (Ning et al, 2009). At present, there is no firm evidence that ADSCs can directly promote tumorigenesis and some works showed an even inhibitory effect of ADSCs when implanted in pre-existing tumours (Cousin et al, 2009). It was thus suggested that reactive cross-talk can take place between ADSCs and other cell types that maintain a proper tissue development and a correct balance between proliferation and differentiation (Casteilla et al, 2011).

Some works addressed the angiogenic capability and suspected that ADSCs respond to chemotactic factors and migrate to the sites of injuries, inflammation, and/or tumour (Kubis et al, 2007; J.M. Kim et al, 2007; Constantin et al, 2009; Lamfers et al, 2009; Lee et al, 2009; Lin, 2010; Gehmert et al, 2010; U. Kim et al, 2011). This property was used in a recent experimental work where engineered ADSCs (able to convert 5-fluorocytosine into the 5-fluorouracil) engrafted into tumours and micro-metastases, activating prodrugs directly within the neoplastic mass (Cavarretta et al, 2010). The secretion of anti-apoptotic factors, and the T cell-mediated immune response suppression have been blamed for a tumour-supporting role (Jones & McTaggart, 2008; Fox et al, 2007; Wels et al, 2008). ADSCs can be found everywhere in the body and their ability to migrate is not a peculiarity of transplanted cells. So, any ADSC in the body could migrate and promote cancer growth and not only transplanted ones. In irradiated patients very few ADSCs can be found in the site of possible residual tumour cells due to radiotherapy itself. So fat grafts implanted directly in the irradiated site could restore a tumour-supporting environment. But this could happen also with flap reconstructions where the ADSCs present in the subcutaneous fat of the flap are transferred to the irradiated areas. Much concern could be raised by *in vitro* stimulated ADSCs. Anyhow, a potential different behaviour between native and cultured cells remains an open question. A recent limited clinical study with a good follow up found no increase in the recurrence rates in patients treated with fat grafts (Petit et al, 2011). A single case of a late osteosarcoma recurrence 18 months after free fat graft was reported (Perrot et al, 2010). In any case, the risk for possible cancer promotion in the context of cancer related diseases cannot still be ruled out at present.

4. The free fat grafts

Free fat grafts were first described by Neuber (Neuber, 1893). In 1914, Bruning (Bruning, 1914) was the first to inject autologous fat into the subcutaneous tissue. Liposuction provided large volumes of autologous fat that could be re-injected. Since 1985 the first works about fat re-implantation from liposuction were published (Illouz, 1985, 1986a, 1986b; Chajchir & Benzaquen, 1986).

4.1 Techniques for fat harvesting

The keystone of fat graft is to transplant as many vital cells as possible in the best survival conditions, while injecting more (nonviable) graft material is useless. The keys for graft survival are well known: adequate donor site, atraumatic harvesting, short time between collection and re-implantation, suitable host bed and adequate stabilization.

As far as regards the best donor site, there is no clear evidence in the literature. In a recent survey, the most preferred site for fat harvest was the abdomen (89%), followed by thighs (34%), flanks (25%), gluteal regions (12%), and knees (9%) (Kaufman et al, 2010). Rohrich found no significant difference in the viability of fat cells collected from the abdomen, flank, thigh, and medial knee (Rohrich et al, 2004). Similar conclusions were obtained by other authors using preadipocytes from the abdomen, breast, and buttock (Von Heimburg, 2004) or from thigh, abdomen, and breast (Ullmann et al, 2005). The donor site choice seems to play a negligible role in graft take. When they are used as fillers, site choice should be based on ease and safety of access, fat distribution and abundance, and patient's preference. When treating critical host beds (as irradiated tissue) or when ADSCs are paramount (as in regenerative surgery), donor site choice could be more significant. Some animal model works showed that the potential of ADSCs differs according to the location of adipose tissue from which they are purified (Prunet-Marcassus et al, 2006). In a recent experimental study, we reported function related structural specializations of adipose tissue, depending on the harvesting site. Large cells and few blood vessels with rare stem niches are present in deposit adipose tissue (large fatty depots like the abdominal area), while good vascularity and adequate staminality can be found in structural adipose tissue (limbs, hips, knees or the trochanteric areas) (Sbarbati et al, 2010).

Another consideration stems from the possible effects of local or general cancer therapies on the number or the viability of ADSCs. A recent work proved that adipose tissue can be severely damaged by radiotherapy, so that the number of ADSCs is deeply reduced and its potential for use in regenerative therapies is dramatically limited (Poglio et al, 2009). Therefore, the donor site should be chosen distant from irradiated areas. No work studied the effects of chemotherapy, monoclonal antibodies or hormone suppression on the number, viability and functionality of ADSCs. Therapies addressing angiogenic activity of tumours or directly interacting with adipose tissue may be relevant and there may be differences in the regenerative effectiveness of fat grafts in patients treated with such therapies. Specific studies may be advisable.

The possible damage induced by harvesting technique has widely been studied. When maximum vacuum levels were comparable, mechanical suction and handheld syringe aspiration showed no difference in injury to fat cells. But histologic studies of human fat grafts demonstrated that relative vacuum levels greater than -500 hPa caused cell membrane expansion and deformation, while membrane rupture and fat cells vaporization occur with higher levels (Niechajev & Sevcuk, 1994). When using large syringes (20-60 mL), extraction normally produces less than -600 hPa vacuum levels and rapidly decreases as the fluid and fat are pulled. Fournier (Fournier, 1988a, 1988b, 1990a, 1990b, 1996, 2000) and Coleman (Coleman, 1995, 1997, 2001) clinically showed that relatively high level suction decreased viable cells concentrations compared to manual aspiration; therefore, they underlined the need for atraumatic harvesting. Tholen observed that very few viable fat cells were present in fat from standard liposuction (large cannula, high vacuum) due to a significant damage (mainly cell membranes rupture) in a large number of lipocytes. On the contrary, a significantly higher rate of intact and viable adipocytes was found when fat was harvested with atraumatic, low-vacuum syringe technique. (Tholen et al, 2010).

Surface adipocytes are nourished from the surrounding recipient bed before vascular in-growth from the bed occurs, while the core cells rely on diffusion only. So the distance between the core and the surface is critical and therefore fat particles dimensions are vital for graft take as larger particles are more prone to central necrosis (Carpaneda & Ribeiro, 1993; Niechajev & Sevcuk, 1994). This is significant only when excisional harvesting is compared to liposuction. On the contrary, smaller liposuction cannulas provide less viable fat grafts (Erdim et al, 2009) probably due to higher cell damage or to damage to the microvascular structure and to the niche.

Some liposuction techniques including ultrasonic emulsification, power- or laser-assisted lipoplasty, or high volume fluid administration ("tumescent" or "super-wet" technique) are blamed to additionally damage the aspirate thus reducing the viable cell rate. Our preference goes to syringe aspiration (20 cc) with a wet technique via open tip or 1-hole bullet tip, 3 mm large cannulas.

4.2 Fat processing

The rationale for fat processing before re-injection stems first of all from the need to remove blood, fluids, debris and free lipid fractions in order to improve the actual volume of viable fat, and to reduce the inflammatory reaction which may jeopardize long term uptake. Secondarily, processing can improve graft take by adding promoting agents or by *in vitro* activation. Finally, some studies are trying to preserve the adipocytes for future uses.

The most common processing techniques are centrifugation (Asken, 1988; Toledo, 1991; Coleman, 1995, 1997, 2001; Fulton et al, 1998; R. Amar, 1999; Locke & de Chalain, 2008), sedimentation and washing/rinsing. In a recent consensus survey, various spin rates centrifugation was preferred by 47% of the respondents, 29% favoured fat washings, 12% opted for "other" unspecified treatment techniques, whereas 12% used no preparation (Kaufman et al, 2010). The concentration of viable fat cells in centrifuged vs. sedimented samples seems to be similar. A reliably high concentration of fat cells after centrifugation was seen (Boschert et al, 2002), but maybe the cell damage was underestimated due to the low centrifugation spin rate. An improved long term graft persistence with decanted samples compared to centrifuged ones (1,500 rpm for 5 min) was suggested (Ramon et al, 2005). A recent work showed interesting results with the "squeezing centrifugation lipotransfer system" to concentrate healthy fat cells, the ADSCs, the patient's own peptides (growth factors), and scaffolds (extracellular matrix) through a combination of squeezing, centrifugation and filtration (Yang & Lee, 2011).

Sample washing after centrifugation (Chajchir & Benzaquen, 1986) or sedimentation (Toledo, 1991; Klein, 1993; Niechajev & Sevcuk, 1994; Fagrell et al, 1996; R. Amar, 1999) or in place of either (Rubin & Hoefflin, 2002) was proposed. Its rationale stems from the dilution of detrimental substances combined to an improved sedimentation. In particular, serial washing with saline can reduce cellular remnants and free lipids (Alexander, 2010). Different washing solutions were proposed: sterile water (Rubin & Hoefflin, 2002), 5% glucose solution (Fournier, 2000) or saline (Carpaneda & Ribeiro, 1993; Niechajev & Sevcuk, 1994). A decrease in the survival of normal saline washed grafts vs. unwashed ones was found (Baran et al, 2002). Moreover, sample washing removes fibrin (Chajchir & Benzaquen, 1986) that could be important in stabilizing adipocytes within the wound bed.

Different processing methods significantly correlated with neither viable adipocytes rates nor grafts longevity (Sommer & Sattler, 2000), while other works (Rose et al, 2006) found that sedimentation was associated to almost double the mean concentration of intact cells than centrifugation (3,000 rpm for 3 min) with or without washing. The limit of almost all these *in vitro* studies is the assumption that morphologically intact cells are viable and that viable adipocytes rate correlates to graft survival.

Lidocaine was proved to reversibly inhibit glucose transport, causing lipolysis as the cells fully regain their function after washing (Moore et al, 1995) or centrifugation (Shoshani et al, 2005), regardless of exposure duration. Serial rinsing with normal saline can also significantly reduce the intracellular lidocaine concentration (Alexander, 2010).

Another reason for fat processing is to add substances that may increase graft take. Even if somewhat controversial, insulin can stabilize cell membrane and enhance the survival rate by increasing intracellular glycogen and lipid formation (Asaadi et al, 1993; Yuksel et al, 2000). Bovine fibroblastic growth factor in an animal model was shown to improve weight retention of the grafts (Eppley et al, 1992); IL-8 reduced fat necrosis due to its angiogenic action, cellular proliferation stimulation, and cytokine and growth factor synthesis (Shoshani et al, 2005). A higher survival rate was noted suspending the aspirate in enriched cell culture medium (Har-Shai et al, 1999) or in vascular endothelial growth factor (Nishimura et al, 2000). Platelet-rich plasma was added to the grafts by some authors with quite contradictory results: some works observed an effective reduction of the inflammatory response and a fat survival improvement (Pires Fraga et al, 2010; Nakamura et al, 2010), while others found no significant positive effect (Por et al, 2009; Salgarello et al, 2011). Freezing aspirate for later use causes the adipocytes rupture, further decreasing viable cell counts: after 8 weeks the cell survival rate is only 5% (Son et al, 2010).

Our preference goes to serial washing and decantation. Normal saline is aspired in the harvesting syringe (half filled with fat) that is gently tilted to improve washing and then it is decanted for about five minutes. The heaviest fraction is discarded and the procedure is repeated two or three times until the fat turns to yellow. The upper fraction (free lipids) is also discarded. This technique gave us good results (Panettiere et al, 2009, 2011).

4.3 Techniques for implantation

Interstitial fluids nourish fat grafts for the first 4 days after transplantation, but during this period oxygen supply and nutrition may be insufficient for graft survival. Graft take can be improved by placing small grafts surrounded by as much as possible healthy recipient tissue, thus maximizing the interface between the graft and the recipient bed. This can be achieved by implanting the fat in multiple tunnels or in single spots (less than 0.1 mL), injecting it linearly while withdrawing the cannula or the needle. Large fat clogs can obstruct the needle/cannula during injection and morre pressure applied to the plunger can cause a large bolus to be inadvertently delivered. Injection guns were therefore proposed to improve control and precision of delivery (Agris, 1987; Newman & Levin, 1987; Niechajev, 1992; Asaadi & Haramis, 1993; Niechajev & Sevcuk, 1994; Berdeguer, 1995; Fulton et al, 1998; Niamtu, 2002, 2010).

Subcutaneous tension should also be always prevented. More than one session of fat grafting is advisable in large defects (Tholen et al, 2010) or when tissue fibrosis is significant (Panettiere et al, 2011), but no sound evidence is available about the minimum interval between them. There is some evidence that newformed blood vessels are similar to normal ones 21 days after free fat graft (Missana et al, 2007). In our experience (Panettiere et al, 2009) a 20 days interval between sessions is generally safe and efficient.

Local anaesthetics should be injected only at the injection point in order to preserve the positive effects of sample washing (Shiffman, 2010). The injection site should be chosen far enough from the recipient area to prevent fat extrusion. In our experience, there is usually no need for suturing the injection point, while sterile taping is advisable. The diameter of the delivery cannula or needle should be at least as large as the one used for harvesting in order to limit graft damage. Although infection of the transplanted fat is not a common event (Valdatta et al, 2001; Dessy et al, 2006; Delay et al, 2009; Talbot et al, 2010), absolute sterility is imperative and antibiotic prophylaxis may be advised.

Our preference goes to large diameter (18-14G) needles for delivery. We gently mould the graft with the fingers to improve its uniform distribution and we place Steri-Strips® to encircle the grafted area in order to limit graft's dislocation. Compression dressings can worsen graft take (blood flow reduction) and cause graft's displacement. On the other hand, mostly when using needles, local bleeding in the recipient site can occur thus hindering graft's survival. In our experience adhesive soft pads (Reston® by 3M®) applied for five days can balance the risks from both recipient site bleeding and graft ischemia.

4.4 The survival rates of fat grafts

The differences in the method of harvest, processing, storage and so on created a great confusion and an extreme variability in the reported results and resorption rates which, mostly in the early lipofilling era, were extremely high, up to 70% (Fournier, 1988, 2000; Carpaneda & Ribeiro, 1993; Coleman, 1995, 1997). But many studies relied on subjective evaluations that cannot provide comparable results. In an MR study, the long-term volume persistence of autologous fat grafts in facial defects was 51% 3 months after the implant and 45% at 6 months. Nine - twelve months after implantation the volume was stabile. Therefore, a one stage overcorrection protocol was suggested to balance the resorption rate (Horl, 1991). CT scan studies found a 47.5% survival rate nine months after injection (O. Amar et al, 2008). In a recent MR study by our group, eight months after the last session of serial fat grafting the fat survival rate was about 62% (Panettiere et al, 2011).

Several techniques were also proposed to improve grafts survival rates (Hiragun et al, 1980; Bircoll & Novack, 1987; Eppley et al, 1992; Niechajev & Sevcuk, 1994). An experimental study proved that fat resorption was lower with excised fat compared to lipoaspirate (Fagrell et al, 1996). It was suggested that the preservation of fat microvascular structure could improve adipocyte viability and subsequently graft take. In a very recent work, the survival rate of ADSCs was significantly improved when they were implanted along with their collagen scaffold (Mojallal et al, 2011).

Some considerations are crucial in our opinion about the concept itself of fat survival rate. The first ambiguous point is how many are the elements whose survival is about to be calculated. All the studies generally assume that the total injected volume is the same as the graft volume. But, while non-viable adipocytes contribute to the total injected volume, their persistence is obviously null, so they cannot contribute to the long term implanted volume at all. Another undetermined variable is the amount of fluids injected (and accounted) with fat (Alexander, 2010), so it is arduous to discriminate between carrier fluids extraction and fat resorption. In other terms, if the first term of a proportion is uncertain, what will it be the meaning of the proportion itself? Consequently, real fat survival rates (i.e. how many implanted vital cells survive) in *in vivo* studies are unpredictable in our opinion, and the comparison of such data between different studies is aleatory.

5. Applications of lipofilling to irradiated breast: personal experience

The personal experience with three different applications of free fat grafts to irradiated breasts is presented. Data are expressed as mean±95% confidence interval. Statistical evaluations were made using the Kruskal-Wallis test for rank variables, the Student's t test for continuous data and the Fisher's exact test for proportions.

5.1 The salvage of pre-exposed prostheses and expanders

Exposition is the worst adverse effect of radiotherapy in implant breast reconstruction. In the present preliminary study we hypothesize a possible role for free fat grafts in the rescue of pre-exposed expansion flaps and prosthetic reconstructions.

5.1.1 Patients and methods

14 patients presenting with pre-exposed expanders and 19 patients with pre-exposed prostheses were offered free fat grafts to prevent reconstruction failure. 10 patients with expander pre-exposure (expanders active branch, EAB, age: 53.2±5.5 years) and 8 ones with implant pre-exposure (prostheses active branch, PAB, age: 52.5±6.2 years) adhered. The remaining patients (4 pre-exposed expanders, age: 49.6±28.8 years, p=0,53 and 11 pre-exposed prostheses, age: 49.9±6.8 years, p=0,55) who refused were treated with local flaps (control branches). The expanders in the EAB were partially deflated before graft. Fat was harvested by syringe from the abdomen, the hips or the trochanteric areas through a 3 mm open tip cannula, washed with saline and implanted around the pre-exposure area and successively in the thinned area too, through an 18G needle.

5.1.2 Results

The flaps in the EAB received 33.8±5.3 cc (range 12-70 cc) of fat per session (total implanted volume: 90.2±35.9 cc, range: 24-161 cc in 2.5±0.7 sessions per patient, range: 1-4 sessions in 2.9±1.3 months). The flaps in the PAB received 24.9±2.9 cc (range 14-40 cc) of fat per session (total implanted volume: 80.9±31.7 cc, range: 27-135 cc in 4.1±1.6 sessions per patient, range: 1-7 sessions in 9.3± 5.5 months). In the active branches, the prosthesis could not be saved in 1 case (failure rate: 12.5%, 0.3-52.7%), while all the expansion flaps were saved (failure rate: 0, 0-30.8%). On the contrary all the expansion flaps (failure rate: 100%, 39.8-100%, p=0.001) and 6 of the prosthetic reconstructions in the control groups failed (failure rate: 54.5%, 23.4-83.3%, p=0.14).

5.1.3 Discussion

Expansion is undoubtedly critical in irradiated patients because even modest volumes can cause high tension, severe ischemia and a high exposition risk, due to flap stiffness. The present study demonstrates that free fat grafts can play an interesting role in expansion flaps salvage, while a significant positive effect in prosthetic reconstruction rescue failed to be proved. In our opinion, the key is that all expanders were at least partially deflated, while the same could not obviously be done with prostheses. This is a limited preliminary study, so the results should not be generalized. The main advantage of free fat grafts is that they are a closed procedure minimizing the risk of expander/prosthesis infection or further flap loss. The main risk is inadvertent expander/prosthesis rupture.

5.2 Aesthetic and functional improvements in reconstructed irradiated breasts

5.2.1 Patients and methods

137 irradiated breast implant reconstructed patients were offered free fat grafts. 48 of them (active branch, AB, mean age 50.6±2.8 years) adhered, while the remaining 89, who refused (control branch, CB, mean age 51.5±2.4 years, p=0.32), received a conservative treatment. The autologous fat was harvested by syringe from the abdomen, the hips or the trochanteric areas using a 3 mm cannula (1-hole, bullet tip) and processed by gentle washing with saline. Then it was implanted using a 14G needle in depressed areas (10-15% overcorrection), under the scars, and in dystrophic sites. Functional results were compared using the LENT-SOMA score, while a five-points scale (5: very good, 1: very poor) was used to compare the aesthetic results.

5.2.2 Results

The patients in the AB received 28.2±2.0 cc of fat per session (range: 8-70 cc) in 3.3±0.6 sessions (range: 1-9) with a 86.0±14.6 days interval (range: 20-392 days) between sessions. The initial LENT-SOMA scores in the two branches were comparable, but they significantly improved in the AB after lipograft (fig. 1). 3 months after the last fat graft all the parameters except oedema were better in the AB than in the CB (table 1). A significant improvement was recorded also comparing homogeneous subgroups with similar initial LENT-SOMA ranks (excluding only breast oedema in the lower rank subgroup) as reported in table 2. Two patients in the AB presenting with Bk3 capsular contracture downgraded to Bk1 after respectively 2 and 4 fat graft sessions (fig. 2). The initial aesthetic outcome was similar in the two branches (2.5±0.2 vs. 2.5±0.2, p=0.624), while it significantly improved in the AB 3 months after the last fat graft session (2.5±0.2 vs. 2.9±0.2, p=0.00137). In particular, a great improvement in superficial irregularities and scars, reduction of fibrosis related deformities, and a general improvement of skin appearance and trophism were observed. The aesthetic result in the CB was significantly worse (2.5±0.2) than in the AB 3 months after the last session (2.9±0.2, p=0.00274).

	Initial evaluation			Active branch			Three months after graft		
	Active	Control	p	Before	3 m. after	p	Active	Control	p
P	0.8±0.3	1.0±0.2	0.09	0.8±0.3	0.4±0.2	**0.02**	0.4±0.2	1.0±0.2	**0.00003**
T	1.0±0.3	1.0±0.2	0.93	1.0±0.3	0.6±0.3	**0.01**	0.6±0.3	1.0±0.2	**0.007**
A	1.5±0.3	1.6±0.2	0.97	1.5±0.3	0.9±0.3	**0.002**	0.9±0.3	1.6±0.2	**0.0004**
O	0.9±0.2	0.8±0.2	0.58	0.9±0.2	0.5±0.2	**0.03**	0.5±0.2	0.8±0.2	0.108
F	1.5±0.3	1.7±0.2	0.20	1.5±0.3	1.0±0.2	**0.01**	1.0±0.2	1.7±0.2	**0.00002**

Table 1. The LENT-SOMA ranks comparison between the two groups at initial evaluation, in the AB before and 3 months after the last fat graft, and between CB and AB 3 months after the last fat graft (P: Pain, T: Teleangiectasias, A: Atrophy, O: Oedema, F: Fibrosis). Statistically significant results are in bold characters.

	Lower ranks subgroup (initial score 0-1)			Higher ranks subgroup (initial score 2-3)		
	Before	3 m. after	p	Before	3 m. after	p
Pain	0.4±0.2	0.2±0.1	**0.007**	2.3±0.4	1.6±0.4	**0.01**
Teleangiectasias	0.6±0.2	0.3±0.1	**0.001**	2.6±0.4	2.0±0.5	**0.04**
Atrophy	0.7±0.2	0.3±0.3	**0.002**	2.5±0.2	1.5±0.3	**0.00007**
Oedema	0.5±0.2	0.3±0.2	0.06	2.1±0.2	1.4±0.6	**0.014**
Fibrosis	0.8±0.1	0.6±0.2	**0.03**	2.6±0.3	1.6±0.3	**0.0002**

Table 2. The LENT-SOMA ranks comparison in homogeneous subgroups of the AB before and 3 months after the last fat graft. Statistically significant results in bold.

Local recurrence occurred in 3 patients in the AB (6.3%, 1.3-17.2%) after a mean interval of 16.0 months (range: 8.2-29.1 months) from fat graft (33.8 months after cancer treatment, range: 23.8-53.5 months) and in 4 patients in the CB (4.5%, 1.2-11.1%, p=0.805) after a mean of 136.0 months (range: 49.7-235.6 months, p=0.109) from mastectomy. Distant metastases were observed in 2 patients in the AB (4.2%, 0.5-14.3%) respectively 10.7 and 21.4 months after fat graft (35.3 months after mastectomy, range: 20.9-50.0 months) and in 3 patients in the CB (3.4%, 0.7-9.5%, p=0.779) 22.4 months (range: 17.0-29.4 months, p=0.350) after mastectomy. The mean follow up after mastectomy was 41.2±9.8 months in the AB and 36.6±11.2 months in the CB (p=0.587).

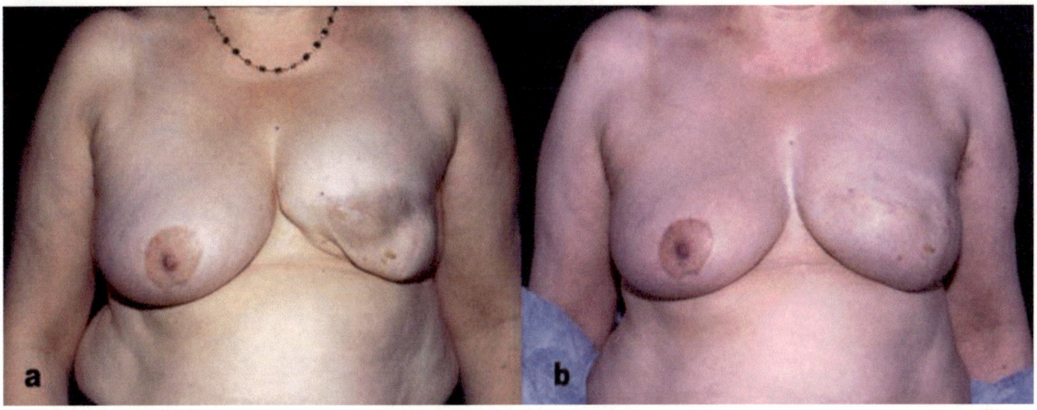

Fig. 1. a: initial severe atrophy and fibrosis; b: dramatic improvement of both parameters 6 months after lipofilling (106 cc in 3 sessions)

5.2.3 Discussion

The present study substantially confirms the results of our previous, more limited published series (Panettiere et al, 2009), but as the present series is more than two folds larger than the previous one, the results appear even more convincing. In particular, a reduced effect of lipofilling on the oedema was confirmed. A possible explanation could be that oedema depends more significantly on the axillary nodes status (sentinel node vs. total dissection, axillary radiotherapy) than on the local tissues. So, a reduced beneficial effect of free fat grafts can be expected. Anyhow, a significant improvement was observed in the subgroup where oedema was initially more severe. Improvement in tissue vascularization and reduction of local inflammatory factors could explain it. In 2 cases a significant improvement of capsular contracture was observed after fat graft. This may be an interesting option for breast augmentation too and, maybe, also to help understand the physiopathology of this challenging adverse event. A possible action mechanism is that ADSCs interact with the inflammatory response as leukotriene antagonists do. Such a hypothesis should obviously be addressed by specific studies. In one case, an accidental prosthetic rupture occurred, due to an inadvertent patient's movement during lipofilling. This was the only procedure-related complication observed, but it should be prevented mostly when dealing with very thin coverage tissues. The data about local and distant recurrence in the present series show no significant difference between the patients who received free fat grafts and those who did not, as far as regards neither incidence, nor distance from cancer surgery. The current series presents some possible biases besides the relatively small number of patients. First of all, 15 patients in the CB (16.9%) were lost at follow up before 3 months. So a higher recurrence rate in the CB could be expected. Secondarily, this study was not specifically designed to address oncologic data. In particular, the patients were not actively and uniformly studied in search for recurrences, and the data here reported relied only on their individual oncologic follow up programs. So, these results should be considered with caution and specific prospective studies should address the relationship between free fat grafts and cancer recurrence.

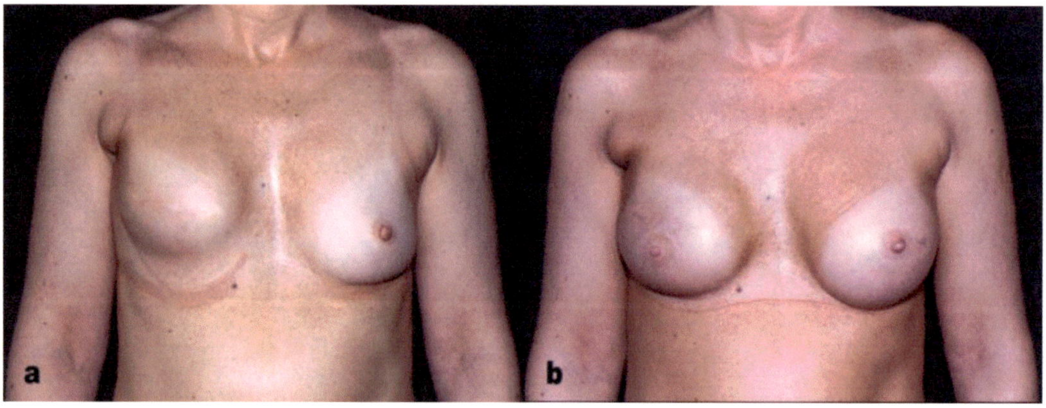

Fig. 2. a: severe fibrosis with Bk3 capsular contracture; b: 4 months after lipofilling (56 cc in 4 sessions), nipple-areola complex reconstruction and contralateral augmentation.

In our opinion, autologous free fat grafts should be routinely offered to all the irradiated implant reconstructed breasts because they can greatly improve both functional and aesthetic results and reduce the incidence of complications.

5.3 The total breast reconstruction with fat grafts only: case reports

Prostheses and autologous flaps are the most common options in breast reconstruction after mastectomy. Autologous flaps are the gold standard in reconstruction failures, but when they are contraindicated, no validated option is available.

5.3.1 Case 1

A 36-year-old patient underwent prophylactic bilateral nipple sparing mastectomy and immediate prosthetic reconstruction 6 years after a left breast quadrantectomy and radiotherapy. Eight months later, the reconstruction failed due to fatal exposure even if several salvage attempts using local flaps were tried. Three years later, the patient asked for reconstruction, but obesity (BMI: 36), and severe asthma contraindicated general anaesthesia. Free fat graft was thus considered the only viable reconstructive option. This case was particularly tricky because of the large breast and the stiffness due to both radiotherapy and the multiple salvage attempts. 700 cc of fat were implanted in 9 sessions in 13.5 months (40 days minimum interval between sessions). The fat was harvested by syringe through a 3 mm open tip cannula from the abdomen, the hips, the thighs, the buttocks or the trochanteric areas and it was washed with saline. The grafts were then implanted using the same syringes and a 14G needle. In the first 4 sessions, small fat volumes were implanted accurately avoiding any significant skin tension (average volume 42.5 cc) under a quite wide surface, in order to release the scar and regenerate the tissues. A great reduction of fibrosis (LENT-SOMA score 3 before session #1; score 1 before session #4) was observed. In a second phase (the last 5 sessions), larger volumes (average: 106 cc) were implanted to improve volume and shape. The overall fat survival rate was 62% measured at MR eight months after the last grafting session. The aesthetic result was pleasant and stable 14 months after the last session (fig. 3). A great improvement in irradiated skin quality and scars was also achieved (LENT-SOMA score before the first session: 8; 8 months after the last session: 3) with improvements in fibrosis (-2), pain (-1), atrophy (-1) and oedema (-1).

5.3.2 Case 2

A 58-year-old woman underwent modified radical mastectomy and prosthetic reconstruction. During expansion she received radiotherapy, but reconstruction was completed with a good result (total LENT-SOMA score: 0, 6 months after the prosthesis was implanted). 8 months later, an infection occurred (Pseudomonas sp.) imposing implant removal. 2 months later (negative blood and tissue cultures) a new reconstruction procedure was performed, but 15 months later the breast suddenly inflated. Pseudomonas was found, so the implant was removed once again. The patient was asking for breast reconstruction, but she then rejected general anaesthesia and local flaps. Therefore, she was proposed a free fat breast reconstruction. A total 367 cc of fat (52.9% larger than the explanted prosthesis) was implanted in 6 sessions (total time: 11.0 months, 61.2±8.5 cc per session) with a 54.8±10.1 days average interval between the sessions. The aesthetic result was pleasant 10.4 months after the last session (fig. 4), with no sign of infection.

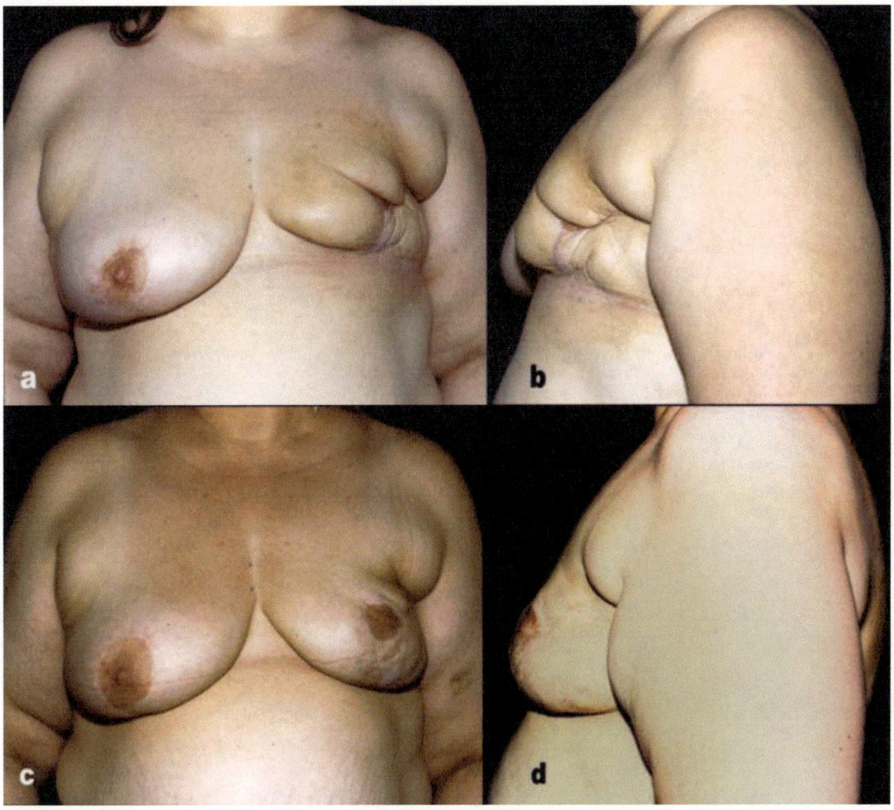

Fig. 3. a, b: case 1, initial status; c, d: 14 months after the last fat graft session

5.3.3 Discussion

The cases here reported offered rather different reconstructive challenges. In the first one, quite a large volume needed to be restored, but a severe fibrosis was present and any attempt to place large volumes of fat under such a stiff skin could cause dangerous tension. In breast reconstruction using free fat only, the grafts usually act as both expanders and vital fillers. Del Vecchio (Del Vecchio, 2009; Khouri & Del Vecchio, 2009) proposed pre-expansion using the BRAVA® system. Even if suction induced by external pre-expansion system was stated to improve blood supply and graft take, in our knowledge, the stiffness observed in the present case was never addressed before with BRAVA® system in published works and its safety on irradiated tissues was not assessed. In case 1, we were concerned about possible risks of pre-expansion as the tissues were extremely thin (mostly in the lower pole). Moreover, we were worried that suction could worsen pain and oedema (both LENT-SOMA score 1). So we opted for a two-step procedure: in the first four sessions we aimed at tissue regeneration, hoping that ADSCs could reduce fibrosis and improve vascularity, so that in the last five sessions larger volumes of fat could be safely implanted. The stable final results demonstrate that this approach is a valuable option.

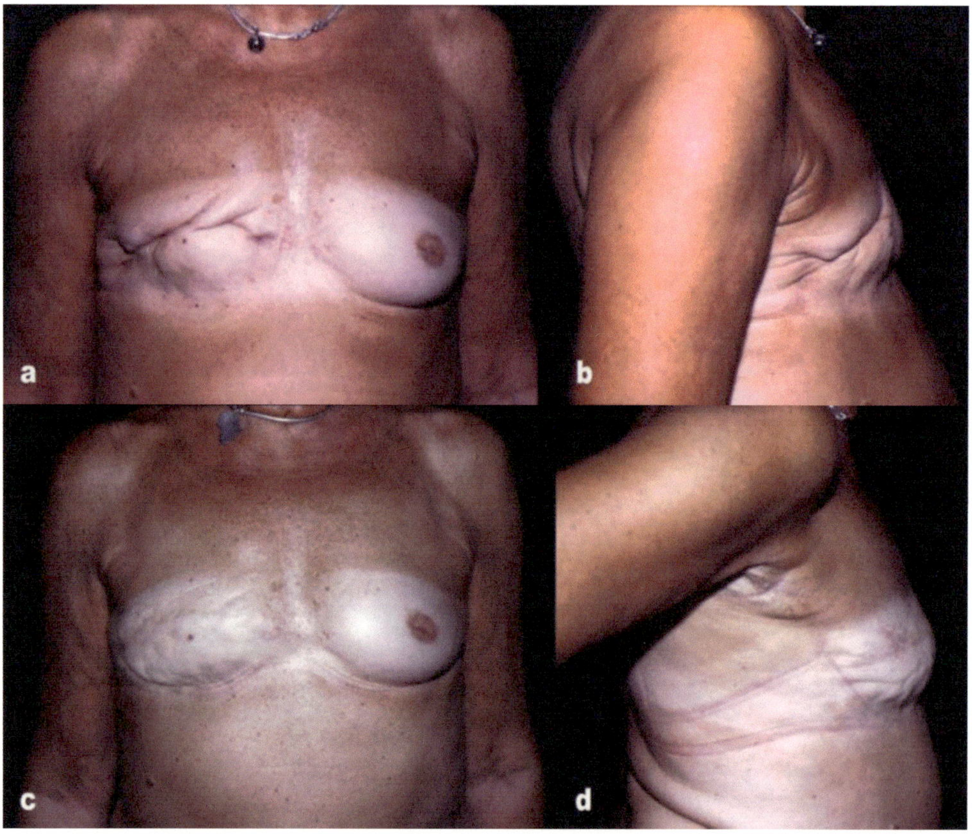

Fig. 4. a, b: case 2, initial status; c, d: 10.4 months after the last fat graft session

In case 2, breast volume was not very large and the tissues showed no significant adverse effect of radiotherapy, but some fibrosis and stiffness developed later due to infections and multiple procedures. So the two-step approach was successfully applied in this case too. But the main concern was possible recurrent infection. In our knowledge there is no specific work addressing fat grafts in potentially infected areas. The patient was administered an antibiogram driven antibiotic treatment to eradicate the infection. A 5-days antibiotic prophylaxis was also empirically administered after the first fat graft session. Standard one-shot prophylaxis was then applied in the following sessions. No sign of re-infection was observed after a 10.4 months follow up. In the present case, free fat grafts proved to be safe also in high infection risk patients.

The long overall reconstruction time is undoubtedly the greatest limit of breast reconstruction using fat grafts. In the present cases respectively 9 sessions in 13.5 months and 6 sessions in 11.0 months were necessary; a mean of 3 sessions were needed in other studies (Delaporte et al, 2009). Moreover, no immediate reconstruction with fat grafts can be planned, even if grafting immediately after mastectomy could probably be an interesting option. Poor donor tissues are other possible limits. The main advantage of breast reconstruction using free fat grafts is the absence of significant contraindications, as it can be performed in almost all patients under local anaesthesia. The technique is undoubtedly easier and extremely less expensive than any other reconstructive option. It can also offer an autologous reconstruction option without major surgeries when other procedures failed.

6. Conclusion

Free fat grafts proved to be a remarkable alternative in irradiated breast reconstruction. Some doubts still remain about the risk of reactivation of dormant cancer cells and further studies should assess chemotherapy, hormone suppression and monoclonal antibodies effects on the regenerated tissues. Advances in adipocyte cryoconservation techniques could further improve the effectiveness by reducing the number of harvesting procedures.

7. References

Agris, J. (1987). Autologous fat transplantation: A 3-year study. *Am J Cosmet Surg,* Vol.4, No.2, (June 1987), pp. 95-102, ISSN 0748-8068

Alexander, R.W. (2010). Fat Transfer with Platelet-Rich Plasma for Breast Augmentation, In: *Autologous Fat Transfer,* Shiffman, M.A. (Ed.), pp. 243-259, Springer-Verlag, ISBN 978-3-642-00472-8, Berlin Heidelberg

Alexander, R.W. (2010). Autologous Fat Grafting: A Study of Residual Intracellular Adipocyte Lidocaine, In: *Autologous Fat Transfer,* Shiffman, M.A. (Ed.), pp. 445-450, Springer-Verlag, ISBN 978-3-642-00472-8, Berlin Heidelberg

Amar, O.; Bruant,-Rodier C.; Lehmann, S.; Bollecker, V. & Wilk A. (2008). Greffe de tissu adipeux: restauration du volume mammaire après traitement conservateur des cancers du sein, aspect clinique et radiologique. *Ann Chir Plast Esthet,* Vol.53, No.2, (April 2008), pp. 169-177, ISSN 0294-1260

Amar, R. (1999). Microinfiltration adipocytaire (MIA) au niveau de la face, ou restructuration tissulaire par greffe de tissu adipeux. *Ann Chir Plast Esthet,* Vol.44, No.6, (December 1999), pp. 593-608, ISSN 0294-1260

Andreassen, C.N.; Alsner, J.; Overgaard, J.; Herskind, C.; Haviland, J.; Owen, R.; Homewood, J.; Bliss, J. & Yarnold, J. (2005). TGFB1 polymorphisms are associated with risk of late normal tissue complications in the breast after radiotherapy for early breast cancer. *Radiother Oncol*, Vol.75, No.1, (April 2005), pp. 18-21, ISSN 0167-8140

Asaadi, M. & Haramis, H.T. (1993). Successful autologous fat injection at 5-year follow-up. *Plast Reconstr Surg*, Vol.91, No.4, (December 1993), pp. 755-756, ISSN 0032-1052

Asken, S. (1988). Facial liposuction and microlipoinjection. *J Dermatol Surg Oncol*, Vol.14, No.3, (March 1988), pp. 297-305, ISSN 0148-0812

Autio, P.; Saarto, T.; Tenhunen, M.; Elomaa, I.; Risteli, J. & Lahtinen, T. (1998). Demonstration of increased collagen synthesis in irradiated human skin in vivo. *Br J Cancer*, Vol.77, No.12 (June 1998), pp. 2331-2335, ISSN 0007-0920

Baran, C.N.; Celebioglu, S.; Sensoz, O.; Ulusoy, G.; Civelek, B. & Ortak, T. (2002). The behavior of fat grafts in recipient areas with enhanced vascularity. *Plast Reconstr Surg*, Vol.109, No.5, (April 2002), pp. 1646-1651, ISSN 0032-1052

Barcellos-Hoff, M.H.; Park, C. & Wright, E.G. (2005). Radiation and the microenvironment-tumorigenesis and therapy. *Nat Rev Cancer*, Vol.5, No.11, (November 2005), pp. 867-875, ISSN 1474-175X

Bentzen, S.M. (2006). Preventing or reducing late side effects of radiation therapy: radiobiology meets molecular pathology. *Nat Rev Cancer*, Vol.6, No.9, (September 2006), pp. 702-713, ISSN 1474-175X

Berdeguer, P. (1995). Five years of experience using fat for leg contouring. *Am J Cosmet Surg*, Vol.12, No.3, (n.d.), pp. 221-229, ISSN 0748-8068

Bircoll, M. & Novack, B.H. (1987). Autologous fat transplantation employing liposuction techniques. *Ann Plast Surg*, Vol.18, No.4, (April 1987), pp. 327-329, ISSN 0148-7043

Boschert, M.T.; Beckert, B.W.; Puckett, C.L. & Concannon, M.J. (2002). Analysis of lipocyte viability after liposuction. *Plast Reconstr Surg*, Vol.109, No.2, (February 2002), pp. 761-765, ISSN 0032-1052

Bruning, P. (1914). Cited by Broeckaert, TJ & Steinhaus, J. Contribution a l'etude des greffes adipueses. *Bull Acad Roy Med Belgique*, Vol.28, (n.d.), pp. 440

Brush, J.; Lipnick, S.L.; Phillips, T.; Sitko, J.; McDonald, J.T. & McBride, W.H. (2007). Molecular mechanisms of late normal tissue injury. *Semin Radiat Oncol*, Vol.17, No.2, (April 2007), pp. 121-130, ISSN 1053-4296

Caplan, A.I. & Dennis, J.E. (2006). Mesenchymal stem cells as trophic mediators. *J Cell Biochem*, Vol.98, No.5, (August 2006), pp. 1076-1084, ISSN 1097-4644

Carpaneda, C.A. & Ribeiro, M.T. (1993). Study of the histologic alterations and viability of the adipose graft in humans. *Aesthetic Plast Surg*, Vol.17, No.1, (Winter 1993), pp. 43-47, ISSN 0364-216X

Casteilla, L.; Planat-Bénard, V.; Cousin, B.; Silvestre, J.S.; Laharrague, P.; Charrière, G.; Carrière, A. & Pénicaud, L. (2005). Plasticity of adipose tissue: a promising therapeutic avenue in the treatment of cardiovascular and blood diseases? *Arch Mal Coeur Vaiss*, Vol.98, No.9, (September 2005), pp. 922-926, ISSN 0003-9683

Casteilla, L.; Planat-Benard, V.; Laharrague, P. & Cousin, B. (2011) Adipose-derived stromal cells: Their identity and uses in clinical trials, an update. *World J Stem Cells*, Vol.3, No.4, (April 2011), pp. 25-33, ISSN 1948-0210

Cavarretta, I.T.; Altanerova, V.; Matuskova, M.; Kucerova, L.; Culig, Z. & Altaner, C. (2010). Adipose tissue-derived mesenchymal stem cells expressing prodrug-converting enzyme inhibit human prostate tumor growth. *Mol Ther*, Vol.18, No.1, (January 2010), pp. 223-231, ISSN 1525-0016

Chajchir, A. & Benzaquen, I. (1986). Liposuction fat grafts in face wrinkles and hemifacial atrophy. *Aesth Plast Surg*, Vol.10, No.2 (February 1986), pp. 115-117, ISSN 1432-5241

Coleman, S.R. (1995). Long-term survival of fat transplants: Controlled demonstrations. *Aesthetic Plast Surg*, Vol.19, No.5, (September-October 1995), pp. 421-425, ISSN 0364-216X

Coleman, S.R. (1997). Facial recontouring with lipostructure. *Clin Plast Surg*, Vol.24, No.2, (April 1997), pp. 347-367, ISSN 0094-1298

Coleman, S.R. (2001). Structural fat grafts: The ideal filler? *Clin Plast Surg*, Vol.28, No.1, (January 2001), pp. 111-119, ISSN 0094-1298

Constantin, G.; Marconi, S.; Rossi, B.; Angiari, S.; Calderan, L.; Anghileri, E.; Gini, B.; Bach, S.D.; Martinello, M.; Bifari, F.; Galiè, M.; Turano, E.; Budui, S.; Sbarbati, A.; Krampera, M. & Bonetti, B. (2009). Adipose-derived mesenchymal stem cells ameliorate chronic experimental autoimmune encephalomyelitis. *Stem Cells*, Vol.27, No.10 , (October 2009), pp. 2624-2635, ISSN 1549-4918

Cousin, B.; Andre, M.; Arnaud, E.; Penicaud, L. & Casteilla, L. (2003). Reconstitution of lethally irradiated mice by cells isolated from adipose tissue. *Biochem Biophys Res Commun*, Vol.301, No.4, (February 2003), pp. 1016-1022, ISSN 0006-291X

Cousin, B.; Ravet, E.; Poglio, S.; De Toni, F.; Bertuzzi, M.; Lulka, H.; Touil, I.; André, M.; Grolleau, JL.; Péron, JM.; Chavoin, JP.; Bourin, P.; Pénicaud, L.; Casteilla, L.; Buscail, L. & Cordelier, P. (2009). Adult stromal cells derived from human adipose tissue provoke pancreatic cancer cell death both in vitro and in vivo. *PLoS One* Vol.4, No.7, (July 2009), pp. e6278, ISSN 1932-6203

Cowan, C.M.; Shi, Y.Y.; Aalami, O.O.; Chou, Y.F.; Mari, C.; Thomas, R.; Quarto, N.; Contag, C.H.; Wu, B. & Longaker, M.T. (2004). Adipose-derived adult stromal cells heal critical-size mouse calvarial defects. *Nat Biotechnol*, Vol.22, No.5, (May 2004), pp. 560-567, ISSN 1087-0156

Delaporte, T.; Delay, E.; Toussoun, G.; Delbaere, M. & Sinna, R. (2009). Reconstruction mammaire par transfert graisseux exclusif: à propos de 15 cas consécutifs. *Ann Chir Plast Esthet*, Vol.54, No.4, (August 2009), pp. 303-316, ISSN 0294-1260

Del Vecchio, D. (2009). Breast reconstruction for breast asymmetry using recipient site pre-expansion and autologous fat grafting: a case report. *Ann Plast Surg*, Vol.62, No.5, (May 2009), pp. 523-527, ISSN 0148-7043

Delay, E.; Garson, S.; Tousson, G. & Sinna, R. (2009). Fat injection to the breast: technique, results, and indications based on 880 procedures over 10 years. *Aesthet Surg J*, Vol.29, No.5 (September-October 2009), pp. 360-376, ISSN: 1090-820X

Dessy, L.A.; Mazzocchi, M.; Fioramonti, P. & Scuderi N. (2006). Conservative management of local Mycobacterium chelonae infection after combined liposuction and lipofilling. *Aesthetic Plast Surg*, Vol.30, No.6, (November-December 2006), pp. 717-722, ISSN 0364-216X

Donnenberg, V.S.; Zimmerlin, L.; Rubin, J.P. & Donnenberg, A.D. (2010). Regenerative therapy after cancer: what are the risks? *Tissue Eng Part B Rev*, Vol.16, No.6, (December 2010), pp. 567-575, ISSN 1937-3376

Ebrahimian, T.G.; Pouzoulet, F.; Squiban, C.; Buard, V.; André, M.; Cousin, B.; Gourmelon, P.; Benderitter, M.; Casteilla, L. & Tamarat, R. (2009). Cell therapy based on adipose tissue-derived stromal cells promotes physiological and pathological wound healing. *Arterioscler Thromb Vasc Biol*, Vol.29, No.4, (April 2009), pp. 503-510, ISSN 1524-4636

Efimenko, A.; Starostina, E.; Kalinina, N & Stolzing, A. (2011). Angiogenic properties of aged adipose derived mesenchymal stem cells after hypoxic conditioning. *J Transl Med*, Vol.18, No.9, (January 2011), pp. 10-24, ISSN 1479-5876

Eppley, B.L.; Sidner, R.A.; Platis, J.M. & Sadove, A.M. (1992). Bioactivation of free-fat transfers: A potential new approach to improving graft survival. *Plast Reconstr Surg*, Vol.90, No.6, (December 1992), pp. 1022-1030, ISSN 0032-1052

Erdim, M.; Tezel, E.; Numanoglu, A. & Sav, A. (2009). The effects of the size of liposuction cannula on adipocyte survival and the optimum temperature for fat graft storage: an experimental study. *J Plast Reconstr Aesthet Surg*, Vol.62, No.9, (September 2009), pp. 1210-1214, ISSN 1748-6815

Faghahati, S.; Delaporte, T.; Toussoun, G.; Gleizal, A.; Morel, F.; Delay, E. (2010). Traitement par transfert graisseux des séquelles postradiques de tumeur faciale maligne de l'enfance. *Ann Chir Plast Esthet*, Vol.55, No.3, (June 2010), pp. 169-178, ISSN 0294-1260

Fagrell, D.; Enestrom, S.; Berggren, A. & Kniola, B. (1996). Fat cylinder transplantation: An experimental comparative study of three different kinds of fat transplants. *Plast Reconstr Surg*, Vol.98, No.1, (July 1996), pp. 90-96, ISSN 0032-1052

Favaro, E.; Amadori, A. & Indraccolo, S. (2008). Cellular interactions in the vascular niche: implications in the regulation of tumor dormancy. *Acta Pathologica Microbiologica et Immunologica Scandinavica*, Vol.116, No. 7-8, (July-August 2008), pp. 648-659, ISSN 1600-0463

Fournier, P.F. (1988). Who should do syringe liposculpturing? *J Dermatol Surg Oncol*, Vol.14, No.10, (October 1988), pp. 1055-1056, ISSN 0148-0812

Fournier, P.F. (1988). Why the syringe and not the suction machine? *J Dermatol Surg Oncol*, Vol.14, No.10, (October 1988), pp. 1062-1107, ISSN 0148-0812

Fournier, P.F. (1990). Facial recontouring with fat grafting. *Dermatol Clin*, Vol.8, No.3, (July 1990), pp. 523-537, ISSN 0733-8635

Fournier, P.F. (1990). Reduction syringe liposculpturing. *Dermatol Clin*, Vol.8, No.3, (July 1990), pp. 539-551, ISSN 0733-8635

Fournier, P.F. (1996). A simplified procedure for locking the plunger during syringe-assisted liposculpturing. *Plast Reconstr Surg*, Vol.98, No.3, (September 1996), pp. 569-570, ISSN 0032-1052

Fournier, P.F. (2000). Fat grafting: My technique. *Dermatol Surg*, Vol.26, No.12, (December 2000), pp. 1117-1128, ISSN 1076-0512

Fox, J.M.; Chamberlain, G.; Ashton, B.A. & Middleton, J. (2007). Recent advances into the understanding of mesenchymal stem cell trafficking. *Br J Haematol*, Vol.137, No.6, (June 2007), pp. 491-502, ISSN 0007-1048

Erickson, G.R.; Gimble, J.M.; Franklin, D.M.; Rice, H.E.; Awad, H. & Guilak, F. (2002). Chondrogenic potential of fat derived stromal cells. *Biochem Biophys Res Comm*, Vol.290, No.2, (January 2002), pp. 763-769, ISSN 0006-291X

Fulton, J.E.; Suarez, M.; Silverton, K. & Bames, T. (1998). Small volume fat transfer. *Dermatol Surg*, Vol.24, No.8, (August 1998), pp. 857-865, ISSN 1076-0512

Garcia-Olmo, D.; Garcia-Arranz, M. & Herreros, D. (2008). Expanded adipose-derived stem cells for the treatment of complex perianal fistula including Crohn's disease. *Expert Opin Biol Ther*, Vol.8, No.9, (September 2008), pp. 1417-1423, ISSN 1744-7682

Garcia-Olmo, D.; Herreros, D.; Pascual, I.; Pascual, JA.; Del-Valle, E.; Zorrilla, J.; De-La-Quintana, P.; Garcia-Arranz, M. & Pascual, M. (2009). Expanded adipose-derived stem cells for the treatment of complex perianal fistula: a phase II clinical trial. *Dis Colon Rectum*, Vol.52, No.1, (January 2009), pp. 79-86, ISSN 1530-0358

Gehmert, S.; Gehmert, S.; Prantl, L.; Vykoukal, J.; Alt, E. & Song, Y.H. (2010). Breast cancer cells attract the migration of adipose tissue-derived stem cells via the PDGF-BB/PDGFR-beta signaling pathway. *Biochem Biophys Res Commun*, Vol.398, No.3, (July 2010), pp. 601-605, ISSN 1090-2104

Gimble, J. & Guilak, F. (2003). Adipose-derived adult stem cells: Isolation, characterization, and differentiation potential. *Cytotherapy*, Vol.5, No.5, (n.d.), pp. 362-369, ISSN 1465-3249

Gimble, J.M.; Katz, A.J. & Bunnell, B.A. (2007). Adipose-derived stem cells for regenerative medicine. *Circ Res*, Vol.100, No.9, (May 2007), pp. 1249-1260, ISSN 1524-4571

Giotopoulos, G.; Symonds, R.P.; Foweraker, K.; Griffin, M.; Peat, I.; Osman, A. & Plumb, M. (2007). The late radiotherapy normal tissue injury phenotypes of telangiectasia, fibrosis and atrophy in breast cancer patients have distinct genotype-dependent causes. *Br J Cancer*, Vol.96, No.6, (March 2007), pp. 1001-1007, ISSN 0007-0920

González, M.A.; Gonzalez-Rey, E.; Rico, L.; Büscher, D. & Delgado, M. (2009). Treatment of experimental arthritis by inducing immune tolerance with human adipose-derived mesenchymal stem cells. *Arthritis Rheum*, Vol.60, No.4, (April 2009), pp. 1006-1019, ISSN 0004-3591

Har-Shai, Y.; Lindenhaum, E.S.; Gamliel-Lazarovich, A.; Beach, D. & Hirshowitz, B. (1999). An integrated approach for increasing the survival of autologous fat grafts in the treatment of contour defects. *Plast Reconstr Surg*, Vol.104, No.4, (September 1999), pp. 945-954, ISSN 0032-1052

Hiragun, A.; Sato, M. & Mitsui, H. (1980). Establishment of a clonal cell line that differentiates into adipose cells in vitro. *In Vitro*, Vol.16, No.8, (August 1980), pp. 685-693, ISSN 0073-5655

Horl, H.W.; Feller, A.M. & Biemer, E. (1991). Technique for liposuction fat reimplantation and long-term volume evaluation by magnetic resonance imaging. *Ann Plast Surg*, Vol.26, No.3, (March 1991), pp. 248-258, ISSN 0148-7043

Hoeller, U.; Tribius, S.; Kuhlmey, A.; Grader, K.; Fehlauer, F. & Alberti, W. (2003). Increasing the rate of late toxicity by changing the score? A comparison of RTOG/EORTC and LENT/SOMA scores. *Int J Radiat Oncol Biol Phys*, Vol.55, No.4, (March 2003), pp. 1013-1018, ISSN 0360-3016

Illouz, Y.G. (1985). De l'utilisation de la graisse aspire pour combler les défets cutanés. *Rev Chir Esth Langue Franc*, Vol.10, No.40, (n.d.), pp. 13

Illouz, Y.G. (1986). The fat cell "graft". A new technique to fill depressions. *Plast Reconstr Surg*, Vol.78, No.1, (July 1986), pp. 122-123, ISSN 0032-1052

Illouz, Y.G. & Pflug, M.E. (1986). Die selektive lipektomie oder lipolyse nach IIlouz. *Handchir Mikrochir Plast Chir*, Vol.18, No.3, (May 1986), pp. 118-121, ISSN 0722-1819

Indraccolo, S.; Favaro, E. & Amadori, A. (2006). Dormant tumors awaken by a short-term angiogenic burst: the spike hypothesis. *Cell Cycle*, Vol.5, No.16, (August 2006), pp. 1751-1755, ISSN 1538-4101

Jones, B.J. & McTaggart, S.J. (2008). Immunosuppression by mesenchymal stromal cells: from culture to clinic. *Exp Hematol*, Vol.36, No.6, (June 2008), pp. 733-741, ISSN 0301-472X

Kang, S.K.; Jun, E.S.; Bae, Y.C. & Jung, J.S. (2003). Interactions between human adipose stromal cells and mouse neural stem cells in vitro. *Brain Res Dev Brain Res*, Vol.145, No.1, (October 2003), pp. 141-149, ISSN 0165-3806

Kaufman, M.R.; Bradley J.P.; Dickinson B.; Heller J.B.; Wasson K. O'Hara C.; Huang C.; Gabbay J.; Ghadjar K.; Miller T.A. & Jarrahy R. (2010). Autologous Fat Transfer National Consensus Survey: Trends in Techniques and Results for Harvest, Preparation, and Application, In: *Autologous Fat Transfer*, Shiffman, M.A. (Ed.), 451-458, Springer-Verlag, ISBN 978-3-642-00472-8, Berlin Heidelberg

Mojallal, A.; Lequeux, C.; Shipkov, C.; Rifkin, L.; Rohrich, R.; Duclos, A.; Brown, S. & Damour, O. (2011). Stem Cells, Mature Adipocytes, and Extracellular Scaffold: What Does Each Contribute to Fat Graft Survival? *Aesthetic Plastic Surgery*, DOI: 10.1007/s00266-011-9734-8, (May 2011), pp. 1-12, ISSN 1432-5241

Khouri, R. & Del Vecchio, D. (2009). Breast reconstruction and augmentation using pre-expansion and autologous fat transplantation. *Clin Plast Surg*, Vol.36, No.2, (April 2009), pp. 269-280, ISSN 1558-0504

Kim, J.M.; Lee, S.T.; Chu, K.; Jung, K.H.; Song, E.C.; Kim, S.J.; Sinn, D.I.; Kim, J.H.; Park, D.K.; Kang, K.M.; Hyung Hong, N.; Park, H.K.; Won, C.H.; Kim, K.H.; Kim, M.; Kun Lee, S. & Roh, J.K. (2007). Systemic transplantation of human adipose stem cells attenuated cerebral inflammation and degeneration in a hemorrhagic stroke model. *Brain Res*, Vol.1183, (December 2007), pp. 43-50, ISSN 0006-8993

Kim, U.; Shin, D.G.; Park, J.S.; Kim, Y.J.; Park, S.I.; Moon, Y.M. & Jeong, K.S. (2011). Homing of adipose-derived stem cells to radiofrequency catheter ablated canine atrium and differentiation into cardio-myocyte-like cells. *Int J Cardiol*, Vol.146, No.3, (February 2011), pp. 371-378, ISSN 1874-1754

Kim, Y.; Kim, H.; Cho, H.; Bae, Y.; Suh, K. & Jung, J. (2007). Direct comparison of human mesenchymal stem cells derived from adipose tissues and bone marrow in mediating neovascularization in response to vascular ischemia. *Cell Physiol Biochem*, Vol.20, No.6, (n.d.), pp. 867-876, ISSN 1015-8987

Klein, J.A. (1993). Tumescent technique for local anesthesia improves safety in large-volume liposuction. *Plast Reconstr Surg*, Vol.92, No.6, (November 1993), pp. 1085-1098, ISSN 0032-1052

Kubis, N.; Tomita, Y.; Tran-Dinh, A.; Planat-Benard, V.; Andre, M.; Karaszewski, B.; Waeckel, L.; Penicaud, L.; Silvestre, J.S.; Casteilla, L.; Seylaz, J. & Pinard, E. (2007). Vascular fate of adipose tissue-derived adult stromal cells in the ischemic murine brain: A combined imaging-histological study. *Neuroimage*, Vol.34, No.1, (January 2007), pp. 1-11, ISSN 1053-8119

Lamfers, M.; Idema, S.; van Milligen, F.; Schouten, T.; van der Valk, P.; Vandertop, P.; Dirven, C. & Noske, D. (2009). Homing properties of adipose-derived stem cells to intracerebral glioma and the effects of adenovirus infection. *Cancer Lett*, Vol.274, No.1, (February 2009), pp. 78-87, ISSN 1872-7980

Lee, D.H.; Ahn, Y.; Kim, S.U.; Wang, K.C.; Cho, B.K.; Phi, J.H.; Park, I.H.; Black, P.M.; Carroll, R.S.; Lee, J. & Kim, S.K. (2009). Targeting rat brainstem glioma using human neural stem cells and human mesenchymal stem cells. *Clin Cancer Res*, Vol.15, No.15, (August 2009), pp. 4925-4934, ISSN 1078-0432

Lin, G.; Yang, R.; Banie, L.; Wang, G.; Ning, H.; Li, L.C.; Lue, T.F. & Lin, C.S. (2010). Effects of transplantation of adipose tissue-derived stem cells on prostate tumor. *Prostate*, Vol.70, No.10, (July 2010), pp. 1066-1073, ISSN 1097-0045

Locke, M.B. & de Chalain, T.M. (2008). Current practice in autologous fat transplantation: Suggested clinical guidelines based on a review of recent literature. *Ann Plast Surg*, Vol.60, No.1, (January 2008), pp. 98-102, ISSN 0148-7043

Mazo, M.; Planat-Bénard, V.; Abizanda, G.; Pelacho, B.; Léobon, B.; Gavira, J.J.; Peñuelas, I.; Cemborain, A.; Pénicaud, L.; Laharrague, P.; Joffre, C.; Boisson, M.; Ecay, M.; Collantes, M.; Barba, J.; Casteilla, L. & Prósper, F. (2008). Transplantation of adipose derived stromal cells is associated with functional improvement in a rat model of chronic myocardial infarction. *Eur J Heart Fail*, Vol.10, No.5, (May 2008), pp. 454-462, ISSN 1388-9842

Missana, M.C.; Laurent, I.; Barreau, L. & Balleyguier, C. (2007). Autologous fat transfer in reconstructive breast surgery: indications, technique and results. *Eur J Surg Oncol*, Vol.33, No.6, (August 2007), pp. 685-690, ISSN 0748-7983

Moore, J.H.Jr.; Kolaczynski, J.W.; Morales, L.M.; Considine, R.V.; Pietrzkowski, Z.; Noto, P.F. & Caro, J.F. (1995). Viability of fat obtained by syringe suction lipectomy: Effects of local anesthesia with lidocaine. *Aesthetic Plast Surg*, Vol.19, No.4, (July-August 1995), pp. 335-339, ISSN 0364-216X

Moseley, T.A.; Zhu, M. & Hedrick, M.H. (2006). Adipose-derived stem and progenitor cells as fillers in plastic and reconstructive surgery. *Plast Reconstr Surg*, Vol.118, No.3 supp, (September 2006), pp. 121S-128S, ISSN 0032-1052

Murohara, T.; Shintani, S. & Kondo, K. (2009). Autologous adipose-derived regenerative cells for therapeutic angiogenesis. *Curr Pharm Des*, Vol.15, No.24, (n.d.), pp. 2784-2790, ISSN 1873-4286

Nakamura, S.; Ishihara, M.; Takikawa, M.; Murakami, K.; Kishimoto, S.; Nakamura, S.; Yanagibayashi, S.; Kubo, S.; Yamamoto, N. & Kiyosawa, T. (2010). Platelet-rich plasma (PRP) promotes survival of fat-grafts in rats. *Ann Plast Surg*, Vol.65, No.1 (July 2010), pp. 101-106, ISSN 0148-7043

Naumov, G.N.; Akslen, L.A. & Folkman J. (2006). Role of angiogenesis in human tumor dormancy: animal models of the angiogenic switch. *Cell Cycle*, Vol.5, No.16, (August 2006), pp. 1779-1787, ISSN 1538-4101

Neuber F. (1893). Fettransplantation. *Chir Kongr Verhandl Deutsche Gesellsch Chir*, Vol.22, (n.d.), pp. 66

Newman, J. & Levin, J. (1987). Facial lipo-transplant surgery. *Am J Cosmet Surg*, Vol.4, No.2, (n.d.), pp. 131-140, ISSN 0748-8068

Niamtu, J. (2002). Fat transfer gun used as a precision injection device for injectable soft tissue fillers. *J Oral Maxillofac Surg*, Vol.60, No.7, (July 2002), pp. 838-839, ISSN 0278-2391

Niamtu, J. (2010). Injection Gun Used as a Precision Device for Fat Transfer, In: *Autologous Fat Transfer*, Shiffman, M.A. (Ed.), 397-401, Springer-Verlag, ISBN 978-3-642-00472-8, Berlin Heidelberg

Niechajev, I. (1992). Autologous transplantation of fat (lipofilling) for the improvement of the cheek contour, long-term results. In *Plastic Surgery*, Hinderer, V.T. (Ed.), Vol. II, 747-748, Excerpta Medica, Amsterdam

Niechajev, I. & Sevcuk, O. (1994). Long-term results of fat transplantation: Clinical and histologic studies. *Plast Reconstr Surg*, Vol.94, No.3, (September 1994), pp. 496-506, ISSN 0032-1052

Nomoto-Kojima, N.; Aoki, S.; Uchihashi, K.; Matsunobu, A.; Koike, E.; Ootani, A.; Yonemitsu, N.; Fujimoto, K. & Toda, S. (2011). Interaction between adipose tissue stromal cells and gastric cancer cells in vitro. *Cell Tissue Res*, Vol.344, No.2, (May 2011), pp. 287-298, ISSN 0302-766X

Panettiere, P.; Marchetti, L. & Accorsi, D. (2009). The serial free fat transfer in irradiated prosthetic breast reconstructions. *Aesthetic Plast Surg*, Vol.33, No.5, (September 2009), pp. 695-700, ISSN 0364-216X

Panettiere, P.; Accorsi, D.; Marchetti, L.; Sgrò, F. & Sbarbati, A. (2011) Large-Breast Reconstruction Using Fat Graft Only after Prosthetic Reconstruction Failure. *Aesthetic Plast Surg*, Vol.128, No.5, (October 2011), pp. 703-708, ISSN 0364-216X

Pavy, J.J.; Denekamp, J.; Letschert, J.; Littbrand, B.; Mornex, F.; Bernier, J.; Gonzales-Gonzales, D.; Horiot, J.C.; Bolla, M. & Bartelink, H. (1995). EORTC Late Effects Working Group. Late effects toxicity scoring: the SOMA scale. *Radiother Oncol*, Vol.35, No.1 (April 1995), pp. 11-15, ISSN 0167-8140

Percec, I. & Bucky, L.P. (2008). Successful prosthetic breast reconstruction after radiation therapy. *Ann Plast Surg*, Vol.60, No.5, (May 2008), pp. 527-531, ISSN 0148-7043

Perrot, P.; Rousseau, J.; Bouffaut, A.L.; Rédini, F.; Cassagnau, E.; Deschaseaux, F.; Heymann, M.F.; Heymann, D.; Duteille, F.; Trichet, V. & Gouin, F. (2010) Safety concern between autologous fat graft, mesenchymal stem cell and osteosarcoma recurrence. *PLoS One*, Vol.5, No.6, (June 2010), pp. e10999, ISSN 1932-6203

Petit, J.Y.; Botteri, E.; Lohsiriwat, V.; Rietjens, M.; De Lorenzi, F.; Garusi, C.; Rossetto, F.; Martella, S.; Manconi, A.; Bertolini, F.; Curigliano, G.; Veronesi, P.; Santillo, B. & Rotmensz, N. (2011), Locoregional recurrence risk after lipofilling in breast cancer patients. *Ann Oncol*, doi: 10.1093/annonc/mdr158, (May 2011), ISSN 1569-8041

Phinney, D.G. & Prockop, D.J. (2007). Concise review: mesenchymal stem/multipotent stromal cells: the state of transdifferentiation and modes of tissue repair - current views. *Stem Cells*, Vol.25, No.11, (November 2007), pp. 2896-2902, ISSN 1549-4918

Phulpin, B.; Gangloff, P.; Tran, N.; Bravetti, P.; Merlin, J.L. & Dolivet G. (2009). Rehabilitation of irradiated head and neck tissues by autologous fat transplantation. *Plast Reconstr Surg*, Vol.123, No.4, (April 2009), pp. 1187-1197, ISSN 0364-216X

Pires Fraga, M.F.; Nishio, R.T.; Ishikawa, R.S.; Perin, L.F.; Helene, A.Jr. & Malheiros, C.A. (2010). Increased survival of free fat grafts with platelet-rich plasma in rabbits. *J Plast Reconstr Aesthet Surg*, Vol.63, No.12 (December 2010), pp. e818-822, ISSN 1748-6815

Planat-Benard, V.; Silvestre, J.S.; Cousin, B.; André, M.; Nibbelink, M.; Tamarat, R.; Clergue, M.; Manneville, C.; Saillan-Barreau, C.; Duriez, M.; Tedgui, A.; Levy, B.; Pénicaud, L. & Casteilla, L. (2004). Plasticity of human adipose lineage cells toward endothelial cells: physiological and therapeutic perspectives. *Circulation*, Vol.109, No.5, (February 2004), pp. 656-663, ISSN 1524-4539

Poglio, S.; Galvani, S.; Bour, S.; André, M.; Prunet-Marcassus, B.; Pénicaud, L.; Casteilla, L. & Cousin, B. (2009). Adipose tissue sensitivity to radiation exposure. *Am J Pathol*, Vol.174, No.1, (January 2009), pp. 44-53, ISSN 1525-2191

Por, Y.C.; Yeow, V.K.; Louri, N.; Lim, T.K.; Kee, I. & Song, I.C. (2009). Platelet-rich plasma has no effect on increasing free fat graft survival in the nude mouse. *J Plast Reconstr Aesthet Surg*, Vol.62, No.8, (August 2009), pp. 1030-1034, ISSN 1748-6815

Prantl, L.; Muehlberg, F.; Navone, N.M.; Song, Y.H.; Vykoukal, J.; Logothetis, C.J. & Alt, E.U. (2010). Adipose tissue-derived stem cells promote prostate tumor growth. *Prostate*, Vol.70, No.15, (November 2010), pp. 1709-1715, ISSN 1097-0045

Prunet-Marcassus, B.; Cousin, B.; Caton, D.; André, M.; Pénicaud, L. & Casteilla, L. (2006). From heterogeneity to plasticity in adipose tissues: site-specific differences. *Exp Cell Res*, Vol.312, No.6, (April 2006), pp. 727-736, ISSN 0014-4827

Puissant, B.; Barreau, C.; Bourin, P.; Clavel, C.; Corre, J.; Bousquet, C.; Taureau, C.; Cousin, B.; Abbal, M.; Laharrague, P.; Penicaud, L.; Casteilla, L. & Blancher, A. (2005). Immunomodulatory effect of human adipose tissue-derived adult stem cells: comparison with bone marrow mesenchymal stem cells. *Br J Haematol*, Vol.129, No.1, (April 2005), pp. 118-129, ISSN 0007-1048

Quarmby, S.; Fakhoury, H.; Levine, E.; Barber, J.; Wylie, J.; Hajeer, A.H.; West, C.; Stewart, A.; Magee, B. & Kumar, S. (2003). Association of transforming growth factor beta-1 single nucleotide polymorphisms with radiation-induced damage to normal tissues in breast cancer patients. *Int J Radiat Biol*, Vol.79, No.2, (February 2003), pp. 137-143, ISSN 0955-3002

Ramon, Y.; Shoshani, O.; Peled, I.J.; Gilhar, A.; Carmi, N.; Fodor, L.; Risin, Y. & Ulmann, Y. (2005). Enhancing the take of injected adipose tissue by a simple method for concentrating fat cells. *Plast Reconstr Surg*, Vol.115, No.1, (January 2005), pp. 197-201, ISSN 0032-1052

Rehman, J.; Traktuev, D.; Li, J.; Merfeld-Clauss, S.; Temm-Grove C.J.; Bovenkerk, J.E.; Pell C.L.; Johnstone, B.H.; Considine, R.V. & March, K.L. (2004). Secretion of angiogenic and antiapoptotic factors by human adipose stromal cells. *Circulation*, Vol.109, No.10, (March 2004), pp. 1292-1298, ISSN 1524-4539

Riekki, R.; Parikka, M.; Jukkola, A.; Salo, T.; Risteli, J. & Oikarinen, A. (2002). Increased expression of collagen types I and III in human skin as a consequence of radiotherapy. *Arch Dermatol Res*, Vol.294, No.4, (July 2002), pp. 178-184, ISSN 0340-3696

Rigotti, G.; Marchi, A.; Galiè, M.; Baroni, G.; Benati, D.; Krampera, M.; Pasini, A. & Sbarbati, A. (2007). Clinical treatment of radiotherapy tissue damage by lipoaspirate transplant: a healing process mediated by adipose-derived adult stem cells. *Plast Reconstr Surg*, Vol.119, No.5, (April 2007), pp. 1409-1422, ISSN 0032-1052

Rigotti, G.; Marchi, A.; Stringhini, P.; Baroni, G.; Galiè, M.; Molino, AM.; Mercanti, A.; Micciolo, R. & Sbarbati, A. (2010). Determining the oncological risk of autologous lipoaspirate grafting for post-mastectomy breast reconstruction. *Aesthetic Plast Surg*, Vol.34, No.4, (August 2010), pp. 475-480, ISSN 0364-216X

Roberts, D.L.; Dive, C. & Renehan, A.G. (2010). Biological mechanisms linking obesity and cancer risk: new perspectives. *Annu Rev Med*, Vol.61, (n.d.), pp. 301-316, ISSN 1545-326X

Rodemann, H.P. & Blaese, M.A. (2007). Responses of normal cells to ionizing radiation. *Semin Radiat Oncol*, Vol.17, No.2, (April 2007), pp. 81-88, ISSN 1053-4296

Rohrich, R.J.; Sorokin, E.S. & Brown, S.A. (2004). In search of improved fat transfer viability: A quantitative analysis of the role of centrifugations and harvest site. *Plast Reconstr Surg*, Vol.114, No.1, (January 2004), pp. 391-395, ISSN 0032-1052

Rose, J.G.Jr.; Lucarelli, M.J.; Lemke, B.N.; Dortzbach, R.K.; Boxrud, C.A.; Obagi, S. & Patel, S. (2006). Histologic comparison of autologous fat processing methods. *Ophthal Plast Reconstr Surg*, Vol.22, No.3, (May-June 2006), pp. 195-200, ISSN 0032-1052

Rubin, A. & Hoefflin, S. (2002). Fat purification: Survival of the fittest. *Plast Reconstr Surg*, Vol.109, No.4, (April 2002), pp. 1463-1464, ISSN 0032-1052

Salgarello, M.; Visconti, G. & Farallo, E. (2010). Autologous fat graft in radiated tissue prior to alloplastic reconstruction of the breast: report of two cases. *Aesthetic Plast Surg*, Vol.34, No.1, (February 2010), pp. 5-10, ISSN 0364-216X

Salgarello, M.; Visconti, G. & Rusciani A. (2011) Breast fat grafting with platelet-rich plasma: a comparative clinical study and current state of the art. *Plast Reconstr Surg*, Vol.127, No.6, (June 2011), pp 2176-2185, ISSN 0032-1052

Sarfati, I.; Ihrai, T.; Kaufman, G.; Nos, C. & Clough, K.B. (2001). Adipose-tissue grafting to the post-mastectomy irradiated chest wall: Preparing the ground for implant reconstruction. *J Plast Reconstr Aesthet Surg*, Vol.64, No.9, (September 2011)

Sbarbati, A.; Accorsi, D.; Benati, D.; Marchetti, L.; Orsini, G.; Rigotti, G. & Panettiere P. (2010). Subcutaneous adipose tissue classification. *European Journal of Histochemistry* Vol.54, No.4, (November 2010), pp. e48, ISSN 2038-8306

Shiffman, M.A. (2010) Editor's commentary, In: *Autologous Fat Transfer*, Shiffman, M.A. (Ed.), 463-465, Springer-Verlag, ISBN 978-3-642-00472-8, Berlin Heidelberg

Shoshani, O.; Berger, J.; Fodor, L.; Ramon, Y.; Shupak, A.; Kehat, I.; Gilhar, A. & Ullmann, Y. (2005). The effect of lidocaine and adrenaline on the viability of injected adipose tissue - an experimental study in nude mice. *J Drugs Dermatol*, Vol.4, No.3, (May-June 2005), pp. 311-316, ISSN 1545-9616

Shoshani, O.; Livne, E.; Armoni, M.; Shupak, A.; Berger, J.; Ramon, Y.; Fodor, L.; Gilhar, A.; Peled, I.J. & Ulmann, Y. (2005). The effect of interleukin-8 on the viability of injected adipose tissue in nude mice. *Plast Reconstr Surg*, Vol.115, No.3, (March 2005), pp. 853-859, ISSN 0032-1052

Sommer, B. & Sattler, G. (2000). Current concepts of fat graft survival: Histology of aspirated adipose tissue and review of the literature. *Dermatol Surg*, Vol.26, No.12, (December 2000), pp. 1159-1166, ISSN 1076-0512

Son, D.; Oh, J.; Choi, T.; Kim, J.; Han, K.; Ha, S. & Lee, K. (2010). Viability of fat cells over time after syringe suction lipectomy: the effects of cryopreservation. *Ann Plast Surg*, Vol.65, No.3, (September 2010), pp. 354-360, ISSN 0148-7043

Talbot, S.G.; Parrett, B.M. & Yaremchuk, M.J. (2010) Sepsis after autologous fat grafting. *Plast Reconstr Surg*, Vol.126, No.4 (October 2010), pp. 162e-164e, ISSN 1529-4242

Tholen, R.H.; Jackson, I.T.; Simman, R. & Di Nick, V.D. (2010). Recontouring Postradiation Thigh Defect with Autologous Fat Grafting In: *Autologous Fat Transfer*, Shiffman, M.A. (Ed.), 341-346, Springer-Verlag, ISBN 978-3-642-00472-8, Berlin Heidelberg

Toledo, L.S. (1991). Syringe liposculpture: A two-year experience. *Aesthetic Plast Surg*, Vol.15, No.4, (Fall 1991), pp. 321-326, ISSN 0364-216X

Uccelli, A.; Moretta, L & Pistoia, V. (2008). Mesenchymal stem cells in health and disease. *Nat Rev Immunol*, Vol.8, No.9, (September 2008), pp. 726-736, ISSN 1474-1733

Ullmann, Y.; Shoshani, O.; Fodor, A.; Ramon, Y.; Carmi, N.; Eldor, L. & Gilhar, A. (2005). Searching for the favorable donor site for fat injection: in vivo study using the nude mice model. *Dermatol Surg*, Vol.31, No.10, (October 2005), pp. 1304-1307, ISSN 1076-0512

Valdatta, L.; Thione, A.; Buoro, M. & Tuinder S. (2001). A case of life-threatening sepsis after breast augmentation by fat injection. *Aesthetic Plast Surg*, Vol.25, No.5 (September-October 2001), pp. 347-349, ISSN 0364-216X

Vessella, R.L.; Pantel, K. & Mohla, S. (2007). Tumor cell dormancy: an NCI workshop report. *Cancer Biol Ther*, Vol.6, No.9, (September 2007), pp. 1496-1504, ISSN 1555-8576

Von Heimburg, D.; Hemmerich, K.; Haydarlioglu, S.; Staiger, H. & Pallua, N. (2004). Comparison of viable cell yield from excised versus aspirated adipose tissue. *Cells Tissues Organs*, Vol.178, No.2, (2004), pp. 87-92, ISSN 1422-6405

Wang, P.; Mariman, E.; Renes, J. & Keijer, J. (2008). The secretory function of adipocytes in the physiology of white adipose tissue. *J Cell Physiol*, Vol.216No.1, (July 2008), pp. 3-13, ISSN 1097-4652

Weil, B.R.; Markel, T.A.; Herrmann, J.L.; Abarbanell, A.M. & Meldrum, D.R. (2009). Mesenchymal stem cells enhance the viability and proliferation of human fetal intestinal epithelial cells following hypoxic injury via paracrine mechanisms. *Surgery*, Vol.146, No.2, (August 2009), pp. 190-197, ISSN 1532-7361

Wels, J.; Kaplan, R.N.; Rafii, S. & Lyden, D. (2008). Migratory neighbors and distant invaders: tumor-associated niche cells. *Genes Dev*, Vol.22, No.5, (March 2008), pp. 559-574, ISSN 0890-9369

Wickham, M.Q.; Erickson, G.; Gimble, J.; Vail, T. & Guilak, F. (2003). Multipotent stromal cells derived from infrapatellar fat pat of the knee. *Clin Orthop*, Vol.412, (July 2003), pp. 196-212, ISSN 0009-921X

Yañez, R.; Lamana, M.L.; García-Castro, J.; Colmenero, I.; Ramírez, M. & Bueren, J.A. (2006). Adipose tissue-derived mesenchymal stem cells have in vivo immunosuppressive properties applicable for the control of the graft-versus-host disease. *Stem Cells*, Vol.24, No.11, (November 2006), pp. 2582-2591, ISSN 1066-5099

Yang, H.; Lee, H. (2011). Successful use of squeezed-fat grafts to correct a breast affected by Poland syndrome. *Aesthetic Plast Surg*, Vol.35, No.3, (June 2011), pp. 418-425, ISSN 0364-216X

Yuksel, E.; Weinfeld, A.B.; Cleek, R.; Wamsley, S.; Jensen, J.; Boutros, S.; Waugh, J.M.; Shenaq, S.M. & Spira, M. (2000). Increased free fat graft survival with the long-term, local delivery of insulin, insulin-like growth factor-1, and basic fibroblast growth factor by PLGA/PEG microspheres. *Plast Reconstr Surg*, Vol.105, No.5, (April 2000), pp. 1712-1729, ISSN 0032-1052

Zhang, Y.; Daquinag, A.; Traktuev, D.O.; Amaya-Manzanares, F.; Simmons, P.J.; March, K.L.; Pasqualini, R.; Arap, W. & Kolonin, M.G. (2009). White adipose tissue cells are recruited by experimental tumors and promote cancer progression in mouse models. *Cancer Res*, Vol.69, No.12, (June 2009), pp. 5259-5266, ISSN 1538-7445

Zhao, B.C.; Zhao, B.; Han, J.G.; Ma, H.C. & Wang, Z.J. (2010). Adipose-derived stem cells promote gastric cancer cell growth, migration and invasion through SDF-1/CXCR4 axis. *Hepatogastroenterology*, Vol.57, No.104, (November-December 2010), pp. 1382-1389, ISSN 0172-6390

Zheng, D.N.; Li, Q.F.; Lei, H.; Zheng, S.W.; Xie, Y.Z.; Xu, Q.H.; Yun, X. & Pu, L.L. (2008) Autologous fat grafting to the breast for cosmetic enhancement: experience in 66 patients with long-term follow up. *J Plast Reconstr Aesthet Surg*, Vol.61, No.7, (July 2008), pp. 792-798, ISSN 1748-6815

Zimmerlin, L.; Donnenberg, A.D.; Rubin, J.P.; Basse, P.; Landreneau, R.J. & Donnenberg, V.S. (2011). Regenerative therapy and cancer: in vitro and in vivo studies of the interaction between adipose-derived stem cells and breast cancer cells from clinical isolates. *Tissue Eng Part A*, Vol.17, No.1-2, (January 2011), pp. 93-106, ISSN 1937-335X

Zuk, P.A.; Zhu, M.; Ashjian, P.; De Ugarte, D.A.; Huang, J.I.; Mizuno, H.; Alfonso, Z.C.; Fraser, J.K.; Benhaim, P. & Hedrick, M.H. (2002). Human adipose tissue is a source of multipotent stem cells. *Mol Biol Cell*, Vol.13, No.12, (December 2002), pp. 4279-4295, ISSN 1059-1524

6

Correction of Inverted Nipple: Comparison of Techniques with Novel Approaches

Ercan Karacaoglu
Yeditepe University/School of Medicine Department of Plastic Surgery
Turkey

1. Introduction

The nipple is of tremendous importance as a visual and sexual focus of the female body. As a third focus, the nipple has a nutritive function as in breastfeeding basis. That is why body image, sexuality and breastfeeding are adversely affected by its abnormal conditions.

In order to achieve a successful breast-feeding, an infant needs to suck the whole bulk of nipple and almost hundred to eighty percentage of the areola. That is why abnormal nipple conditions such as inverted nipple may result in problems with starting, establishing and maintaining breast-feeding (Hytten 1954). Nipple inversion may cause cosmetic, functional, and psychological problems. Some of the physical signs may be irritation, inflammation, and interference with breast-feeding (Kim et al., 2003).

Inverted nipple is defined as a non-projectile nipple (Sanghoo & Yoon, 1999; Kim et al., 2003; Stevens et al., 2004) (Fig 1).The nipple is located on a plane lover than the areola. The nipple is invaginated and instead of pointing outward, is retracted into the breast parenchymal and stromal tissue.

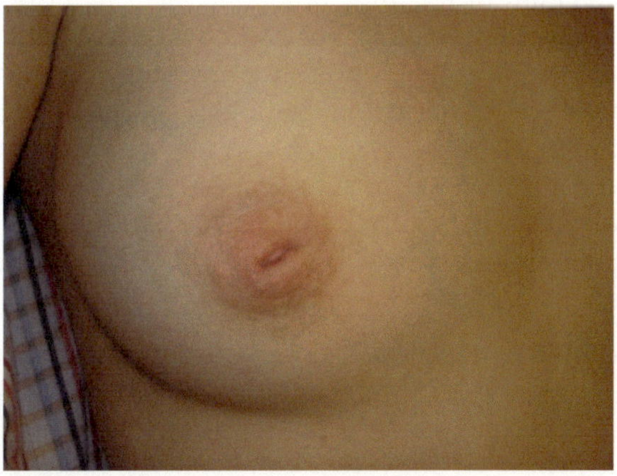

Fig. 1. A 24year-old nulliparous woman with a history of congenital inverted nipple is seen. AP view.

The terms retraction and inversion often are used interchangeably, but such usage is inexact. Retraction is properly applied when only a slit shape area is pulled inward, whereas inversion applies to cases in which the entire nipple is pulled inward occasionally, far enough to lie below the surface of the breast (Nicholson et al, 2009). Inverted nipple may be seen in different forms and structures related to the severity of fibrosis, lack of soft tissue bulk, and lactiferous ductus. In some cases, the nipple may be temporarily protruded if stimulated, but in others, the inversion remains regardless of stimulus.

Inverted nipple is not an uncommon deformity. It was first described by Cooper in 1849 and surgical repair of the inverted nipple was first described by Kehrer in 1888 (Sanghoo & Yoon, 1999, 4).

The nipple is the symbol of the female body with the breast. It is why nipple inversion adversely affects a woman's self-esteem and why they often seek correction of it.

2. Anatomy of the nipple and areola: Nipple-areolar complex

The anatomy of nipple-areola is complex. It is therefore not surprising that the detection of disorders of the nipple-areolar region may be challenging. Although the scope of this chapter is inverted nipple a thorough understanding of anatomic variants of this complex, and the imaging features specific to each is the necessary basis for a comprehensive and appropriate imaging assessment, diagnosis, and treatment. It should also be kept in mind that concurrent benign and pathologic conditions of this complex could be a fact of possibility.

Age is also a variant of nipple areola complex anatomy. It is key to understand the maturation of breast in order to evaluate the abnormal consequences of nipple areola complex. During puberty, the breast mound increases in size. Subsequent enlargement and outward growth of the areola result in a secondary mound (Seltzer, 1994). Eventually, the areola subsides to the level of the surrounding breast tissue, leaving a single breast mound (Seltzer, 1994; Michael, 1991). At full development, the nipple-areolar complex overlies the area between the 2nd and 6th ribs, with a location at the level of the 4th intercostal space being typical for a breast that is not ptotic. The adult breast consists of approximately 15–20 segments demarcated by mammary ducts that converge at the nipple in a radial arrangement. Like the number of segments, the number of mammary ducts may vary. The collecting ducts that drain each segment, which typically measure about 2 mm in diameter, coalesce in the subareolar region into lactiferous sinuses approximately 5–8 mm in diameter (Kopans, 2007). Women occasionally detect a normal lactiferous sinus as a palpable finding at self-examination. In the typical breast, there are 9–20 orifices that drain the segments at the nipple (Kopans 2007, Love 2004).

The nipple-areolar complex contains the Montgomery glands, large or intermediate-stage sebaceous glands that are embryologically transitional between sweat glands and mammary glands and are capable of secreting milk (Kopans, 2007). The Montgomery glands open at the Morgagni tubercles, which are small (1–2-mm-diameter) raised papules on the areola . The nipple-areolar complex also contains many sensory nerve endings, smooth muscle, and an abundant lymphatic system called the subareolar or Sappey plexus. Because the skin of the nipple is continuous with the epithelium of the ducts, cancer of the ducts may spread to the nipple (Kopans 2007).

3. Classification, grading and pathologic basis of the deformity

Nipple inversion can be either acquired or congenital.

Acquired inverted nipple: Nipple inversion secondary to the previous breast surgery, infiltrating ductal carcinoma, and mastitis are examples of the acquired types.

Congenital inverted nipple: Congenital inverted nipple is the most frequent type. The prevalance is reported as 2-10% (Lee et al., 2003; Alaxander & Campbell 1997).

Congenital inverted nipple is clinically classified into three groups:

1. Grade I nipple can be easily pulled out manually and maintains its projection quite well without traction. The nipple is popped out by gentle palpation around the areola. The soft tissue is intact in this form and the lactiferous ducts are normal.
2. Grade II nipple is also popped out by palpation but not as easily as in grade I. The nipple tends to retract. The nipple has moderate fibrosis and the lactiferous ductus is mildly retracted but does not need to be cut to release the fibrosis. These nipples have been shown to have rich collagenous stromata with numerous bundles of smooth muscle.
3. Grade III nipple is a severe form in which inversion and retraction are significant. Manually popping out the nipple is extremely difficult. A traction suture is needed to keep these nipples protruded. The fibrosis beneath the nipple is significant and the soft tissue is markedly insufficient. On histologic examination, the terminal lactiferous ductus and lobular units are atrophic and replaced with severe fibrosis (Sanghoo & Yoon, 1999, Kim et al., 2003)

4. Management

Numerous techniques have been reported to correct the inverted nipple (Alaxander & Campbell, 1997; Kim et al., 2006; Serra-Renom et. Al, 2004; Jiang et al., 2008; Yamada et al., 2004; Ritz et al., 2005; Huang , 2003; Crestinu, 2001; Pompei & Tedesco, 1999) It was also reported that no single technique is appropriate for correcting all types of nipple deformities because different grades of inverted nipple have different levels of fibrosis, soft tissue bulk, and lactiferous ductus stucture (Lee et al., 2003).

The best approach for correction is described as simple and reliable. In addition, a technique with low recurrence rate, with less or no scar, that requires no bulky or special dressing, and that preserves lactiferous ductus function is desirable (Kim et al., 2003).

Here, you will find the most useful techniques used to correct inverted nipple.

4.1 Antenna flap technique (Karacaoglu, 2009)

In this chapter a novel technique for the repair of recurrent grade III inverted nipple is also described in detail. In this technique, dermoadipose flaps that were generated within the area of de-epithelialization during mastopexy were used. The flap is called the ''antenna flap'' because of its way of design.

*Preoperative Marking:*Preoperative planning started with the patient standing. The preliminary marking was identical to that for circumvertical mastopexy. The midline, breast meridian with its extrapolation on the chest wall, and the inframammary fold were marked. The lateral and medial markings were made while pushing the breast laterally and medially with an slight upward rotation, in accordance with the vertical axis drawn below the breast. The new areola was then marked in a classical dome shape. Finally, the lower marking was made. This joined the medial and lateral markings at a level 2 cm above the preexisting fold. The marked area below the areola was used to mark the antenna flap. Marking was done to optimally use the existing de-epithelialization area (Fig. 2, 3).

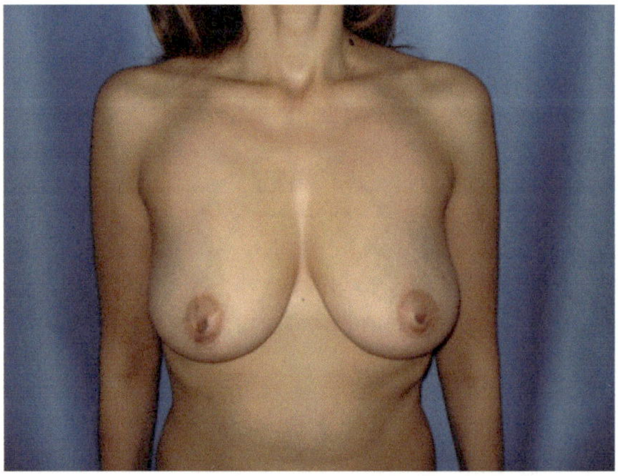

Fig. 2. A woman with a history of congenital inverted nipple is seen. AP view.

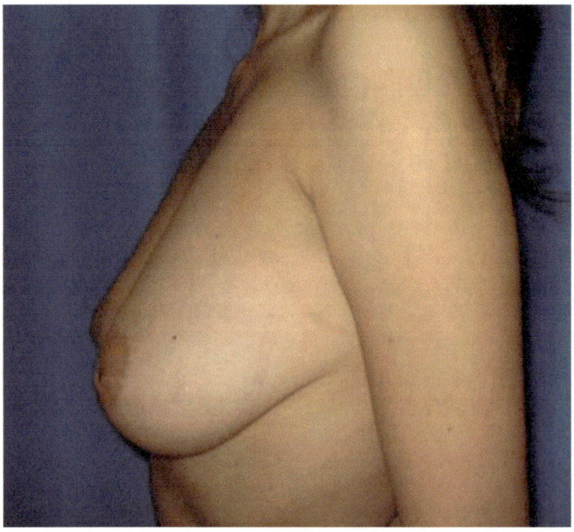

Fig. 3. Lateral view of the same woman in Fig 2.

Surgical Technique: The operative sequence for augmentation mammoplasty was more straightforward. The marked area below the areola was de-epithelialized. Antenna flaps were marked on this area (Fig. 4).

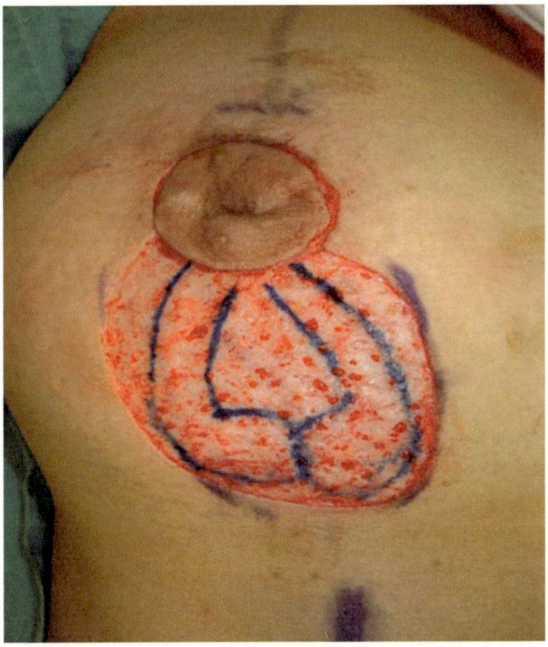

Fig. 4. The marked area below the areola was de-epithelialized. Antenna flaps were marked on this area.

Flaps were elevated to include dermis and 5 mm of fat tissue beneath and attached to the dermal flap using an electrocautery (Fig. 5).

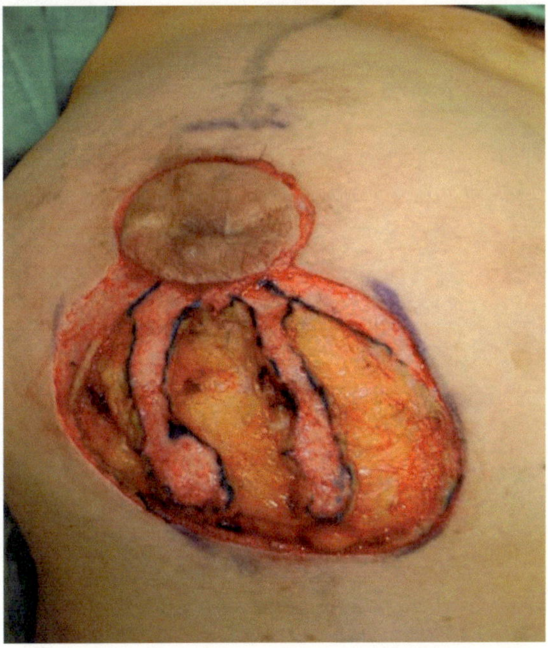

Fig. 5.

These flaps were left intact and the procedure went on with augmentation mastopexy. The breast parenchyma and adipose tissue below the nipple-areola complex were removed within the limits of the markings. A pocket was created in the submuscular space. Once the implant was placed in the pocket, the preliminary markings around the areola and the lateral and medial markings below the areola were reevaluated. Once the implant was in place the nipple position and planned vertical breast closure are tailor-tacked with staples with the patient in a sitting position. A slight flattening of the lower pole was allowed for parenchyma and skin accommodation postoperatively. The edges of the vertical temporary closure were marked and staples removed. The amount of excess skin that could be comfortably removed in the vertical closure was thus determined. At this stage, the de-epithelialization of the skin around the areola and within the medial and lateral markings was completed. Vertical incisions were closed by using 3-0 Monocryl suture (Ethicon Inc., Somerville, NJ).A pocket was created for the transposition of the antenna flaps. For that purpose a 0.5-cm vertical incision was made at the 6 o'clock position at the base of the areola. A tunnel was dissected at and through the areola and extended to the base of the nipple. The tissue beneath the nipple was dissected and the fibrosis was released. The retracting lactiferous ducts were cut mainly from the central portion of the nipple. All the fibrosis and retracting ducts were released until the nipple could maintain its eversion by itself without any traction. Two legs of the antenna flap were inserted into the created pocket (Fig. 6). A satisfactory projection of the nipple was seen at the end of the procedure.

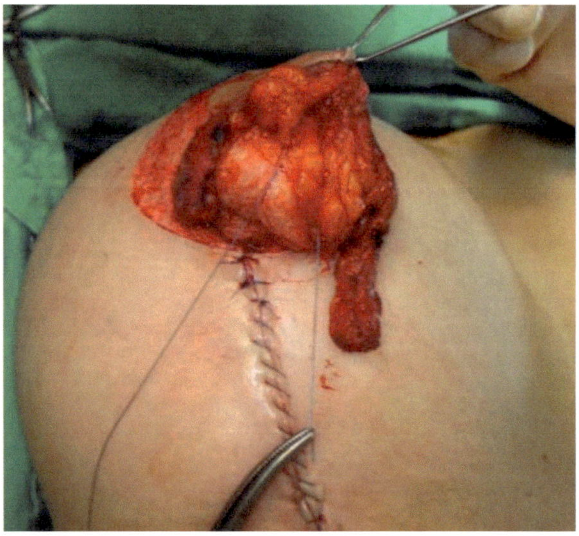

Fig. 6. A satisfactory projection of the nipple was seen at the end of the procedure.

Finally, the periareolar incisions were closed in layers. The periareolar portion was closed in a purse-string fashion by using 3–0 Gore-Tex suture (Gore & Assoc. Inc., Elkton, MD) (Fig. 7). After placement of Steri-strip dressing the newly everted nipple was maintained by a thermoplast splint. The patient was kept in a protective splint for 3 months after surgery.

It has been reported that the patients tolerated the procedure well. No major vital complications like major flap or nipple necrosis has been reported with this technique. In this technique, a high rate of success has been reported that no recurrence of nipple inversion after one and a half-year reported. As of patient satisfaction the technique seems promising that the shape and projection of the patient's nipple was deemed satisfactory (Fig. 8, 9).

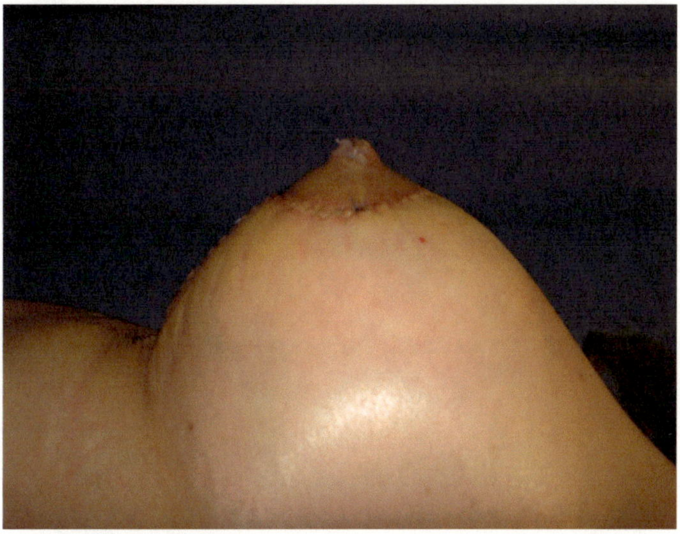

Fig. 7. Early postoperastive result is seen.

The surgical approach presented in this chapter is even an option for correcting a recurrent, congenital inverted nipple. It also should be emphasized that even an alloplastic material could not have corrected the deformity in this particular case. As two other techniques had already been used to correct this deformity in previous surgeries, a new technique named the antenna flap was used. This technique entails transposition of bulky dermoadipose flaps harvested from the de-epithelialized area of the mastopexy into the pocket created beneath the nipple.

In this technique the dead space was filled with autologous tissue where possible complications such as extrusion that is seen with alloplastic materials were avoided. One of the advantages of this technique was the lack of scar in the areola. The disadvantage of the technique is that is it limited to those patients who are candidates for mastopexy.

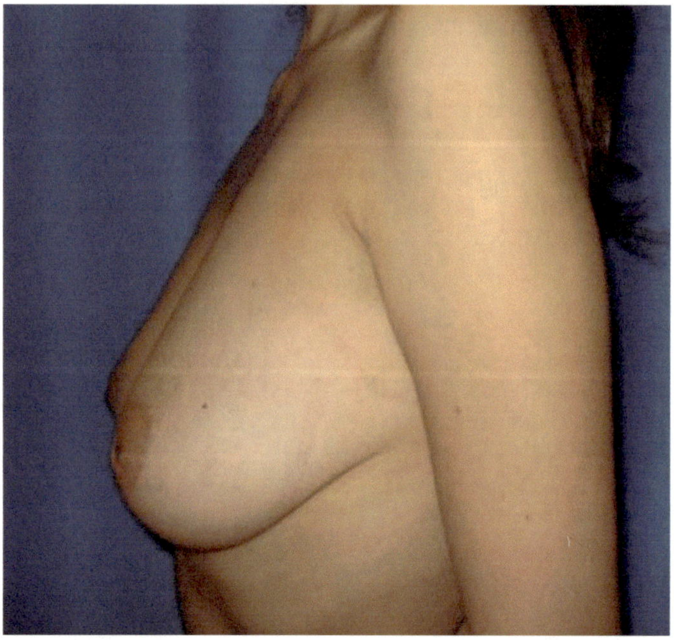

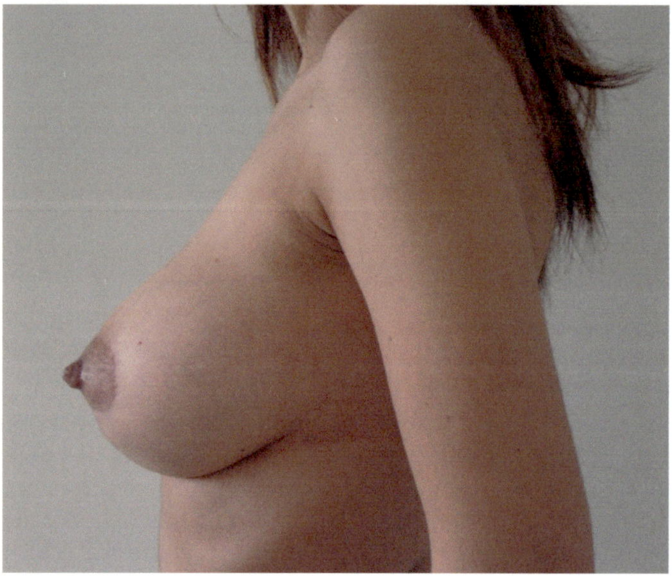

Fig. 8 and 9. As of patient satisfaction the technique seems promising that the shape and projection of the patient's nipple was deemed satisfactory. Patient's lateral view before and 3 years after surgery

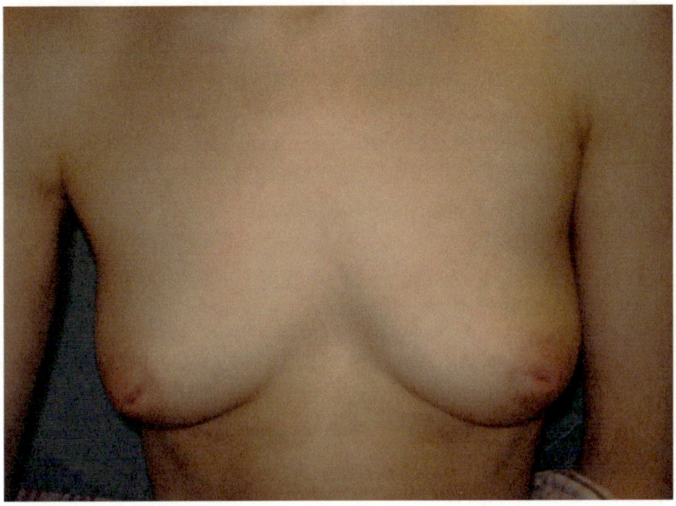

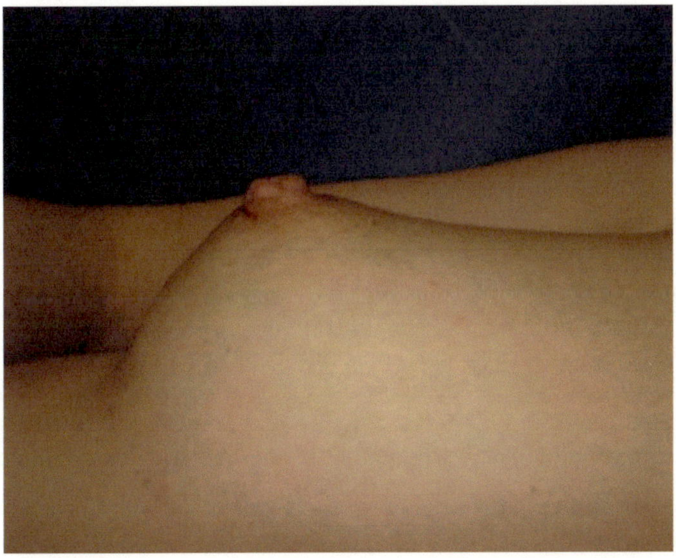

Fig. 10 and 11. A 24year-old nulliparous woman with a history of congenital inverted nipple is seen before and 4 years after surgery.

Author was used this technique in fourteen cases since its description. All patients were happy with the results. No major complications were reported. Only in two cases suture abcesses formation was reported.

As a conclusion, new vascularized tissue brought under the nipple-areola complex to correct recurrent inverted nipple yields a safe and better projection. This technique yields a satisfactory result without recurrence of inversion in fourteen cases. It is strongly recommended that the technique should be considered by the surgeon for any patient contemplating correction of inverted nipple and mastopexy.

4.2 Twisting and locking technique (Kim et al., 2006)

The corrective operation, based on twisting and locking principles, was described for various patterns of inverted nipple, ranging from the grade 1 to the grade 3 (Kim et al., 2006). One of the disadvantages of this technique is about the restriction fort he color of the areola. Patients with a pale colored areola or an areola with smaller diameter are not consireded appropriate fort his technique as a quite a decent amount of areolar tissue is required for the operative technique.

Preoperative Marking: Three diamond-shaped patterns are marked on three concentric circles drawn at the areola, with intervals of 120 degrees.

Surgical Technique: The inner tip of each diamond design is expected to be a margin of the nipple tip, and its width could be controlled for primary closure after nipple protrusion. With closure of the diamond design, the lateral wall of the nipple is formed from the inner side of the design. Therefore, the height of the nipple is determined by the length of the inner side, and the degree of nipple protrusion depends on the inner acute angle of the design. The designed pattern is mostly diamond shaped, and the inner sides are shorter than the outer sides. The lengths of the inner sides should be designed to be equal to the outer sides to make a prominent nipple with a small areola. The exact measurements of the design depends on the size of the nipple and areola of each individual patient. Deepithelialization is performed on the designed area. Three triangular dermal flaps are created and elevated from each deepithelialized area with their bases attached to the nipple. In addition, with temporary traction of the nipple apex provided by a stay suture, the fibrotic bands underneath the nipple base are sufficiently but cautiously released to make a tunnel to minimize injury to the lactiferous ducts. The elevated dermal flaps are passed through the space released underneath the nipple base, pulled out, and sutured firmly with an absorbable suture to the opposite dermis of the neighboring deepithelialized defect.

With this key fixation suture, a twisting effect is created at the nipple base to keep the nipple protruded, and the omega shape of the nipple is finally formed. It is considered that each dermal flap acted as a locking barrier at the nipple base to prevent reinversion. Each deepithelialized defect is easily closed without tension by minimal undermining because of the twisting effect. In some cases, modification is available for easier closure of the defect with a small triangular skin flap that remained during the deepithelialization procedure. The twisting effect created by anchoring dermal fixation makes it possible to form the desirable omega-shaped nipple with a narrow nipple neck and also is expecting to prevent flattening of the nipple.

4.3 Triangular areolar dermal flaps technique (Kim et al, 2003)

Kim et al. introduce an alternative, simple method using 2 triangular areolar dermal flaps. Compared with other methods using triangular areolar dermal flaps, each triangle is approximately 1 mm shorter than the diameter of the nipple, and the deepithelialized areolar dermal flaps are lodged at the slit in the bundle of the lactiferous ducts in the grade 2 inverted nipple. Authors were treated 11 patients (16 nipples) where five patients had bilateral inverted nipples. Patient ages were reported as ranged from 18 to 31 years (mean age, 27 years). All nipples were congenital and they had no previous operation. Thirteen nipples were grade 2 and 3 were grade 3. The mean follow-up period was 8.7 months (range, 3-12 months). Follow-up examinations revealed no evidence of recurrence of inversion. There was no complication associated with surgery, such as infection, hematoma, permanent sensory disturbance, or nipple necrosis. The resulting scars were minimal. All patients were satisfied with their results. The authors conclude that their procedure is reliable, preserves the lactiferous ducts in grade 2 inverted nipple, requires no special postoperative care, and leaves minimal scars and no recurrence of inversion. This technique can be applied to any type of inverted nipple as a primary surgical procedure.

Preoperative marking: The width of the nipple is measured and the design is marked with methylene blue. A circle is drawn around the nipple neck and two triangular flaps- where the bases of which are located on the circle around the nipple neck, are designed at 3 o'clock and 9 o'clock. The marking is completed to assure the following key points: the base of the triangle is approximately 9 to 12 mm, depending on the diameter of the nipple. Each triangle is usually within the areoalar margin, is approximately 1 mm shorter than the diameter of the nipple.

Surgical Technique: A traction suture is place to the nipple strong enough to perform the procedure. The incisions are made at the triangles. On the side of the triangles, the incisions are deepened into the subcutaneous fatty tissue, but limited to the upper dermal layer on the bases of the triangles so the areolar dermal flap is based medially. The triangles are then deepithelized, and the areolar dermal flaps are raised leaving the subcutaneous fat to the flaps. While traction is applied to the nipple the tethering fibrous tissue bands are identified and transected to free the nipple. A non-absorbable suture is put into the tip of each areolar dermal flap. Using a small pick up each suture is pulled out through the slit under the opposite areolar dermal flap. Pulling tha absorbable sutures the areolar dermal flaps are turned down and pulled through the slit so that they cross each other within it. The sutures are stitched to the lower dermis of the nipple base just beside each of the opposite elevated triangular flaps. The donor areas are closed without undermining with the two layers and then the traction suture is removed from the nipple.

4.4 Internal 5-point star suture technique (Serra-Renom et al, 2004)

Some of the methods reported for the surgical treatment of the inverted nipple include insertion of autologous or heterologous material to provide volume and projection to the nipple, thereby avoiding recurrence.In this technique, the authors described the use of a surgical technique for grade III inverted nipple in which the nipple remains protruded when it is pulled out, and sectioning of the lactiferous ducts and an internal 'star' stitch to avoid both nipple collapse and introduction of heterologous filling material.

Surgical technique: In cases of severely inverted nipple with severe fibrosis and shortening of the lactiferous ducts, the authors' technique combines the pulling out of the nipple and the release of the fibrosis and retracting ducts with the introduction of a stitch of polyglactin as filling material, performing an internal star suture in only one surgical intervention, without the need for using graft material, or local flaps that introduce scars around the nipple. The technique is simple.The results are deemed satisfactory.

4.5 Other techniques

-Nipple aspirator (Jiang et al, 2008):

A self-designed instrument for inverted nipple was described by Jiamg et al.

-Correcting an inverted nipple with an artificial dermis (Yamada et al, 2004):

This report describes and incorporates a new concept of using artificial dermis for tissue augmentation and is performed without sacrificing any donor site and complex design. It was applied to four nipples in two nulliparous cases. For all four corrected inverted nipples, good results were reported with no complications. No deformities of the nipple or the areola were reported and as an advantage of the technique the surgical scars were reported as inconspicuous.

-Internal sidewall suturing technique: (Lee et al., 2003)

The aouthors described a simple technique for providing long-term correction for the grade III severely inverted nipple without the use of dermal flaps.

Surgical technique: An inferior periareolar incision extending from 5 o'clock to 7 o' clock was made, and a periareolar flap was raised to the nipple. A 3-0 nylon suture was placed through the nipple, after which the nipple was everted through complete release of all fibrous bands and tethering attachments. We accomplished long-term eversion of the nipple by suturing the internal sidewalls of the nipple together. This technique has been performed in 17 patients. No recurrence was reported even 1 year after surgery.

The technique for treatment of the inverted nipple is simple to perform and seems to provide reliable, long-term Correction (Lee et al,. 2003).

-Three Periductal Dermofibrous Flaps (Huang, 2003)

The inverted nipple may be congenital or caused by repeated inflammation and breast surgery. The reported prevalence of congenital inverted nipple ranges from 1.77% (Sanghoo & Yoon, 1999)to 3.26%, and most of them are bilateral and umbilicated (Kim et al., 2003). The inversion has been linked to many aesthetic, functional, and psychological problems. Many methods have been proposed to correct this deformity since the first surgical correction by Kehrer in 1879. I propose a new method with three periductal dermofibrous flaps to add bulk to the nipple base and to form a hammock to prevent recurrence. The design also shortens the circumference of the root of the nipple without compromise of the neurovascular supply. We have corrected 46 nipples of 25 patients with this method successfully since 1996. This method can be applied to all types of inverted nipple without significant complications.

5. Conclusion

Various procedures have been proposed for the repair of inverted nipple since it was first described (Alaxander & Campbell, 1997; Kim et al., 2006; Serra-Renom et. Al, 2004; Jiang et al., 2008; Yamada et al., 2004; Ritz et al., 2005; Huang , 2003; Crestinu, 2001; Pompei & Tedesco, 1999). No single technique is appropriate for correcting all the types of nipple deformities because different grades of inverted nipple have different levels of fibrosis, soft tissue bulk, and lactiferous ductus stucture (Lee et al,. 2003). Some of the techniques include construction at the base of the nipple by using areolar dermal flaps (Kim et al., 2003; Kim et al., 2006; Huang 2003) modified suturing "t" (Stevens et al., 2004; Serra-Renom, 2004) or a combination of these two (Pompei & Tedesco, 1999) to prevent the collapse of the nipple. Other techniques use alloplastic materials, i.e., silicone or PTFE, where extrusion is a potential complication; they have their own limitations (Serra-Renom, 2004).

The novel surgical approach of Karacaoglu, *antenna dermal flap Technique*, presented in this chapter is for correcting a recurrent, congenital inverted nipple. It also should be emphasized that even an alloplastic material could not have corrected the deformity in this particular case. The patient was also asking for breast augmentation and lifting in addition to correction of her recurrent inverted nipple. As two other techniques had already been used to correct this deformity in previous surgeries, a new technique named the antenna flap was used. This technique entails transposition of bulky dermoadipose flaps harvested from the de-epithelialized area of the mastopexy into the pocket created beneath the nipple. The shape and projection of the patient's nipple was deemed satisfactory. In this technique the dead space was filled with autologous tissue where possible complications such as extrusion that is seen with alloplastic materials were avoided. This technique allowed for correction of ptosis and breast augmentation in the same surgical procedure. Combining the three procedures did not adversely affect the results of each procedure. One of the other advantages of this technique was the lack of scar in the areola. The disadvantage of the technique is that is it limited to those patients who are candidates for mastopexy.

As a conclusion, new vascularized tissue brought under the nipple-areola complex to correct recurrent inverted nipple yields a safe and better projection. This technique yields a satisfactory result without recurrence of inversion and is encouraged to use by the surgeons for any patient contemplating correction of inverted nipple and mastopexy.

6. References

Alaxander JM, Campbell MJ. Prevalance of inverted and non-protractile nipples in antenatal women who intend to breastfeed. *Breast* Vol. 6, (1997), pp72–78.

Crestinu JM The correction of inverted nipples without scars: 17 years' experience, 452 operations. *Aesthet Plast Surg,* Vol. 25, No. 3, (2001) p246-248.

Huang WC A new method for correction of inverted nipple with three periductal dermofibrous flaps. *Aesthet Plast Surg, Vol.* 27, No. 4, (2003), pp 301–304.

Hytten F.E. Clinical andchemicalstudies in human lactation; IX breast-feeding in hospital. *Br. Med. J,* Vol. 2, No. 2, (December 1954), pp. 1447-1452.

Jiang HQ, Wei X, Yuan SM, Tang LM Nipple aspirator: a self-designed instrument for inverted nipple. *Plast Reconstr Surg* Vol. 121, No. 3, (2008), pp 141e–143e.

Karacaoglu, E. Correction of Recurrent Grade III Inverted Nipple with Antenna Dermoadipose Flap: Case Report. *Aesth Plast Surg* (2009), Vol. 33, pp 843–848.

Kim JT, Lim YS, Oh JG Correction of inverted nippleswith twisting and locking principles. *Plast Reconstr Surg* Vol. 118, No. 7, (2006), pp 1526–1531.

Kim DY, Jeong EC, Eo SR, Kim KS, Lee SY, Cho BH. Correction of inverted nipple: an alternative method using two triangular areolar dermal flaps. *Ann Plast Surg* Vol 51, No. 6, (2003) pp.636–640.

Kopans D. (2007) Breast anatomy and basic histology, physiology, and pathology. In: *Breast Imaging,* Kopans D, ed.. 3rd ed. 7–43, Lippincott Williams & Wilkins, ISBN: 978-1-4419-1728-7, Philadelphia

Lee MJ, DePolli PA, Casas LA Aesthetic and predictable correction of the inverted nipple. *Aesthet Surg J Vol* 23, (2003), pp 353–356.

Love SM, Barsky SH. Anatomy of the nipple and breast ducts revisited. *Cancer* Vol. 101, (2004), pp1947–1957.

Pompei S, Tedesco M A new surgical technique for the correction of the inverted nipple. *Aesthet Plast Surg,* Vol. 23, No. 5, (1999), pp 371– 374.

Nicholson BT, Harvey JA, Cohen MA.Nipple-areolar complex: normal anatomy and benign and malignant processes.*Radiographics.*Vol.2, No 29, (March-April 2009), pp. 509-523.Doi10.1148/rg.292085128

Osborne MP. (1991) Breast development and anatomy. In: *Breast Diseases* , Harris J, Hellman S, Henderson I, KinneD, eds. 2nd ed. 1-13, Lippincott, ISBN: 978-0-7817-9117-5, Philadelphia

Ritz M, Silfen R, Morgan D, Southwick G Simple technique for inverted nipple correction. *Aesthet Plast Surg,* Vol. 29, No. 1, (2005), pp 24–27.

Sanghoo H, Yoon H. The inverted nipple: its grading and surgical correction. *Plast Reconstr Surg* Vol. 104, No. 2, (1999) pp.389–395.

Seltzer V. The breast: embryology, development, and anatomy. *Clin Obstet Gynecol,* Vol. 37 (1994), pp879–880.

Serra-Renom J, Fontdevila J, Monner J Correction of the inverted nipple with an internal 5-point star suture. *Ann Plast Surg,* Vol. 53, No. 3, (2004), pp 293–296.

Stevens WG, Fellows DR, Vath SD, Stoker DA Anintegrated approach to the repair of inverted nipples. *Aesthet Surg J* Vol. 24, (2004), pp 211–215.

Yamada N, Kakibuchi M, Kitaoshi H, Kurokawa M, Hosokawa K, Hashimoto K. A method for correcting an inverted nipple with an artificial dermis. *Aesthetic Plast Surg*. 2004 Jul-Aug;28(4):233-8.

7

Tuberous Breast: Clinical Evaluation and Surgical Treatment

Giovanni Zoccali and Maurizio Giuliani
Department of Health Sciences, Plastic, Reconstructive and Aesthetic Surgery Section, University of L'Aquila
Italy

1. Introduction

First described in detail by Rees and Aston in 1974, tuberous breast deformity is a pathologic condition of the breast affecting teenage woman either unilaterally or bilaterally. Other names of this deformity include snoopy breast, conical breast, tubular breast deformity, domen nipple, lower pole hypoplasia.

The clinical aspect of this malformation is the base absence or deficient in vertical as well as horizontal dimension.

1.1 Epiphenomenon

Definition of what comprises a tuberous breast have varied since the first description. Most definition have included a range of feature such us:

a. A contracted skin envelop both horizontally and vertically.
b. A constricted breast base.
c. A reduction in the volume of the breast parenchyma.
d. Abnormal elevation of inframammary fold.
e. Peudoherniation of the breast parenchyma into the areola.
f. Areola hypertrophy

Some (or all) of these epiphenomenon appear to be present on first inspection of the patient, see fig.1.

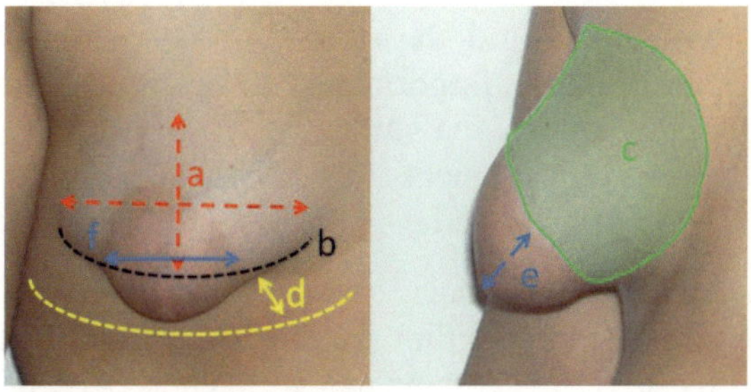

Fig. 1. Clinical epiphenomenon of tuberous breast.

1.2 Epidemiology

The exact incidence has not been properly investigated and remain undetermined and is probably impossible to ascertain because many woman who have mild degree of deformity may not seek help of be aware that a deformity exists. It is generally sporadic with little risk of occurrence in relatives. From a careful literature review the tuberous breast deformity has an high incidence in woman presenting with a breast asymmetry.

2. Pathogenesis

The etiology of tuberous breast remain still unclear. No genetic disorder are been associate to this condition and no hereditary transmission is observed. The pathogenesis of this breast deformity is linked to an aberration in thorax superficial fascia that blocks the normal expansion of glandular tissue, Fig. 2.

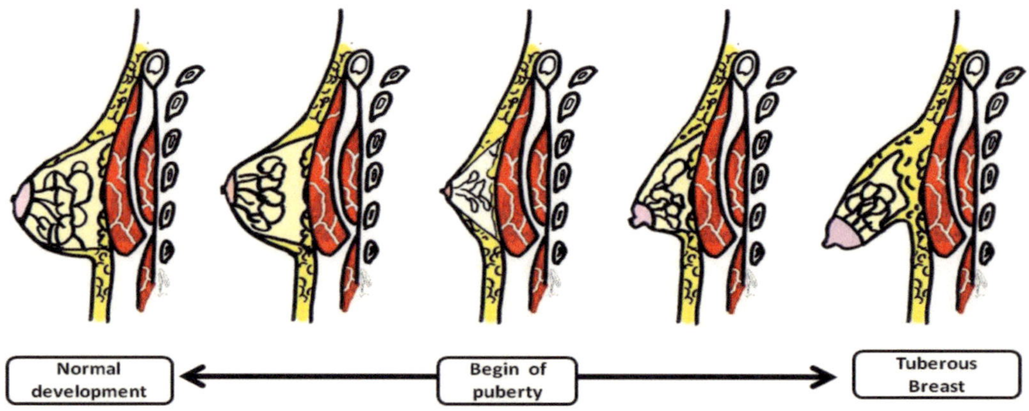

Fig. 2. Pathogenesis of tuberous breast: left side normal breast, right side malformed breast.

Normally the breast glandular tissue originate from the mammary ridge, which develops from ectoderm during the fifth week., most part of this ridge disappear, except for a small portion in the thorax region, which persists and penetrates the underlying mesenchyme around 10 to 14 weeks. The glandular development remain quiescent until puberty.

During puberty, the mammary tissue is contained in the thickness of superficial fascia. This anatomical structure is composed by two layers: the superficial one covering the outer surface of mammary parenchyma and the deeper one separate the posterior aspect of parenchyma from the muscle plane. Important is to underline that the superficial layer doesn't cover all the anterior parenchyma surface, it is absence in the area underneath the areola. With normal breast development this structure allow the peripheral breast expansion.

The onset of tuberous breast is secondary to a constricting fibrous ring at the level of periphery of the nipple- areola complex that inhibit the normal development of the breast and therefore the breast tissue cannot expand sidewards and herniates through the weakest point which is the areola area because of the missing of superficial layer.

3. Classifications

Several classification schemes for tuberous breast have been proposed. The system described by von Heimburg has become the most commonly used. At the end of 20th century Grolleau reported a new classification. (Grolleau et al. 1999)

3.1 von Heimburg classification (von Heimburg et al. 1996)

The first edition of von Heimburg classification was divided in four categories based on the degree of hypoplasia and the size of the skin envelope, fig. 3:

- Type I: hypoplasia of the lower medial quadrant.
- Type II: Hypoplasia of the lower medial and lateral quadrants, sufficient skin in the subareolar region.
- Type III: Hypoplasia of the lower medial and lateral quadrants, deficiency of skin in the subareolar region.
- Type IV: Severe breast constriction, minimal breast base.

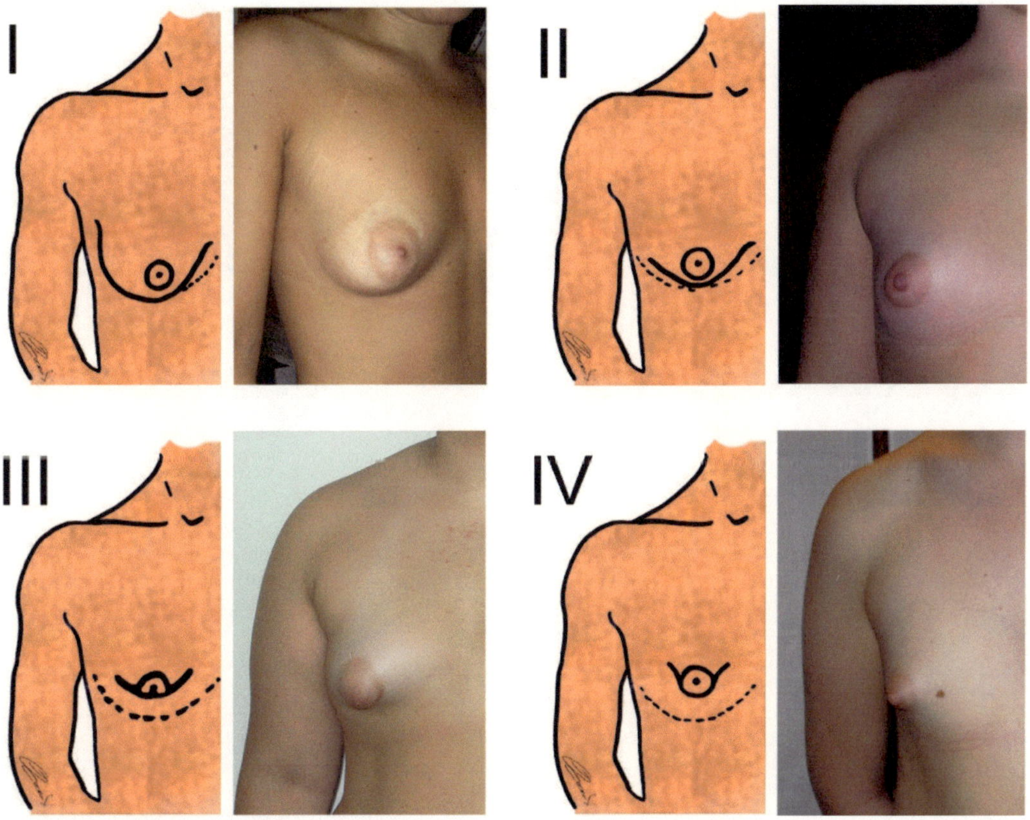

Fig. 3. Von Heimburg classification

It has been argued that type II and III are really the same because the amout of the skin envelope is simply dependent on the size of the glandular tissue itself.

3.2 Grolleau classification (Grolleau et al. 1999)

Following this classification system, the degree of the disorder have been reduced to three classes solely based on the degree of hypoplasia of the base of the breast, fig. 4:

- Type I: Hypoplasia of the lower medial quadrant.
- Type II: Hypoplasia of both lower quadrants.
- Type III: Hypoplasia of all four quadrants.

This classification allows a sufficient preoperative planning to choose the appropriate surgical procedure.

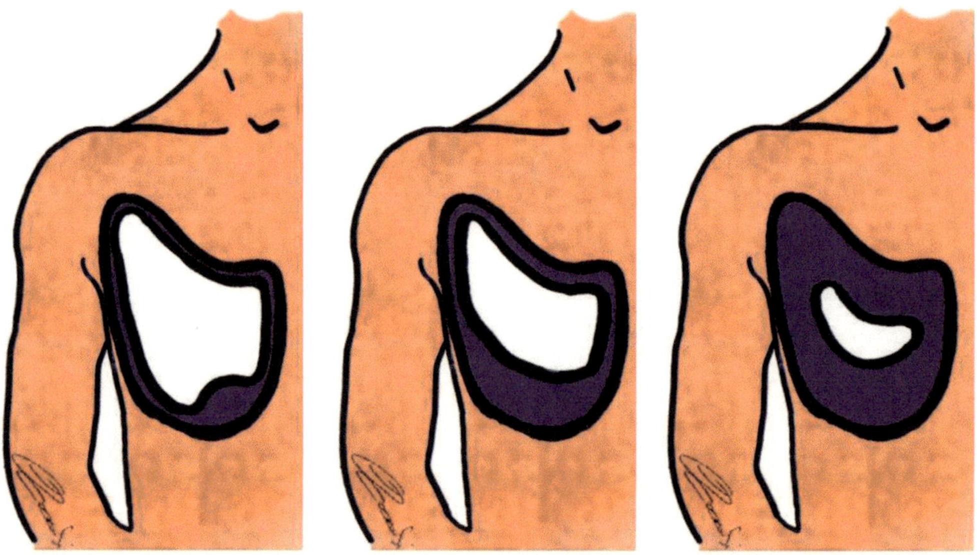

I II III

Fig. 4. Grolleau classification: in violet the theoretical breast size, in white the real amount of glandular tissue.

4. Differential diagnosis

In front of a wild clinical features of tuberous breast, differential diagnosis have to be done with all asymmetry condition and especially with breast ptosis, fig. 5.

The true tuberous breast has a constriction of both diameter, horizontal and vertical; tubular breast have a constriction only of horizontal one. This didactic differentiation of the same disorder is useful only in operative procedure choice. In ptotic breast the glandular parenchyma and areola have a normal structure but their position is wrong being an increase of distance between nipple-areola complex and sternal nock.

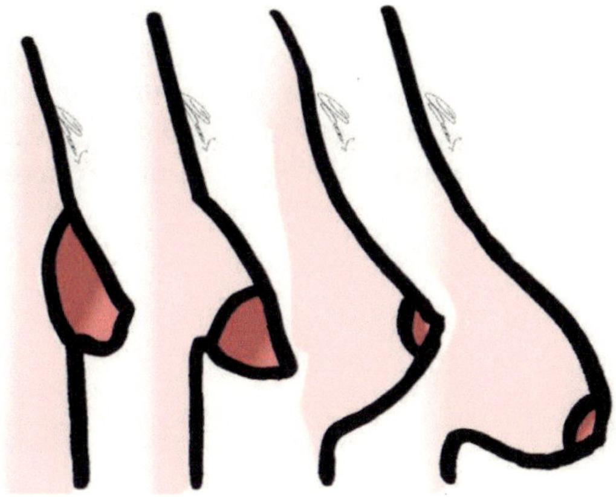

Fig. 5. Differential diagnosis: 1. Tuberous breast, 2. Tubular breast, 3. Normal breast, 4.Ptotic breast.

5. Treatment

Surgery is the only way to treat tuberous breast. In literature numerous technique to correct tuberous breast deformity are reported. There has been no paradigm shift in the approach to the surgery of tuberous breast. The surgical protocol have to be planned on the patient in order to correct all malformation features.

5.1 Therapeutic goal

The surgical correction of tuberous breast deformity and its variants requires a comprehensive and systematic approach. Only after understanding the specific anatomic characteristics of the deformity can the surgeon plan a single stage procedure to treat each anatomic problem. The fundamental pillar to achieve a good reconstruction are:

- Reduce the areola hypertrophy.
- Increase the skin amount in the breast lower pole.
- Take down the infra mammary fold.
- Expand the glandular parenchyma.
- Increase the breast volume.

6. Surgical procedures

In the follow part of this chapter are reported some surgical techniques to correct the tuberous breast deformity and the authors personal experience performing Puckett technique.

6.1 Prosthesis implantation

The attempt to achieve a correction of tuberous deformity with prosthesis implantation is common. Often the device is located behind the glandular parenchyma through an incision in the inframammary fold or trans-areola. This technique not always correct the parenchyma tissue imbalance and the skin envelope deficiency in the inferior breast mound. The double-bubble condition is the result of prosthetic device implantation behind the parenchyma without the expansion of breast tissue, breaking the fibrous ring. Is commonly accept that the placement of an implant as sole treatment may accentuate the appearance of the deformity, fig 6.

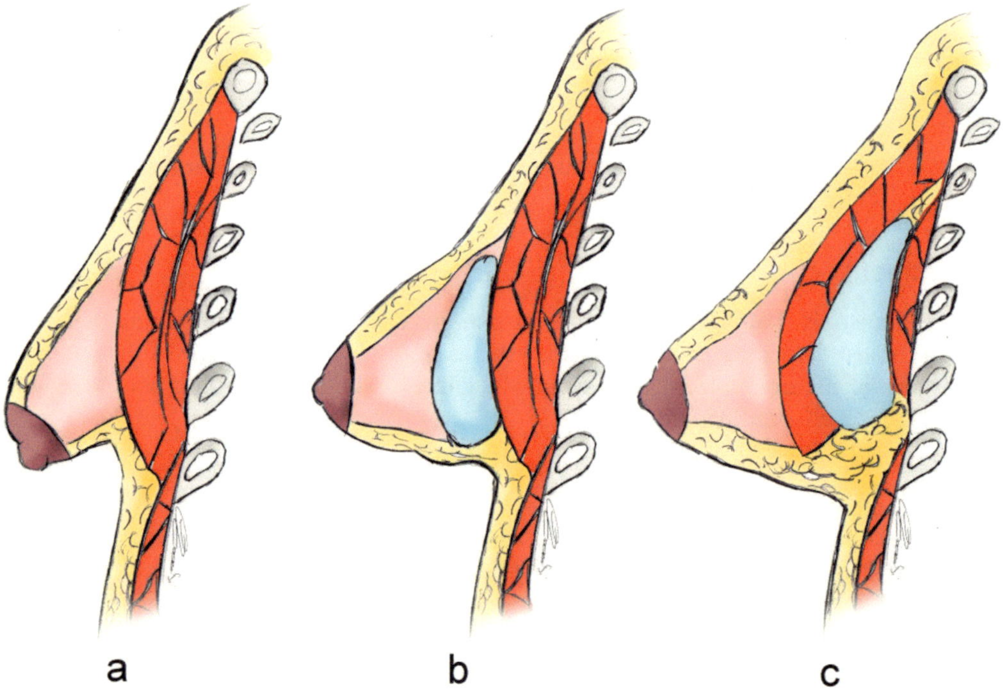

Fig. 6. Double-bubble breast after reconstruction with silicone implant. a: before surgery; b: prosthesis is inserted behind the breast tissue; c: prosthesis is located under the muscle

6.2 Mailalrd Z-Plasty (Maillard, 1986)

The target of this procedure is increase the length of nipple-inframmammary fold distance.

The first step is to plan a circumareolar area in order to correct the macroareola, after peri-areola de-epithelialization, the inferior portion of the breast is extensively mobilized in the subcutaneous plane, dissection is extended inferiorly to the inframammary fold, and the glandular parenchyma is detached from the muscular fascia. The areola is moved superiorly and the breast inferior pole is reshaped performing a Z-plasty, fig 7.

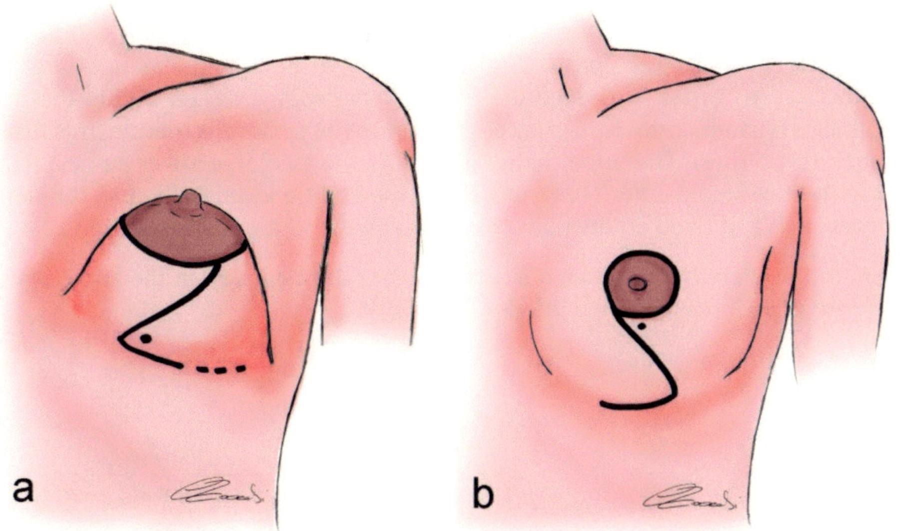

Fig. 7. Millard Z-plasty – a: preoperative planning; b: result.

6.3 Modified thoracoepigastric flap (Dinner & Dowen, 1987)

This procedure is useful in case of deficiency of lower pole tissue especially in III type deformity. The flap is based medially with its blood supply from the lateral branches of the superior epigastric artery. The flap is dissected as thick as possible, the end of the flap is de-epithelialised and fold over itself. The folded part of the flap increase the breast volume supporting the nipple-areola complex. In front of macroareola a circular reduction can be performed, fig. 8.

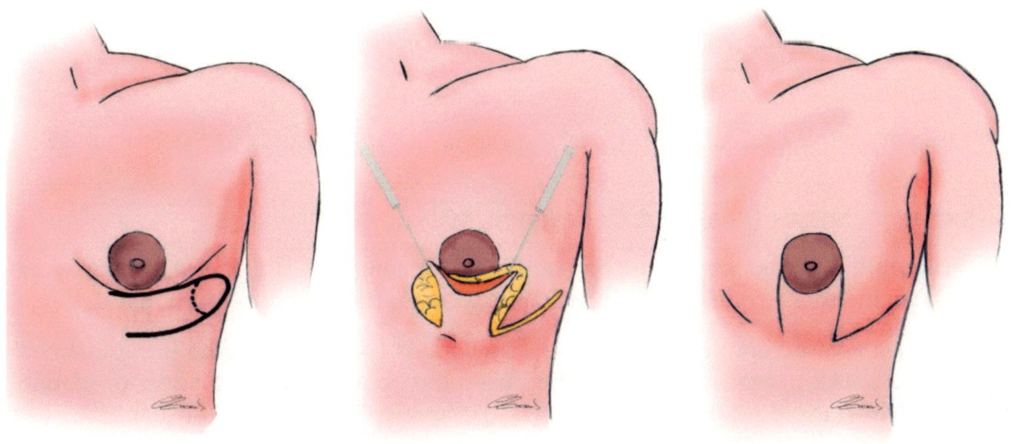

a b c

Fig. 8. Thoracoepigastric flap. a: preoperative planning, b: flap elevation, c: result.

6.4 Ribeiro technique (Ribeiro, 1998)

The most significant element in the technique is crating the glandular flap and positioning it on the thoracic wall. The procedure star with a circumareolar incision and de-epithelialization in order to reduce the areola hypertrophy. Then divide the mammary gland in half with an incision that is perpendicular to the pectoralis muscle (this disrupts the constricting fascia ring). The upper half will contain the areola; a lower pedicle flap will be created with lower half. The flap is mobilized medially and laterally and the flap is then folded over itself and fixed on the thoracic wall to give inferior pole projection.

In patient with severe hypomastia, a silicon implant can be insert in the space between the superior part of the breast and the inferior flap, fig. 9.

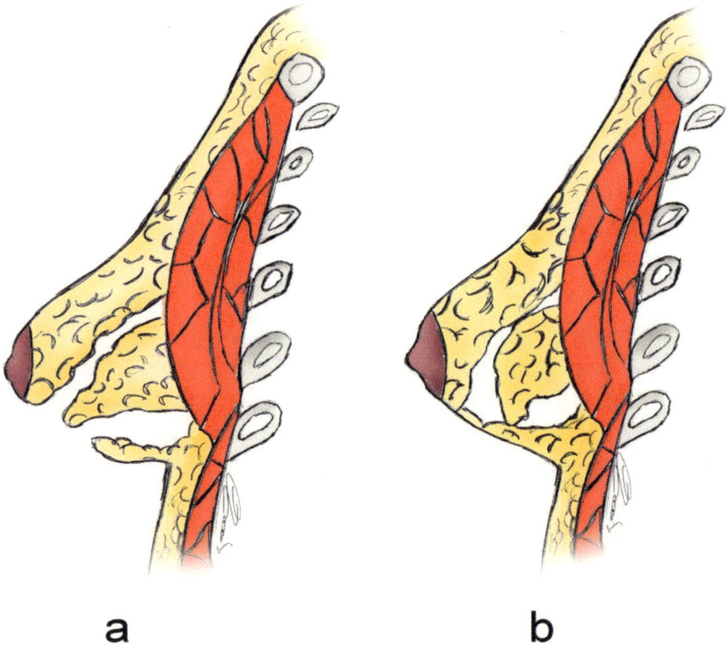

Fig. 9. Ribeiro technique - a: glandular flap elevation, b: final position of flap.

6.5 Puckett technique (Puckett & Concannon, 1990)

This procedure use the same concept of Ribeiro technique. The breast parenchyma is manipulated in order to built a glandular flap to increase the lower pole hypoplasia.

After circumareola de-epithelialization the dissection is conduct until the inframmamamry fold and the breast parenchyma is detached from the pettorali fascia, a superior glandular pedicle is drown dividing the inferior part of the breast. The flap apex is then fixed to the infra mammary fold to prevent the retraction during the healing.

In case of hypoplasia a silicon implant can be placed behind the breast tissue or under the muscular plane, fig. 10.

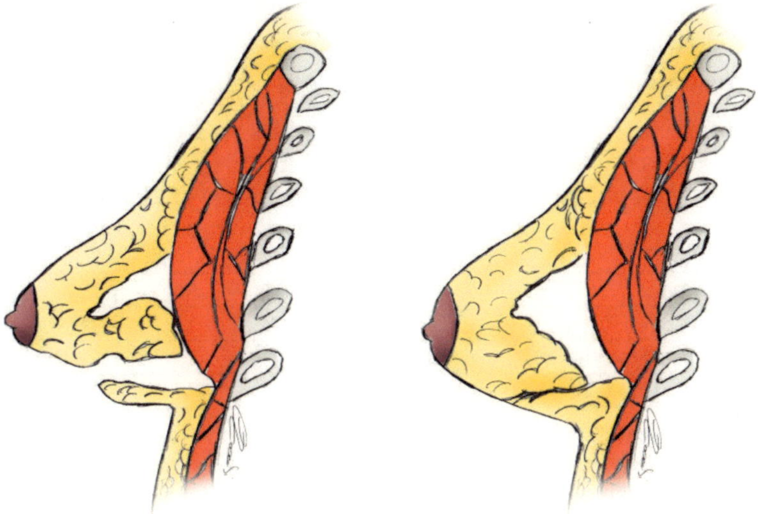

a b

Fig. 10. Puckett technique: a: glandular flap elevation, b: final position of flap. The volume deficiency can be filled with a silicone gel prosthesis placed behind the breast parenchyma or under the pectoralis muscle.

6.6 Lipofilling

Lipofilling also known as fat transfer or fat graft is newer technique to treat touberous breast. In order to improve the breast contour, the fat tissue, obtained by a liposuction and processed using Coleman protocol, is injected in tissues thickness. The fundamental limit of this technique is linked to the low amount of tissue that can be transfer: to survive the fat graft needs the contact with surrounding tissue so the injection of high quantity in the same place not allow the revascularization of fat that gradually become necrotic and absorbed. In order to reach a good result, the patient is bind to repeat several times the surgical procedure. Is Authors opinion that lipofilling may be useful to treat low grade deformity or have to be consider as a refinement procedure.

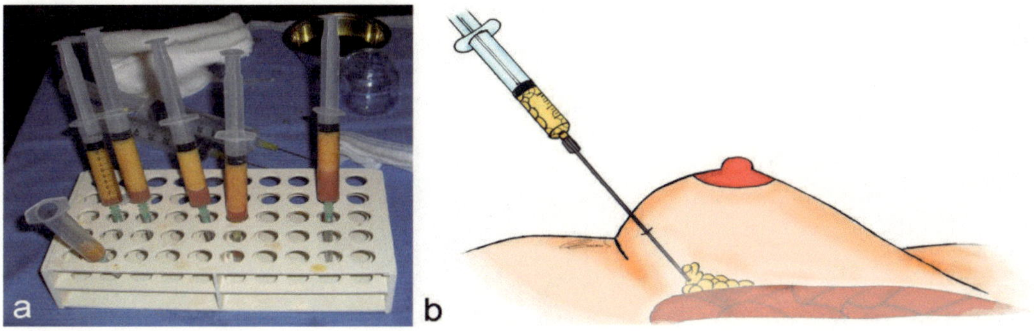

Fig. 11. Lipofilling: a) fat processing; b) Fat injection.

7. Personal experience with Puckett technique

In this section we describe the Puckett surgical technique in detail and our personal experience performing this procedure.

In the period from March 2009 to June 2011, 27 subjects with tuberous breast were referred to the Operative Unit of Plastic, Reconstructive and Aesthetic Surgery of L'Aquila University. Our court was composed by 27 female, with an average age of 21 years old (range 16-37); The deformity was bilateral in 25 patient and in 10 a severe asymmetry was present. Table 1.

Average age	21
Range	16 - 37
N° of patients with bilateral malformation	25 (92.5%)
N° of patients with severe asymmetry	11 (33.4%)

Table 1. Personal casuistry

A total of 52 breasts were treated and in accordance with von Heimburg classification were divided in four groups as follow:

- 7 breasts (13.46%) Type I
- 18 breasts (34.61%) Type II
- 22 breasts (42.3%) Type III
- 5 breasts (9.61%) Type IV

In order to estimate the amount of breast tissue and the contraction severity, all patient received a ecography. After surgery a antibiotic therapy was administered and a compressive dressing (post-surgery bra) was performed for all patients.

7.1 Surgical procedure

In order to better show the new-inframammary fold, the patient is placed in operatory room in semiseated position. To obtain vasoconstriction and hydrodissection, a solution with lidocaine and epinephrine is injected in breast parenchyma, fig. 12a. An areolotome is placed on the areola in order to determine the physiological dimension of NAC, Fig. 12b.

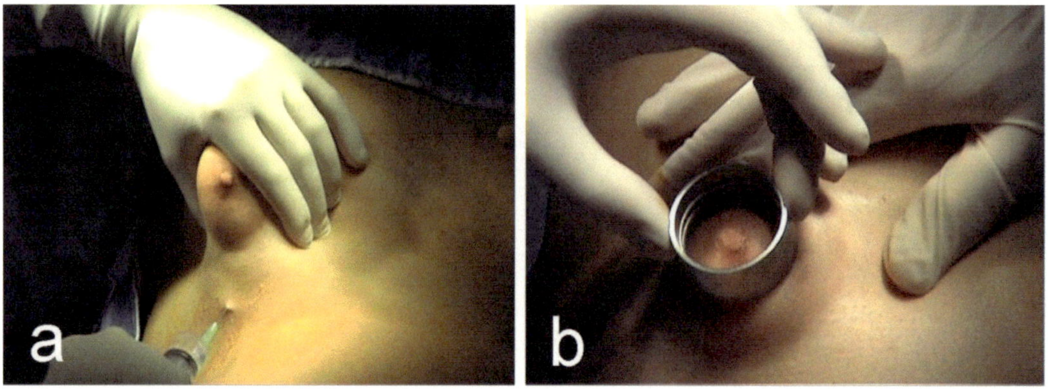

Fig. 12.

The areola outer border and neo-inframamamry fold are then marked, fig. 13a.

The new areolar margin is incised by a scalpel, fig. 13b, and the superabundance of areolar tissue is then removed, fig. 14a. With cautery the deepithelialized area is incised approximately 5 mm from the margin of the skin. The incision is extended from the right side to the left following the previous incision curvature. Just the dermis is discontinued the glandular parenchyma is pulled out through the incision as an hernia, fig. 14b.

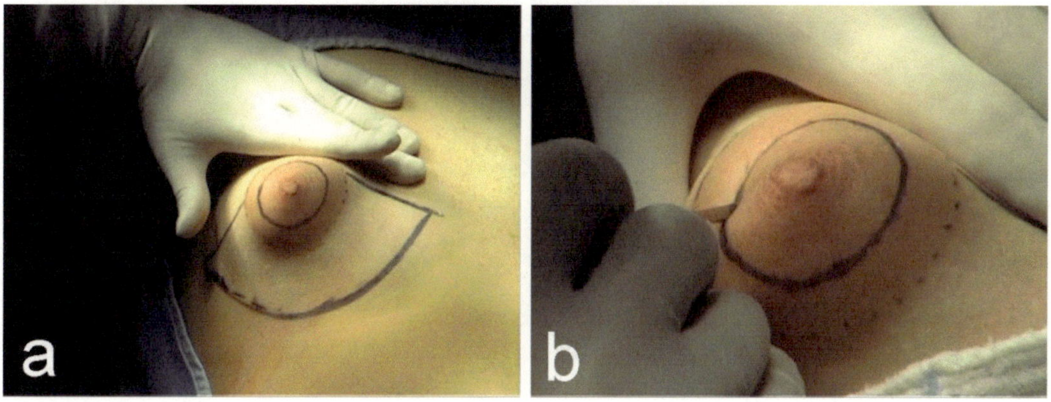

Fig. 13.

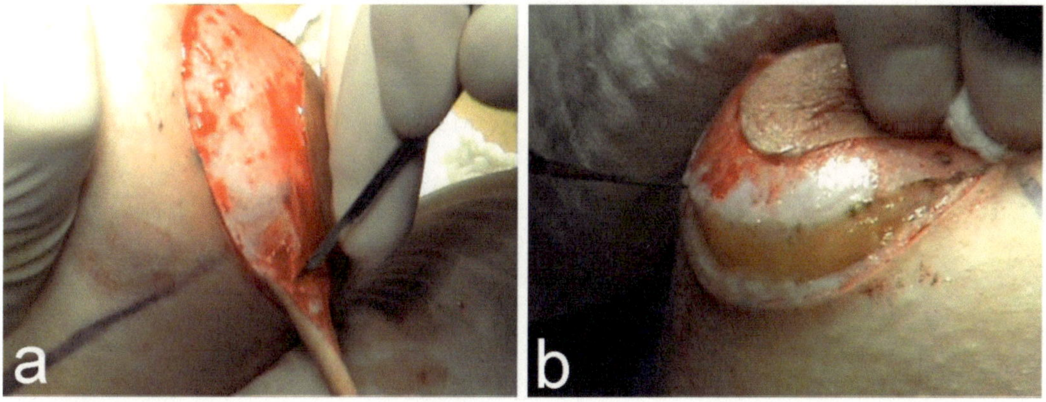

Fig. 14.

The inferior portion of the breast is completely separated from its skin covering. The dissection plain is placed 0.5-1cm from the dermis, fig, 15a. The adherence between the glandular parenchyma and pectoralis muscle fascia are discontinued, fig. 15b.

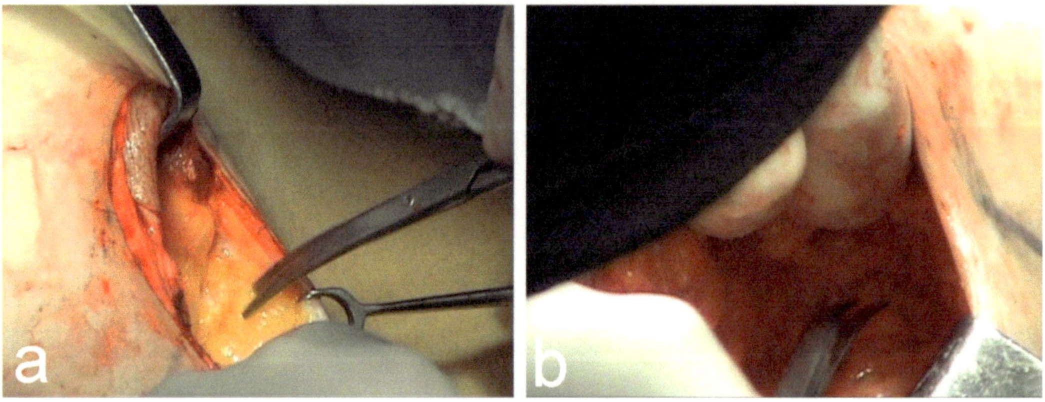

Fig. 15.

Due the delivery of all breast connection from surrounding tissue, the parenchyma can be everted, fig. 16a. Raising the superior pedicle glandular flap allow to create a sub glandular pocket in order to locate a prosthesis if a volume deficiency is present. To discontinue the fibrose ring causing the breast deformity, the glandular posterior wall is incised by the cautery, fig. 16b.

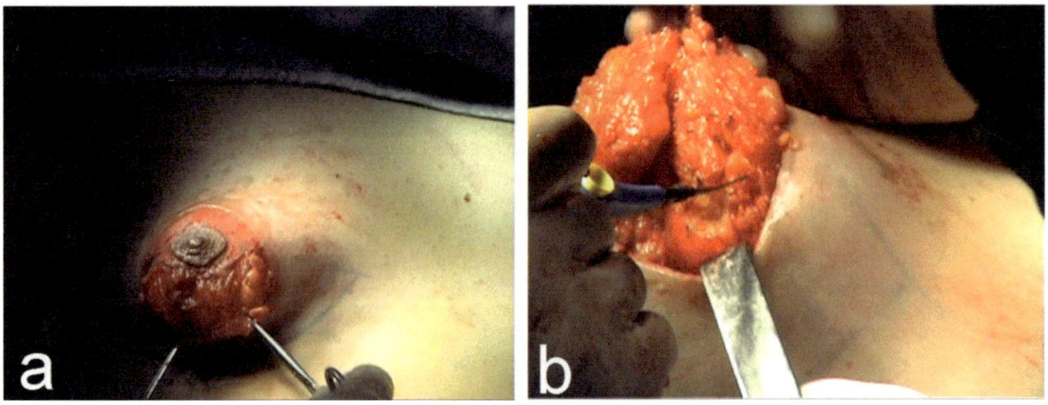

Fig. 16.

A series of incision have to be done to create a V-Y flap in order to eliminate the parenchyma tension, Fig. 17a. If necessary a silicon gel prosthesis is placed, fig. 16b. If the amount of glandular parenchyma doesn't allow to place the implant behind the breast tissue, a pocket under the muscular plane have to be done in order to better dissimulate the device presence.

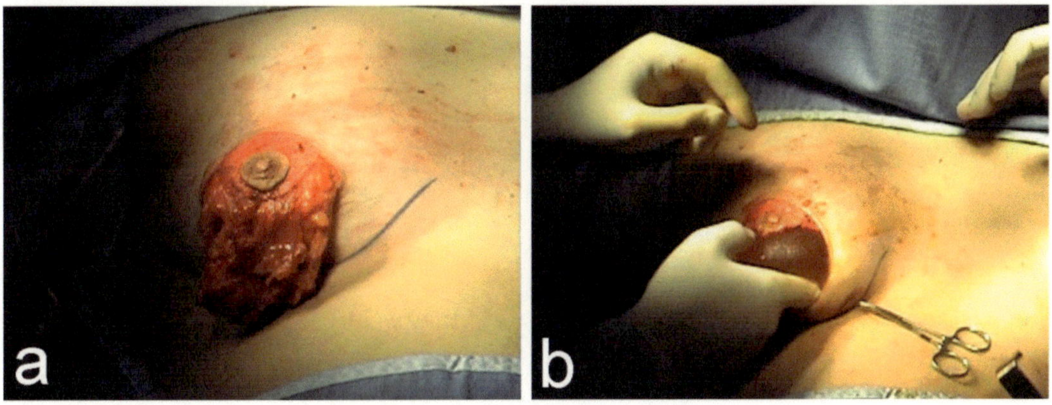

Fig. 17.

After breast tissue expansion is completed, the inferior border of glandular flap has to be lie to the dermis of new-inframammary fold. To eliminate this risk, a series of suture thread go through the skin first and then through the gland, fig 18a. They are pulled by a needle that passes it from the skin surface (at the level of new inframammary fold) into the dissected subcutaneous plane, until it ahchors the caudal border of expanded breast, fig 18b.

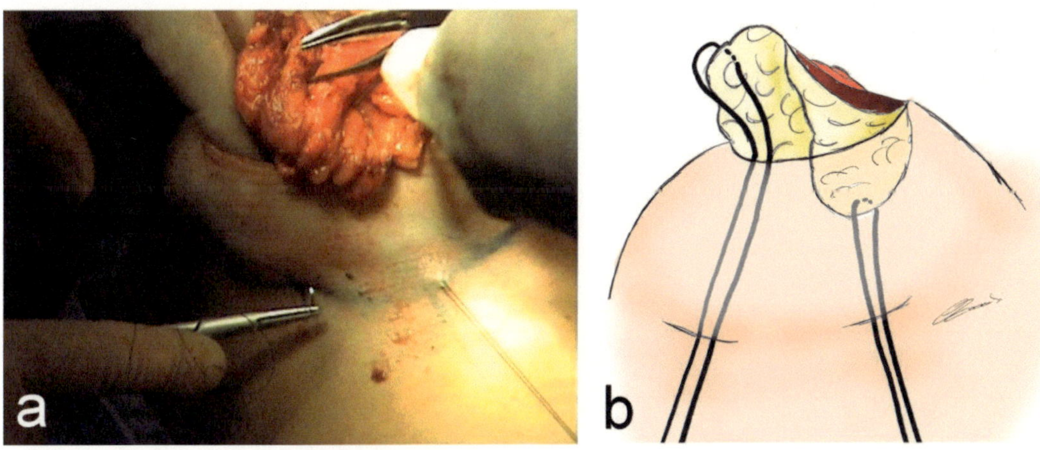

Fig. 18.

Transdermal anchorages of the gland are then tied at their ends around a soft cotton roll, fig 19, this prevent the nock decubitus and breast retraction during the healing process.

The traction system will be removed in 15 days after surgery.

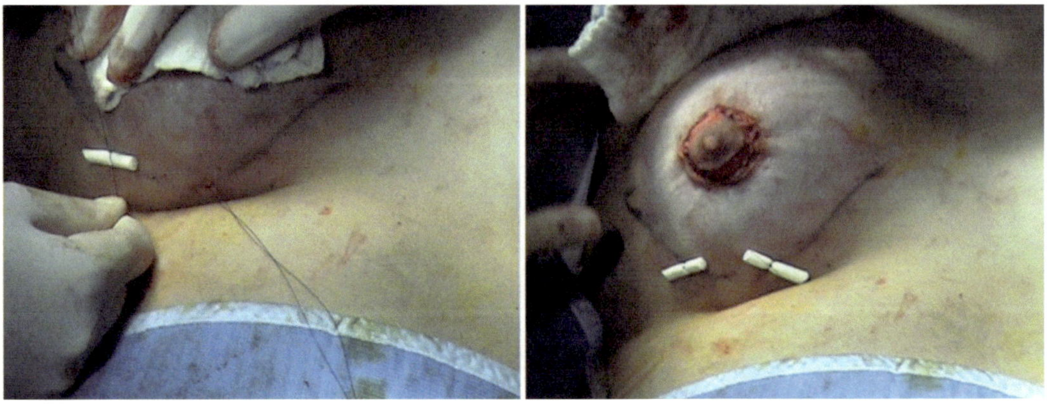

Fig. 19.

The areola is repositioned and a deep suture is performed like in round-block mastopexy and the superficial layer is closed using a continue suture with the cutaneous portion that pass through the dermis and the areolar run on the tissue surface, fig. 20a.

The aim of this suture is to further distribute the small wrinkles which inevitably form when joining two very different length margins, fig. 20b. Finally a dressing is applied.

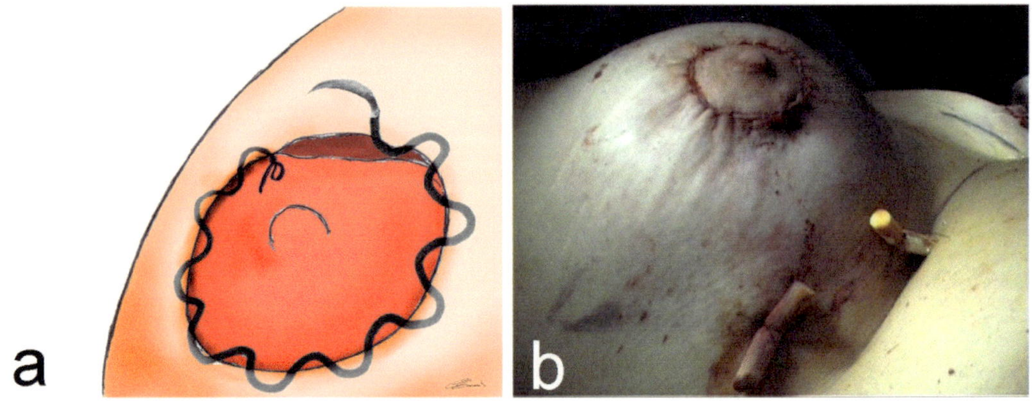

Fig. 20.

8. Results

With a minimum follow-up of 6 month we obtain the complete remission in all patients.

All treated breast received an implant to correct the volume deficiency.

All prosthesis have the same physical characteristics like high cohesive silicone gel, round shape and textured surface.

In four cases, type IV (7.69%),, the prosthesis device was implanted under the muscular plane, a retroglandular plane for the other cases was chosen.

In one patient with severe asymmetry and suffering of hypomastia in which the few glandular tissue was completely replaced by fibrous tissue (maximum ecographic diameter of 1,5cm), in order to avoid a double bubble aspect after implant, we performed a subtotal adenectomy.

In our series the 18,5% (5 patients) of complications were been observed; the high value of adverse events is linked to the inclusion of not complete satisfy patient.

The 7,4% (2 patients) was the real percentage of clinical complications (1 wound infection and partial dehiscence, 1 seroma).

9. Case reports

9.1 Case report no. 1. Fig. 21.

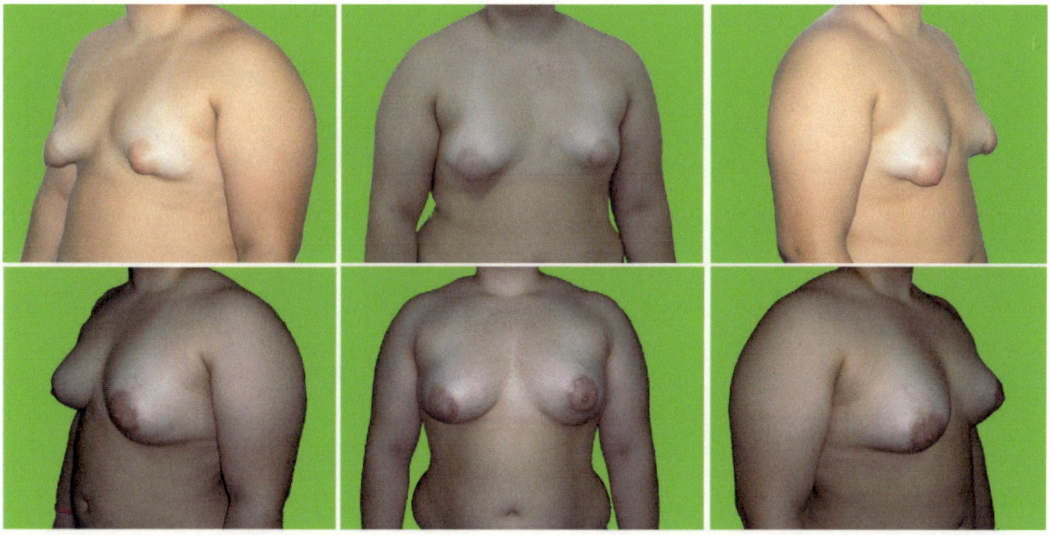

Fig. 21. C.C. - 21yars-holg girl with bilateral tuberous breast Type III, a hypoplasia is also associated. We have a reconstruction performing Puckett technique and the volume deficiency was restored with two silicone implant behind the gland (L: 200cc. R: 180cc). No complication was observed.

9.2 Case report no. 2. Fig. 22.

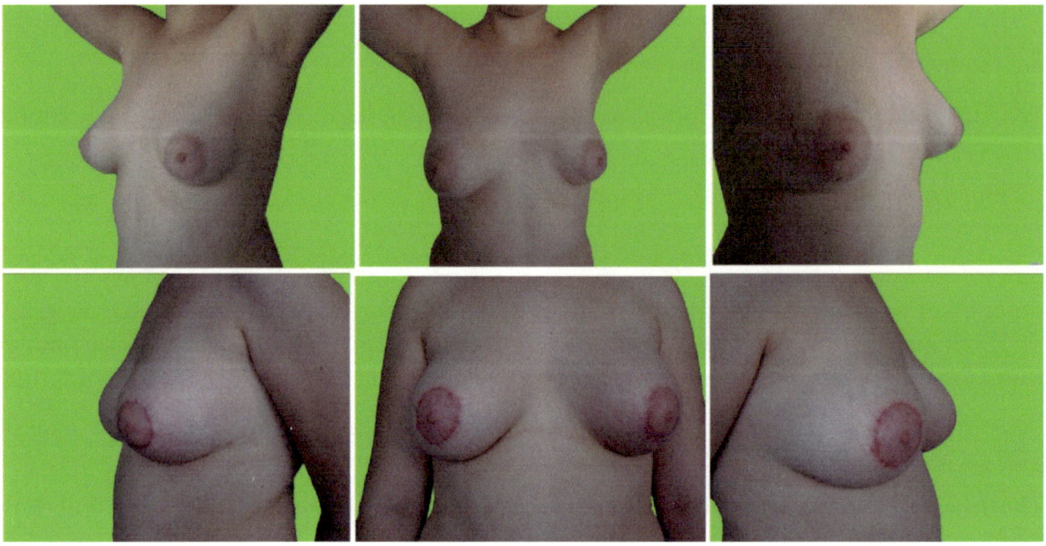

Fig. 22. G.S. – 18years-old girl with left tuberous breast type II with low asymmetry .

The deformity was correct with the Puckett technique and we insert a silicone prosthesis behind the breast parenchyma (140cc). The improve the symmetry we perform a round-block mastopexy on the right breast.

9.3 Case report no. 3. Fig. 23.

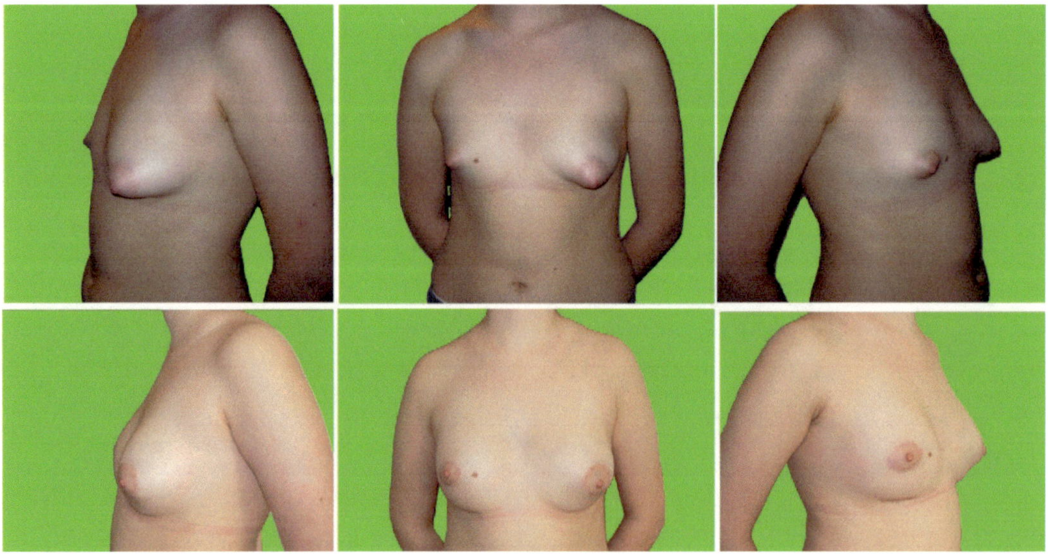

Fig. 23. M.L. 19yars-hold girl with bilateral tuberous breast Type III for left side and type IV for right, severe hypoplasia and asymmetry were The left breast was reconstructed using Puckett technique and positioning a prosthesis behind the gland (190cc). The right presenting a very

few amount of glandular parenchyma, an implant under the muscle was positioned (230cc) and in order to avoid the double-bubble effect, a partial adenectomy was performed.

9.4 Case report no. 4. Fig. 24.

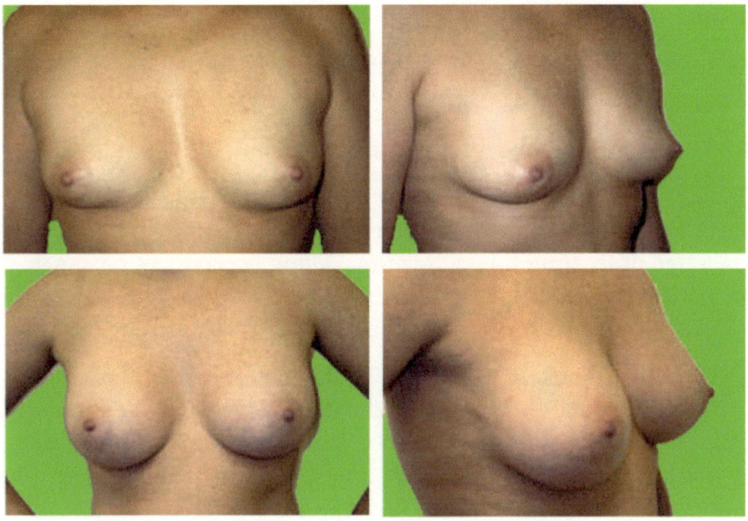

Fig. 24. T.M. - 25yars-holg girl with bilateral tuberous breast Type II. We have a reconstruction performing Puckett technique and retroglandular implant (R=L:190cc).

9.5 Case report no. 5. Fig. 25.

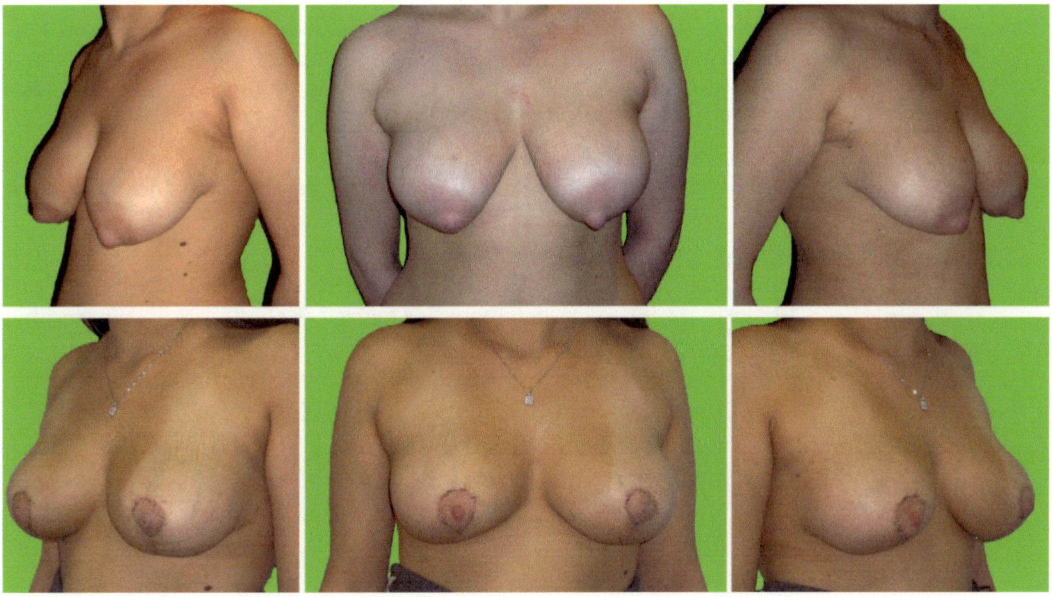

Fig. 25. A.V - 22yars-holg girl with bilateral tuberous breast Type I. hypoplasia of medial quadrant, macroareola and parenchyma hypertrophy are present in both breasts.

A modify Puckett technique was used: after glandular parenchyma expansion a skin remodeling was performed, living only a vertical scar like Lejour procedure.

No prosthesis devices were needed.

10. Conclusions

Tuberous breast can cause major psychological problems in the affected women presenting a surgical challenge for the plastic surgeons.

The management of the tuberous breast syndrome and its variants is best achieved by understanding the essence of the deformity.

The abundance of techniques available in literature for correcting the tuberous breast attests to the great challenge of treating this deformity. Many procedures have same steps and the little variations permit to the surgeon to have a better surgical plan to improve the patient outcome.

Is Authors opinion that Puckett technique is the better way to correct this deformity. Performing a superior pedicle flap of glandular tissue allows to the surgeon to discontinue the fibrous ring and to better expose the thoracic wall during inframammary fold reconstruction, and a good reshaping of glandular parenchyma is also permitted.

Although the results are sometimes not perfect, the psychological impact of such treatment is extremely positive with an augmentation of self-esteem and a progressive normalization of social activities.

11. References

Bach, AD,. Kneser, U., Beier, JP., Breuel, C., Horch, RE., & Leffler, M. (2009). Aesthetic correction of tuberous breast deformity - lessons learned with a single-stage procedure. *The Breast Journal,* Vol. 15, No. 3, (May-June 2009), pp. 279-286, ISSN 0960-9776

De Luca-Pytell, DM., Piazza, RC., Holding, JC., Snyder, N., Hunsicker, LM., & Phillips, LG. (2005). The incidence of tuberous breast deformity in asymmetric and symmetric mammaplasty patients. *Plastic and Reconstructive Surgery,* Vol. 116, No. 7, (December 2005), pp. 1900-1901, ISSN 0032-1052

Mandreakas, AD., & Zambacos GJ,. (2010). Aestetic reconstruction of the tuberous breast deformity: a 10-yar experience. *Aestetic Surgery Journal,* Vol. 30, No. 5, (September 2010), pp. 680-692, ISSN 1090-820X

Pacifico, MD., & Kang, NV.(2007) The tuberous breast revisited. *Journal of Plastic, Reconstructive & Aesthetic Surgery.* Vol. 60, No. 5., (January 2007), ISSN 1748-6815

Rees, TD., & Aston, SJ. (1976). The tuberous breast. *Clinics in Plastic Surgery,* Vol.3, No.4, (April 1976), pp. 339-347, ISSN 0094-1298

Part 3

Aesthetic

8

Combination of Liposuction and Abdominoplasty

Francisco J. Agullo[1,2], Sadri O. Sozer[1,2] and Humberto Palladino[1,2]
[1]*Texas Tech University Health Sciences Center, El Paso, TX*
[2]*El Paso Cosmetic Surgery Center, El Paso, TX*
USA

1. Introduction

Developments in surgical techniques over the past century now allow safe and efficient surgical correction of contour deformities.(Pitanguy, 2000) The abdomen and trunk represent areas of heightened patient interest and surgical technique modification. Consequently, familiarity with the presentation and effective treatment of these patients has become increasingly important.(Aly, 2004; Cardenas-Camarena, 2005) Liposuction and abdominoplasty are both used to address contour deformities of the trunk. Although controversial, the combination of both is seen more and more often.

Abdominoplasty is indicated for abdominal wall laxity, excess skin, striae, and/or diastases of the rectus muscles. It is the only procedure available to remove the excess skin and plicate the muscle layer of the abdomen. Multiple ways of classifying patients for abdominal contour modifying procedures have been described based on the myoaponeurotic layer,(Nahas, 2001) skin and subcutaneous tissue excess,(Nahas, 2001; Bozola, 1988) and the combination of both.(Matarasso, 1991, 1995; Toledo, 2004)

Liposuction, a surgical intervention designed to treat superficial and deep deposits of subcutaneous fat distributed in aesthetically unpleasing proportions, has proven to be a successful method of improving body contour. It is indicated, by itself, in the abdomen, when there is presence of excess subcutaneous fat, without excess skin, stretch marks, or abdominal wall laxity. It is an excellent adjunct to any abdominoplasty procedure providing refined contours and sculpting.

A guide describing guidelines for electing the best procedure for the patient is presented. We utilize recent improvements in abdominoplasty and liposuction in order to combine them safely and effectively according to extent of trunk involvement, excess skin and subcutaneous tissue, lipodystrophy, and abdominal wall laxity. All abdominoplasties should be complemented with liposuction in different degrees.

2. Types of abdominoplasties and indications

After a thorough examination of the abdomen and trunk, patients seeking correction of abdominal contour deformities can be stratified into four treatment groups with the following inclusion criteria and treatment modality (Figure 1):

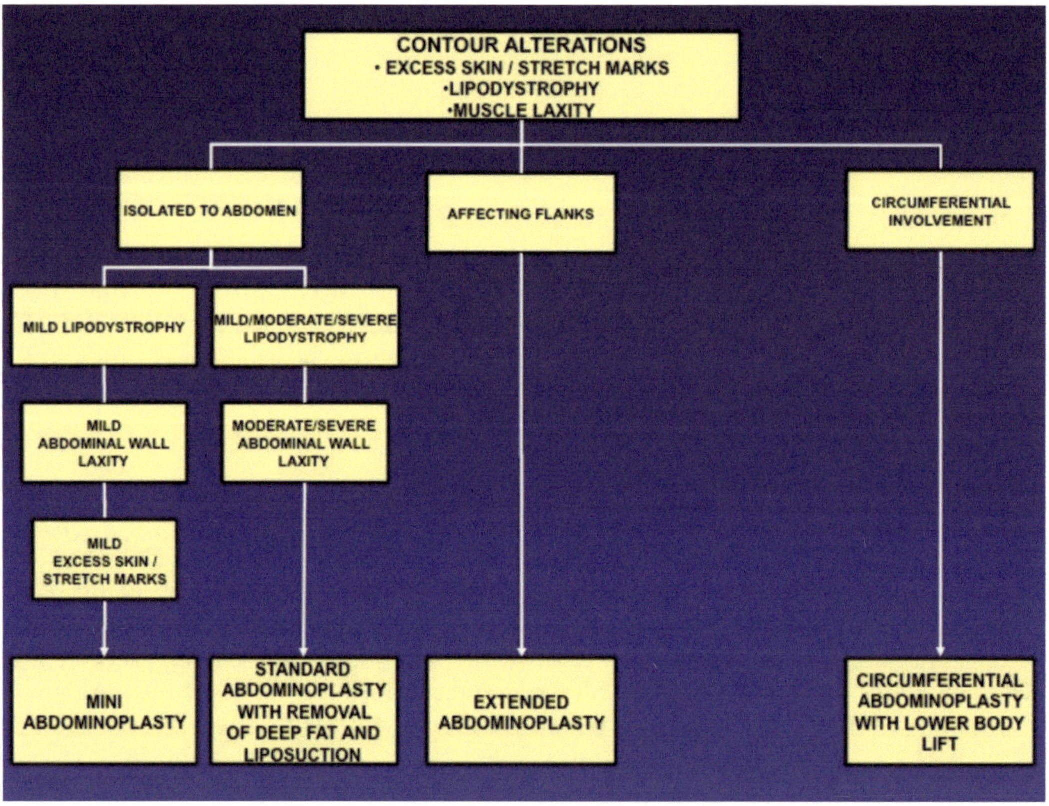

Fig. 1. Algorythm for selecting best abdominoplasty procedure for a patient based on degree of excess skin, lipodystrophy, muscle laxity, and location.

1. **Mini abdominoplasty.** Indicated in patients with mild excess skin and minimal stretch marks, mild lipodystrophy, and mild abdominal wall weakness. The procedure consists of liposuction of the abdomen and flanks in combination with a vertical plication of the rectus fascia from xiphoid to pubis and fusiform plication of the oblique fascias. (Sozer & Agullo, 2006) An M-shaped skin excision is utilized and the abdominoplasty is performed with the aid of a lighted retractor (Figure 2). Plication is performed with absorbable sutures. The procedure is achieved without increasing the standard miniabdominoplasty incision size, and with limited undermining with the aide of a lighted retractor. Unlike the long incision of the traditional abdominoplasty, this incision is short and skin excision is limited. The M-shaped cutaneous incision keeps the distance between the pubis and umbilicus long while putting tension on the sides, and the lateral to medial vector in closure also helps address the waistline. (Ramirez, 2000) We have observed that patients that are candidates for a miniabdominoplasty will invariably obtain a better result if they undergo a traditional abdominoplasty. This is a patient's decision, since there is a tradeoff between incision length and end result.
2. **Standard abdominoplasty.** Included in this treatment group are patients with mild lipodystrophy of the upper abdomen with moderate to severe excess skin and stretch marks and any degree of abdominal wall weakness. The technique follows typical methodology with wide undermining and vertical plication of the rectus fascia from

xiphoid to pubis and fusiform plication of the oblique fascias to enhance the waistline. (Nahas, 2001; Santos, 1998) Deep liposuction of the abdomen below Scarpa's fascia is performed. Liposuction of the flanks is also routinely performed to complement the results. After the abdominoplasty flap is elevated up to the costal margin, the deep fat to Scarpa's fascia is directly excised.

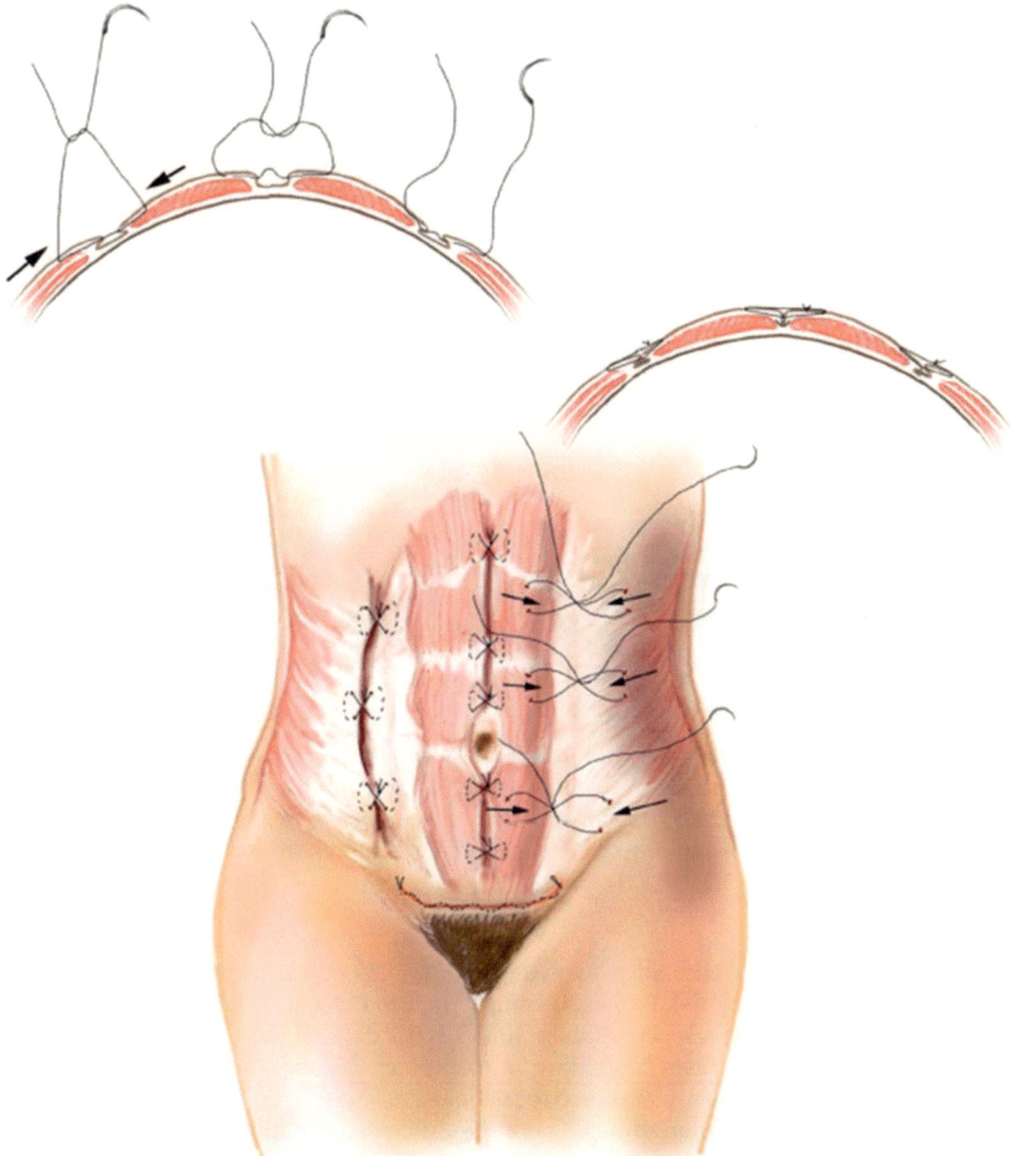

Fig. 2. Miniabdominoplasty with triple plication. A lighted retractor is used to undermine the abdominal midline up to the xiphoid. The midline fascia is plicated from xiphoid to pubis, limited lateral undermining is achieved and bilateral fusiform plications of the oblique fascia made.

3. **Extended Abdominoplasty.** Indicated in any of the patients seeking correction of the abdominal contour deformity which have involvement of excess skin and subcutaneous tissue in the flanks. Also termed a flankplasty.
4. **Circumferential abdominoplasty.** Indicated in patients with moderate to severe excess skin with circumferential involvement of abdomen, thighs, lower back, and buttocks. All degrees of lipodystrophy and abdominal wall laxity are included. Traditional circumferential abdominoplasty with lower body lift is performed.(Lockwood, 1993; Pascal, 2002) Liposuction of the flanks and thighs is standard in most patients. Complementary buttock augmentation with a local dermal fat flap can be performed.(Sozer & Agullo, 2005) This procedure is no longer reserved for the postbariatric patient,(Aly, 2004; Modolin 2003) as patients who are overweight or moderately obese can attain great results.(Morales, 2003)

It is important to note that these recommendations should serve as a guide, as our algorythm itself has changed from our original description in 2007.(Sozer & Agullo, 2007) It is also important to consider the patient's wishes and expectations. Although a patient may have the best results with a circumferential lift, they may only consider abdominoplasty due to scar length, recovery time, or economic considerations.

3. Contraindications

Contraindications for abdominoplasty with liposuction include patients with:

- cardiopulmonary disease
- bowel or bladder dysfunction
- diabetes
- wound-healing problems
- immunodeficiency
- smokers
- morbid obesity

Nicotine use is a significant comorbidity. We insist that our patients achieve complete smoking cessation for at least six weeks preoperatively and six weeks postoperatively. Patients who wish to become pregnant in the future pose a relative contraindication, as much of the results obtained with muscle plication and skin resection will be lost.

4. Precautions

A full physical exam is necessary to evaluate the patient in order to select the ideal procedure and identify any risk factors. It is important to obtain a full history and review of systems and identify the presence of abdominal hernia defects. Most patients benefit from from full laboratory analyses including a complete blood count, electrolyte panel, coagulation studies, chest x-ray and electrocardiogram. These tests are ordered depending on the patient's age and co-morbidities. There should be no hesitation in obtaining clearance by the patient's physician or cardiologist if necessary. Patients are thoroughly educated as to the extent of the procedures, risks, complications, alternatives, and team approach. Photographs are obtained prior to surgery in the standard and appropriate views.

Deep venous thrombosis (DVT) is one of the most feared complications due to its relation to pulmonary embolism (PE) and its fatal consequences. A thorough preoperative evaluation to identify risk factors of thrombosis and the use of preventive measures (stockings, pneumatic intermittent compression systems, etc) together with early mobilization, appropriate hydration and anticoagulation when indicated are sufficient to prevent venous thrombosis in healthy individuals. During the immediate postoperative period (first 24 hours) is imperative to carry out early mobilization (6-8 hours after surgery) as well as the use of compressive garments. Lymphatic drainage and massage could be considered as adjuvant therapies as well. The symptoms of pulmonary embolism include sharp hest pain, shortness of breath, chest pain that worsens with deep breathing or coughing, coughing up blood, tachycardia, sweating and anxiety. Although controversial, we treat all high risk patients with fractionated heparin preoperatively and continue the treatment for five days.

In our practice, ninety percent of the procedures are performed in a fully accredited and certified surgical center; exceptions include patients undergoing concurrent gynecological procedures, large circumferential tissue excisions after weight loss, anticipated greater than 23 hour stay, and anemia with possibility of need for transfusion. All cases are done under general anesthesia by an anesthesiologist.

During surgery, warm tumescent solution, IV fluid warmer, and bear hugger are used for temperature control. Most patients undergoing extended or circumferential abdominoplasties have an overnight stay in the surgical center or hospital respectively. Sequential compression devices are used for deep venous thrombosis prophylaxis during and after the procedure until the patient begins ambulation. Patients are continuously monitored during their stay, and intra and post-operative prophylactic antibiotics are used. An indweling bladder catheter is used to decompress the bladder and facilitate abdominal muscle plication.

5. Surgical technique

All of the different types of abdominoplasty procedures are begun in the same fashion. The patient is first marked in standing position in the preoperative holding area. The abdominoplasty incision is marked low, extending from the midline, approximately 7 cm above the mons cleft and extending laterally towards the flanks. The length of the incison is determined by the type of procedure selected from the algorythm discussed above. For circumferential and extended abdominoplasties, a line is drawn to meet in a V shape at the sacrum at the level of the beginning of the gluteal cleft. The patient is then taken to the operating room, undergoes general endotracheal anesthesia with a paralytic, and is placed in the prone position with gel rolls.

Standard tumescent suction assisted liposuction (SAL) is employed in the flanks and back. Liposuction is performed from multiple port sites and at both the deep and superficial level. Ultrasonic or laser assisted liposuction are helpful when the areas of the back are treated as this fat tends to be more dense. It is also a useful adjunct when the patient has had previous liposuction procedures.

At this point, if a circumferential lift is to be performed, the excisions can be carried out in the traditional manner. We often combine the circumferential lift with an autologous myocutaneous flap in order to achieve buttock fullness.(Sozer & Agullo, 2005) If an extended abdominoplasty is to be carried out, then the excess skin and subcutaneous tissue in the flanks is excised and the defect closed in layered fashion.

The patient in then turned to the supine position. Again, SAL after tumescense is carried out in the flanks at the superficial and deep levels in a 1 to 1 ratio. Thorough liposuction of the abdomen is the carried out after tumescense at the deep level below Scarpa's fascia.

Although there may be controversy in combining thorough liposuction of the abdomen with abdominoplasty, the anatomy supports the safety of the procedure. Once an abdominoplasty is performed, the blood supply to the skin and fat of the abdominal fat shifts from the perforating vessels coursing through the rectus abdominis muscle to the perforating branches of the lateral intercostal arteries. Through the intercostal perforators, the blood supply to the abdomen begins superficially and laterally, and it is terminally perfused centrally and deeply. This is the reason why the fat deep to Scarpa's fascia can be resected or liposuctioned. (Matarasso, 2000; Hunstad, 2011)

After liposuction the abdominoplasty is carried out in the standard surgical fashion. The inferior abdominal incision is made and carried down to the abdominal fascia. The abdominal skin and subcutaneous tissue flap is then raised to the xyphoid and up to but not above the costal margin in order to preserve the intercostal perforators. The umbilicus is left attached to the abdominal wall. Triple plication of the abdominal fascia is carried out (Figure 2). The patient is flexed at the hips and the excess abdominal flap tissue is excised. The fat that remains deep to Scarpa's fascia is then sharply excised. This step is often simplified by the prior liposuction and a plane is often present between Scarpa's fascia and the deep fat. The patient is flexed at the waist and the excess skin and subcutaneous tissue is excised from the abdominal flap. An opening is created in the abdominal flap at the level of the umbilicus. One to two drains are placed and the abdomen is closed in a layered fashion.

6. Postoperative care

Patients ussually return to normal activity within two to three weeks after surgery. During this time mobilization is of upmost importance. Immediately after surgery, a compressive garment is used and kept for four weeks. Patients are encouraged to use knee high compression stockings to decrease edema. Patients are allowed to rest in bed in the most comfortable position for them, usually supine. Ambulation is started the same day or the next morning depending on concurrent procedures. Sitting is not restricted.

Patients are encouraged to straighten up within 4-5 days postoperatively. Drains are left in place until the output is less than 30 mL in 24 hours. This typically takes between 7 and 10 days. External sutures are typically removed after 7 days.

7. Results

In our initial prospective study 151 female patients were treated for abdominal contour and musculoaponeurotic deformities from January 2004 to July 2005 after one year follow up.[16] We found a significant difference in mean BMI between pre and post-abdominoplasty ($p=0.01$), 26 kg/m^2 and 24 kg/m^2 respectively. According to BMI classification, there was a significant difference in the prevalence of overweight and obesity between the pre and post-abdominoplasty procedure (Table 2). The prevalence of overweight and obesity decreased by 8% and 9%, respectively ($p=0.01$). Furthermore, a significant decrease of mean BMI was observed among all types of abdominoplasty ($p=0.01$). The estimated mean weight of tissue excised was 2.6 kg, with a significant correlation between the amount of specimen excised and decrease in BMI post-abdominoplasty ($p < 0.01$). The same results were found when liposuction volume was analyzed (Table 1).

The prevalence of complications after abdominoplasty was 11%, comparable to those previously described.[25-27]. The most common complication was the formation of wound seroma (4%) and delayed wound healing (4%). Four patients (3%) had partial dehiscence of the wound treated with a wound vacuum device. The mean BMI between those women with complications and those without complications was 27.3 kg/m^2 and 26.3 kg/m^2 respectively. A stratified analysis was performed to evaluate an association between BMI classification and the prevalence of complications. Although there was a trend in complications with higher BMI, no statistically significant difference was found between the number of women who had complications and BMI classification ($p= 0.74$). In all cases, the revisions and treatment of the complications resulted in patient acceptance and satisfaction.

Half of all the patients had additional cosmetic procedures (n=73), including breast augmentation (29%), mastopexy (25%), brachioplasty (3%), blepharoplasty (2%), brow lift (2%), fat injections (10%), neck lift (2%), and medial thigh lift (1%). Liposuction was not included as an additional procedure, and circumferential abdominoplasties with lower body lifts were counted as single procedures. In addition, 8% of the patients underwent abdominal hysterectomies at the same time as the abdominoplasty (n=12). The relationship between complications in patients that underwent additional procedures (10%) and those that did not (13%) was not significant ($p=0.5$).

	Pre-abdominoplasty	**Post-abdominoplasty**	***P*-value**
Weight (kg), mean ± SD	71 ± 14	66 ± 14	0.01
BMI (kg/m^2), mean ± SD	26 ± 5	24 ± 4	0.01
WHO BMI (kg/m^2) classification (%)			< 0.05
< 20 (underweight)	2	9	
20-24.9 (normal)	42	54	
25-29.9 (overweight)	37	29	
≥ 30 (obese)	19	8	
Specimen excised (kg)		2.6	0.01*
Liposuction volume (mL)		1998	0.01*

* $p < 0.01$ after linear regression analysis between specimen excised, liposuction volume removed, and BMI after abdominoplasty.

Table 1. Weight and BMI results pre and post-abdominoplasty.

Although, not published yet, our experience with the combination of liposuction and abdominoplasty remains similar to that of our previous study. There have been no incidents of flap necrosis. Hunstad recently published a similar technique without encoutering flap necrosis. (Hunstad, 2011)

Figures 4-8 show results with the different types of abdominoplasty combined with liposuction. I all cases there is an improvement in the abdominal contour, decrease in excess skin and subcutaneous tissue, decrease in amount of stretch marks, improvement in the abdominal wall, and refinement of the waistline.

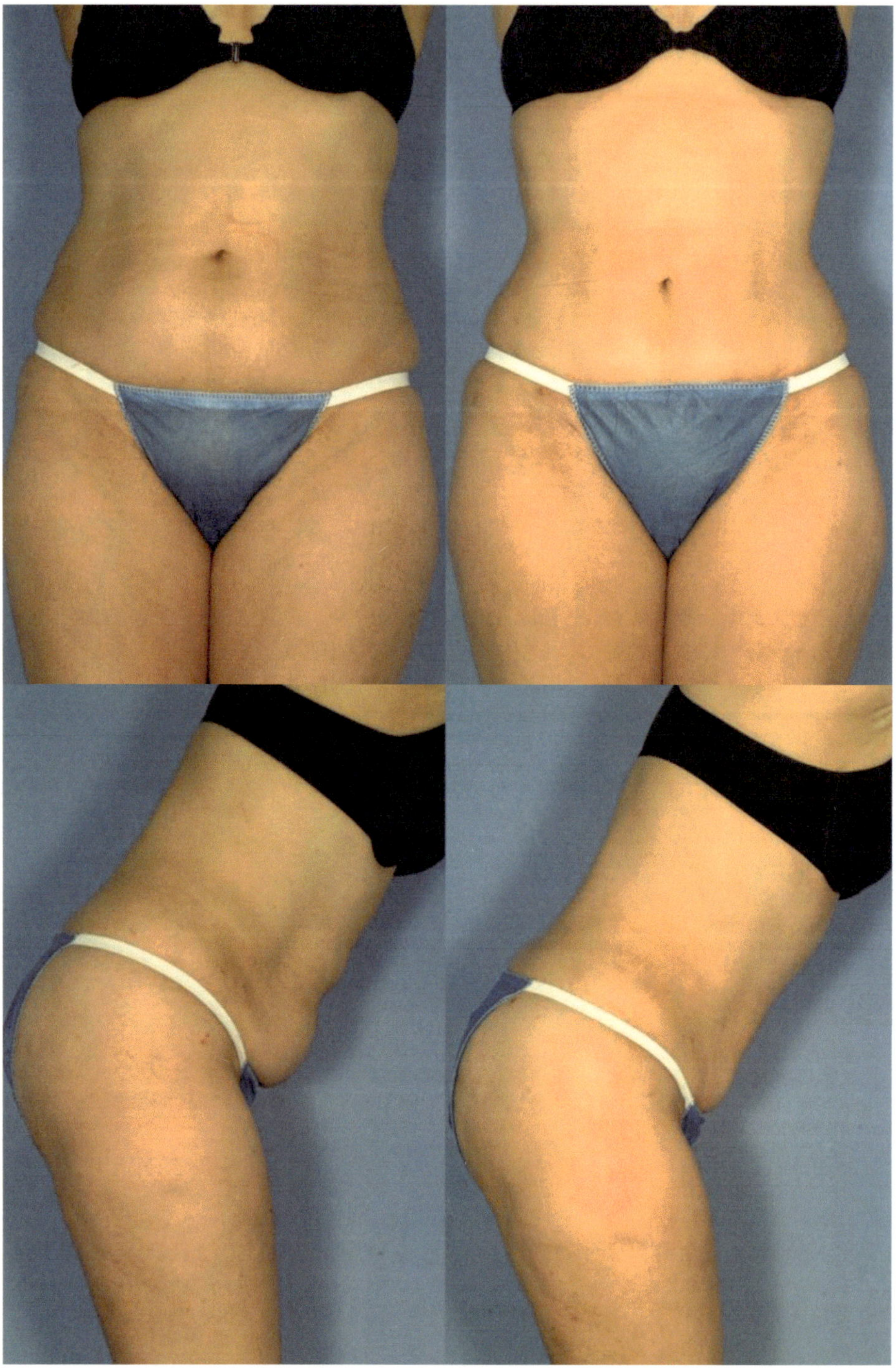

Fig. 4. Patients with mild excess skin and minimal stretch marks, mild lipodystrophy, and mild abdominal wall weakness. A and C are before, and B and D are 8 months after liposuction and triple plication miniabdominoplasty.

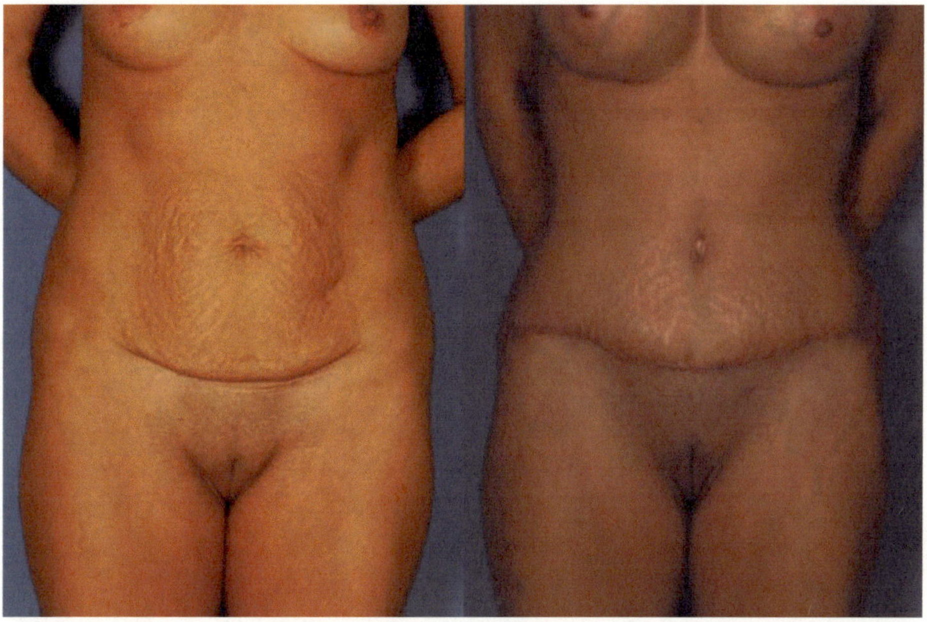

Fig. 5. Patient with excess skin, mild abdominal wall laxity, and marked striae. 8 weeks after abdominoplasty tith tripple plication of the fascia and liposuction of the abdomen and flanks.

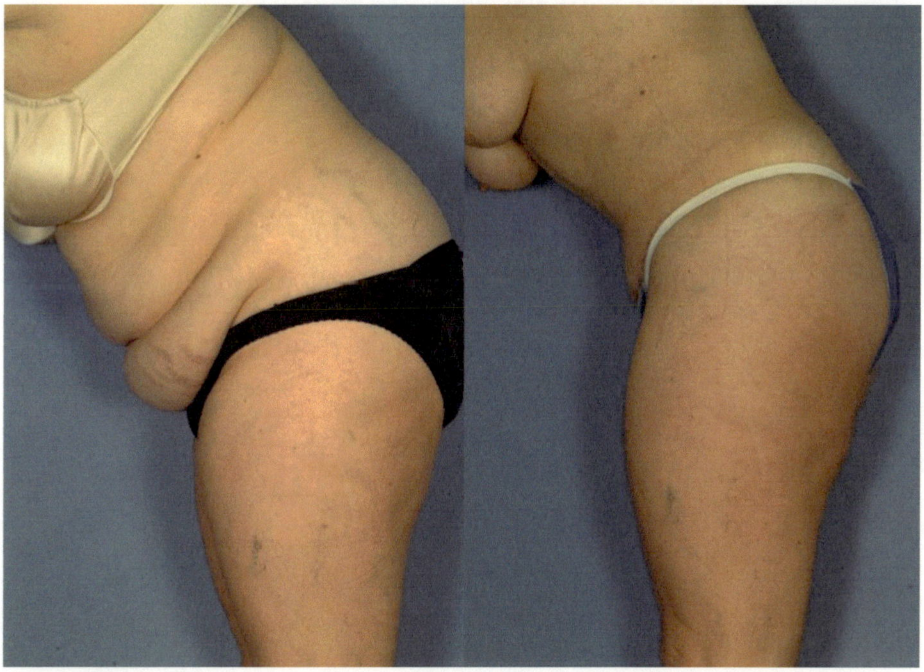

Fig. 6. Patients with mild excessive skin and stretch marks with moderate to severe lipodystrophy and mild abdominal wall laxity. 8 months after abdominoplasty with thorough liposuction of the abdomen.

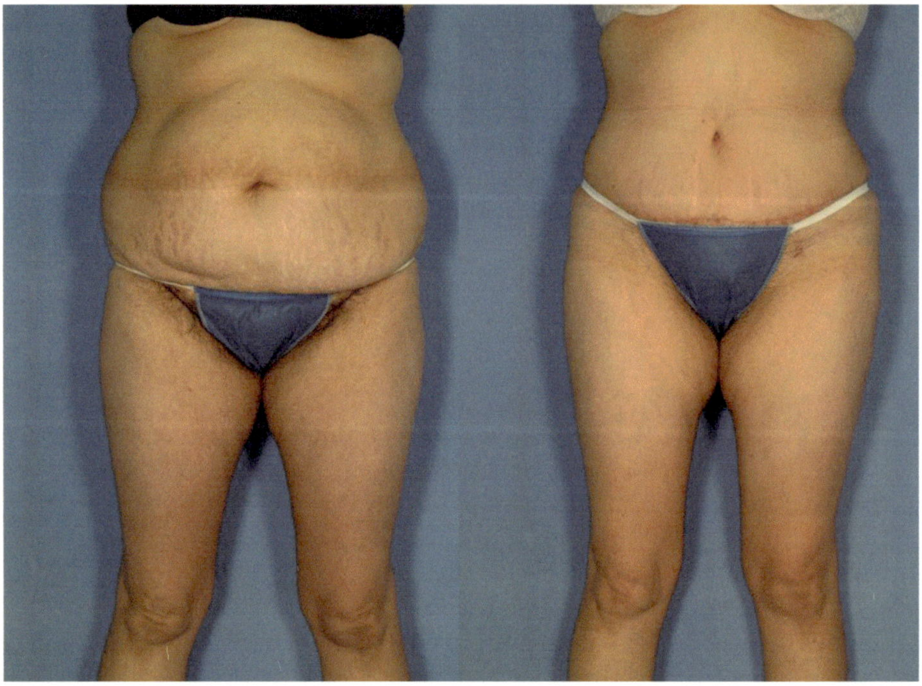

Fig. 7. Patients with moderate excessive skin and stretch marks with moderate to severe lipodystrophy and moderate to severe abdominal wall laxity. 8 months after abdominoplasty with thorough liposuction of the abdomen with removal of deep fat.

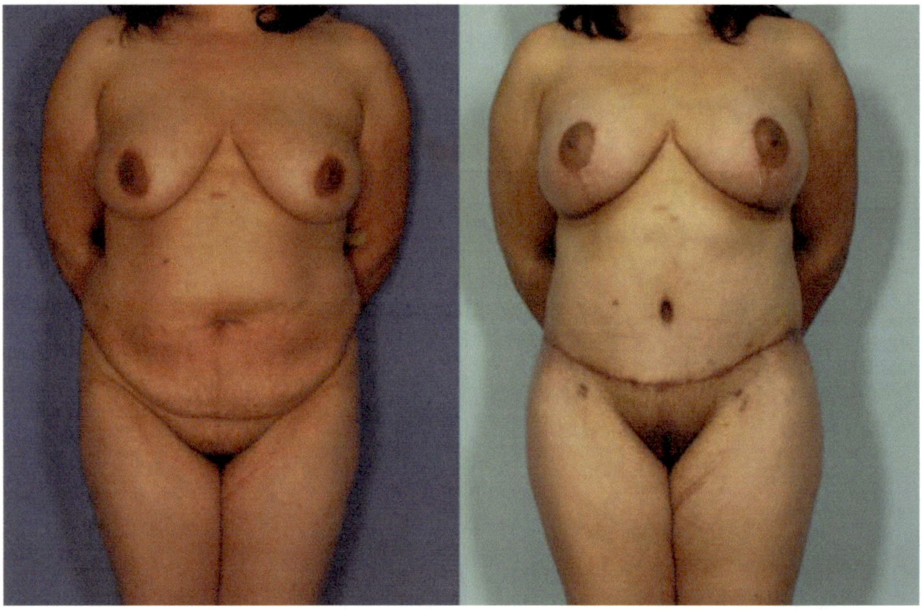

Fig. 8. Patient with excess skin and subcutaneous fat of the abdomen as well as flanks. Moderate abdominal laxity with minimal stretch marks. 8 months after extended abdominoplasty with liposuction of the abdomen and flanks.

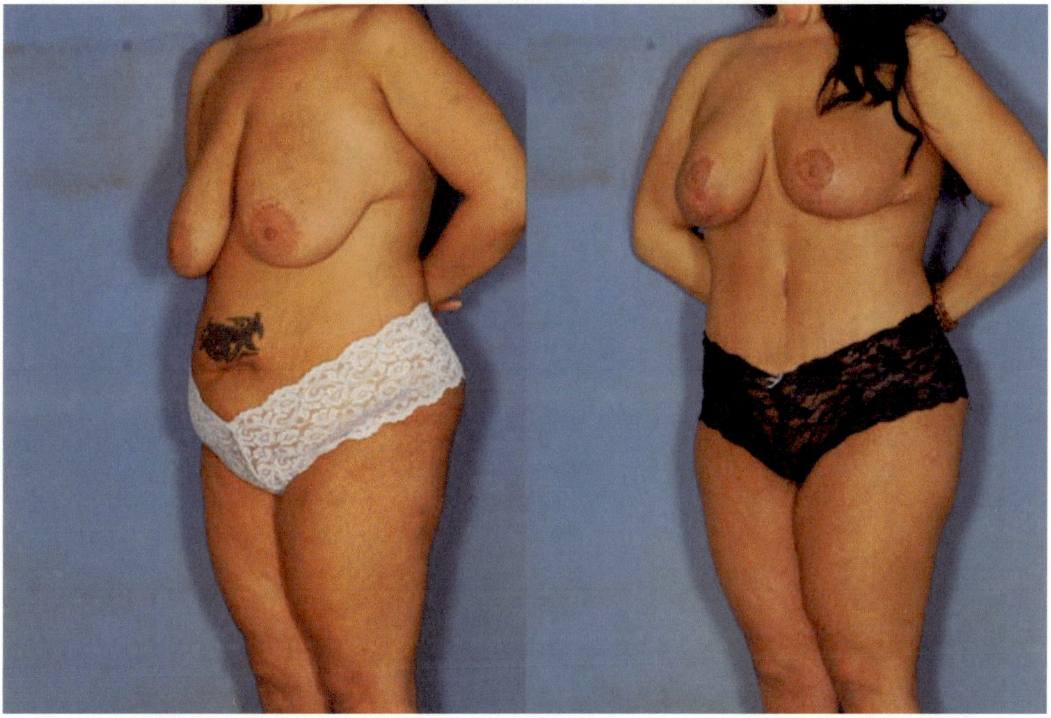

Fig. 9. Patient with excess skin and subcutaneous fat of the abdomen as well as flanks. Marked abdominal laxity and stretch marks. 8 months after extended abdominoplasty with liposuction of the abdomen and flanks.

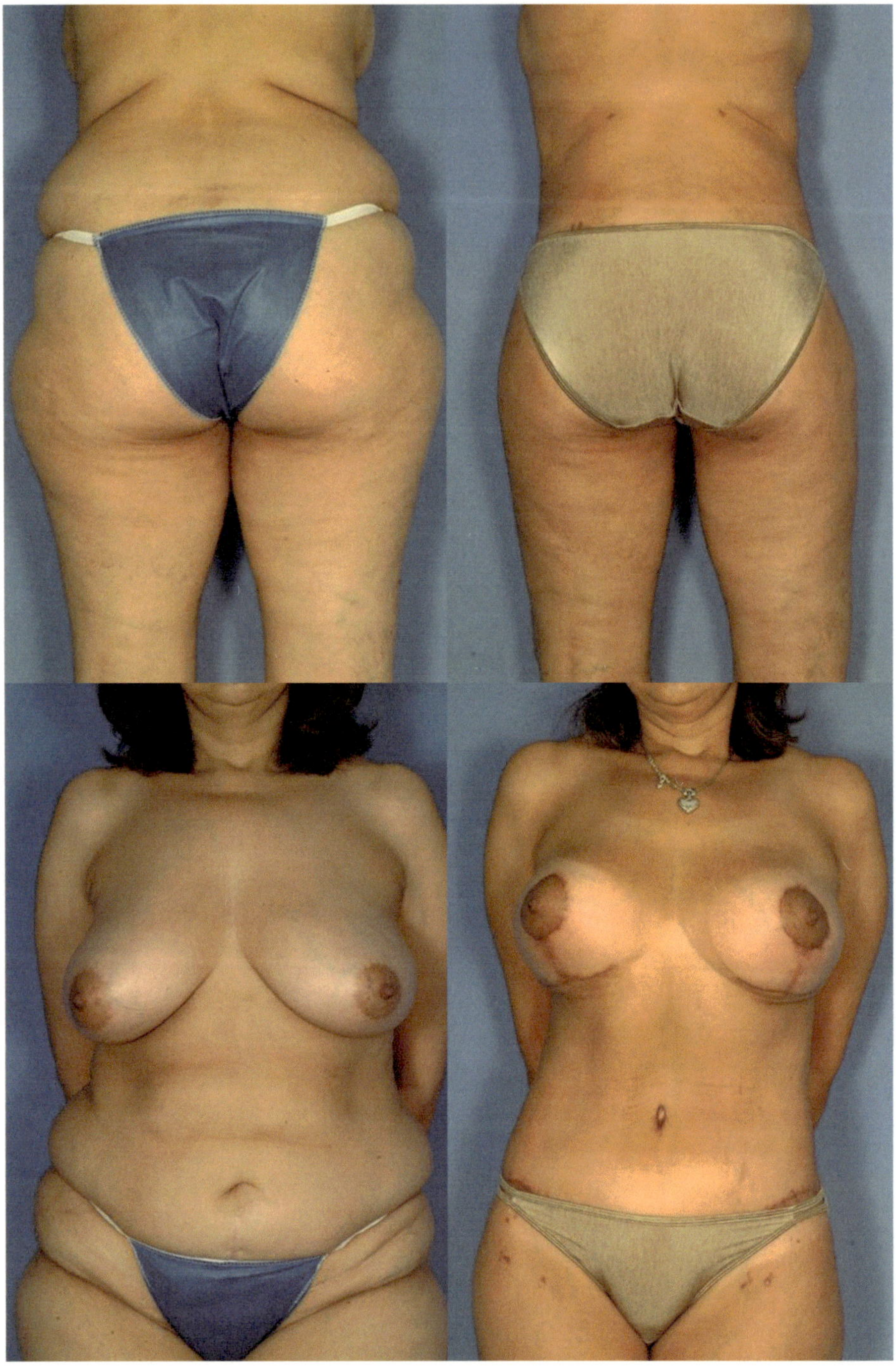

Fig. 10. Patient with moderate excessive skin with circumferential involvement of abdomen, thighs, lower back, and buttocks, and severe lipodystrophy. 8 months after a circumferential abdominoplasty with liposuction and lower body lift with autoprosthesis buttock augmentation with a dermal fat flap.

8. Conclusion

Multiple modifications for performing abdominoplasty have been described. Like any surgical procedure, careful patient selection and procedure selection optimizes the final outcome. We provide an effective and flexible algorithm for selection of the ideal abdominoplasty procedure according to grade of excess skin and stretch marks, lipodystrophy, and musculoaponeurotic looseness. Most important is the combination of abdominoplasty with thorough liposuction of the abdominal wall and flanks. The guidelines provide significant improved tension of the whole abdominal wall, enhancement of the waistline, and improvement in the uniformity of the contour of the abdomen. The final decision is always determined by the surgeon's judgment and the patient's individual preferences. Many patients are excellent candidates for an extended or circumferential abdominoplasty, but may not wish to undergo such an extensive procedure.

9. References

Avelar, M. J. Abdominoplasty without panniculus undermining and resection: Analysis and 3-year follow-up of 97 consecutive cases. *Aesth. Surg.* 22: 16, 2000.

Avelar, J. M. Abdominoplasty combined with lipoplasty without panniculus undermining: Abdominolipoplasty - a safe technique. Clin. Plast. Surg. 33: 79, 2006.

Aly, A., Cram, A., Chao, M., et al. Belt lipectomy for circumferential truncal excess: The University of Iowa experience. *Plast. Reconstr. Surg.* 111: 398, 2003.

Aly, A., Cram, A., and Heddens, C. Truncal body contouring surgery in the massive weight loss patient. Clin. Plast. Surg. 31: 611, 2004.

Bozola, A. R., and Psillakis, J. M. Abdominoplasty: A new concept and classification treatment. *Plast. Reconstr. Surg.* 82: 983, 1988.

Byrd, H. S., Barton, F. E., and Orenstein, H. H, et al. Safety and efficacy in an accredited outpatient plastic surgery facility: A review of 5316 consecutive cases. *Plast. Reconstr. Surg.* 112: 636, 2003.

Cardenas-Camarena, L. Various surgical techniques for improving body contour. *Aesth. Plast. Surg.* 29: 446, 2006.

Hunstad, J.P., Jones, S.R. Abdominoplasty with thorough concurrent circumferential abdominal tumescent liposuction. *Aesth. Plast. Surg.* 31: 572, 2011.

Lockwood, T. Lower body lift with superficial fascial system suspension. *Plast. Reconstr. Surg.* 92: 1112, 1993.

Mast, B. A. Safety and efficacy of outpatient full abdominoplasty. *Ann. Plast. Surg.* 54: 256, 2005.

Matarasso, A. Abdominolipoplasty: A system of classification and treatment for combined abdominoplasty and suction-assisted lipectomy. *Aesth. Plast. Surg.* 15: 111, 1991.

Matarasso, A. Liposuction as an adjunct to a full abdominoplasty revisited. *Plast. Reconstr. Surg.* 106: 1197, 2000.

Matarasso, A. Minimal-access variations in abdominoplasty. *Ann. Plast. Surg.* 34: 255, 1995.

Modolin, M., Cintra, W., Gobbi, C., et al. Circumferential abdominoplasty for sequential treatment after morbid obesity. *Obes. Surg.* 13: 95, 2003.

Morales, G. H. Circular lipectomy with lateral thigh-buttock lift. *Aesth. Plast. Surg.* 27: 50, 2003.

Nahas, F. X. A pragmatic way to treat abdominal deformities based on skin and subcutaneous excess. *Aesth. Plast. Surg.*. 25: 365, 2001.

Nahas, F. X. An aesthetic classification of the abdomen based on the myoaponeurotic layer. Plast. Reconstr. Surg. 108: 1787, 2001.

Pascal, J. F., and Le Louarn, C. Remodeling bodylift with high lateral tension. *Aesth. Plast. Surg.* 26: 223, 2002.

Pitanguy, I. Evaluation of body contouring surgery today: A 30-year perspective. *Plast. Reconstr. Surg.* 105: 1499, 2000.

Ramirez, O. Abdominoplasty and abdominal wall rehabilitation: A comprehensive approach. *Plast. Reconstr. Surg.* 105: 425, 2000.

Santos, E., and Muraira, J. The waist and abdominoplasty. *Aesth. Plast. Surg.* 22: 225, 1998.

Sozer, S. O., Agullo, F. J., Wolf, C. Autoprosthesis buttock augmentation during lower body lift. *Aesth. Plast. Surg.* 29: 133, 2005.

Sozer, S. O., and Agullo, F. J. Triple plication in miniabdominoplasty. *Aesth. Plast. Surg.* 30: 263, 2006.

Sozer, S.O., Agullo, F.J., Santillan, A.A., Wolf, C. Decision making in abdominoplasty. *Aesth. Plast. Surg.* 31: 117, 2007.

Toledo, L. S. The overlap of lipoplasty and abdominoplasty: indication, classification, and treatment. *Clin. Plast. Surg.* 31: 539, 2004.

Vastine, V. L., Morgan, R. F., Williams, G. S., et al. Wound complications of abdominoplasty in obese patients. *Ann. Plast. Surg.* 42: 34, 1999.

Walgenbach, K. J., and Shestak K. C. "Marriage" abdominoplasty: Body contouring with limited scars combining mini-abdominoplasty and liposuction. *Clin. Plast. Surg.* 31: 571, 2004.

9

Gynecomastia and Liposuction

Francisco J. Agullo[1,2], Sadri O. Sozer[1,2] and Humberto Palladino[1,2]
[1]*Texas Tech University Health Sciences Center, El Paso, TX*
[2]*El Paso Cosmetic Surgery Center, El Paso, TX*
USA

1. Introduction

Gynecomastia is derived from the Greek terms gynec (feminine) and mastos (breast). The literal translation, male breasts, relates to any condition that results in excessive development of breast tissue in males.

Galen introduced the term gynecomastia in the second century AD. He defined gynecomastia as an unnatural increase in the breast fat of males. The first recorded description of a reduction mammaplasty was by Paulas of Aegina in the seventh century AD, who referred to the condition as an "effeminacy of men."

Gynecomastia is responsible for a significant amount of emotional and psychological trauma especially in the young population. The treatment of gynecomastia has continued to evolve over the ages and today needs to be designed specifically to address the amount of skin excess, glandular breast tissue, adipose tissue, degree of breast ptosis, and the size of the nipple areolar complex (NAC). Each component should be considered separately to optimize the outcome.

2. Incidence

The increase in breast size due to the accumulation of fatty tissue, as seen in obese patients, is considered pseudogynecomastia. True gynecomastia may or may not be associated with pathologic conditions as this can be the result of the usual physiologic development. Prevalence of asymptomatic gynecomastia is 60%–90% in neonates, 50%–60% in adolescents, and up to 70% in men age 50–69 years. [1-3] Trimodal distribution for asymptomatic gynecomastia is noted (neonatal, pubertal, and in elderly males). Prevalence of symptomatic gynecomastia is markedly lower.

Physiologic gynecomastia is common in adolescents at the time of puberty with published incidence rates of 25 to 65% by the ages of 14. [4] By the time pubertal changes are completed and hormonal levels stabilized the persistence of gynecomastia is uncommon. Different series report between 30% and 50% incidence although in adolescent populations the incidence of bilateral gynecomastia could be even higher.[5]

Previous studies have reported that in an average out-patient clinic you may see 10 to 20 new cases of gynecomastia per year, accounting for up to 80% of all male breast referrals. [2,

3, 6, 7] In a recent study the referrals for specialist evaluation for gynecomastia have increased 500% since 1990's making this pathology more prevalent.[8]

3. Pathophysiology

The hormonal role of estrogen/testosterone ratio has been identified as a cause of gynecomastia although many other reasons were identified as possible causes of gynecomastia (Table 1). Is important to rule out any other pathologic process related to gynecomastia, in particular testicular sources. A thorough interrogation should be performed including family history as well as relevant medications, recreational drugs, etc.

Physiologic	**Androgen deficiency**	**Drugs**
Neonatal	Hypogonadism	Alcohol
Puberty	Primary	Amphetamines
Advance age	Klinefelter's syndrome	Chemotherapeutic agents
Familial	Kallman's syndrome	Cimetidine
	Congenital anorchia	Digitalis
	ACTH deficiency	Haldol
Systemic Conditions / idiopathic	Defects in androgen systhesis	Hydroxyzine
	Secondary	Isoniazid
Obesity	Trauma	Methyldopa
Hyperthyroidism	Orchitis	Marijuana
Hypothyroidism	Cryptorchidism	Opiates
Chronic illness	Irradiation	Phenothiazines
AIDS	Hydrocele	Progestins
	Spermatocele	Reserpine
	Varicocele	Spironolactone
Neoplastic	Renal failure	Tricyclinc antidepressants
Breast carcinoma	Exogenous Androgens	
Liver carcinoma		
Lung carcinoma	Estrogen excess	
Adrenal tumors	Testucular soruces	
	Germ cell tumors	
	Choriocarcinoma	
Infectious	Seminoma	
	Teratoma	
Sparganum or plerocercoid larva of the tapeworm	Non-germ cell tumors	
	Leydig cell tumor	
	Granulaosa-theca tumor	
	Sertoli cell tumor	
	True Hermaphroditism	
	Liver disease	
	Exogenous estrogen	
	Malnutrition	

Table 1. Causes of Gynecomastia

Symmetrical and bilateral breast enlargement is usually the result of both glandular and adipose tissue enlargement. In those cases where a unilateral or asymmetrical involvement is noted a thorough diagnostic investigation should be done to rule out breast carcinoma, where a breast biopsy is indicated.

4. Indications and contraindications

Considering that gynecomastia is a cause of emotional and psychological distress is important to clearly identify the main concern for the patient in the context of development. Many times is just a matter of aesthetic concern but other circumstances such as pain, tenderness, and even the possibility of cancer should be considered. Reassurance and guidance play an important role in the adolescent population during puberty. Watchful waiting during these years is an accepted practice.

All patients undergoing gynecomastia should be optimized to avoid complications. NSAID's should be stopped one week prior to the procedures and resumed one week after the procedure if necessary. No patients on therapeutic anticoagulation should be treated for this condition. Smoking is relative contraindications but is our practice to require smoking cessation for at least two weeks prior to the procedure and four weeks after the procedure. Contraindications for gynecomastia include patients with:

- cardiopulmonary disease
- renal failure
- therapeutic anticoagulation
- wound-healing problems
- immunodeficiency
- active smokers
- morbid obesity

5. Patient evaluation and selection

A complete evaluation is necessary to identify the cause of the pathology, optimize the timing for surgery, rule out neoplastic origin, and avoid unnecessary interventions.

Physical examination should include bilateral breast exams as well as neck and axillary bimanual palpation to rule out any masses or adenopathies. A bilateral testicular examination should be included.

Any palpable mass, especially in asymmetric enlargement should undergo biopsy to rule out malignancy.

Laboratory evaluation should follow physical findings and patients should be appropriately referred to an endocrinologist as needed.

6. Medical management

Neonatal and puberal gynecomastia are usually self limiting and often do not require any type of treatment. Less than 10% of adolescent will experience persistent breast enlargement that will require some kind of intervention. On the other hand, gynecomastia of advanced age does not resolve spontaneously and often requires treatment. Several drugs have been used in the treatment of gynecomastia for different reasons. Clomiphene, an antiestrogen has been utilized and reported since 1970's by multiple authors [9-11]. The androgen Danazole has also been used with success [12-14]. Testosterone supplementation for cases of testosterone deficiency has been used. Most recently Tamoxifen has been used with some success[15-17]. Even radiation has been reported in the past.

Medical treatment of gynecomastia is usually applied during the first stages of the disease as a palliative method to control symptoms such as pain and tenderness while surgical management is usually the method of choice to address the aesthetic concern.

7. Surgical management

The surgical management of gynecomastia has evolved considerably over the last 60 years. Since the first descriptions by Webster in 1946 [18], the subsequent classifications by Simon in 1973[19], and the introduction of liposuctions for gynecomastia in 1983 [20] a broad spectrum of alternatives developed to address the multiple degrees of this condition. The subsequent advances in technologies and minimally invasive techniques allowed for a more refined approach to the condition. Based on this Dr. Rohrich expanded the classification and management alternatives in 2003. [21]

7.1 Considerations

There are certain characteristics that need to be addressed when planning a surgical approach to gynecomastia. These characteristics are:

- Amount of skin excess and skin quality
- Adipose component
- Glandular component
- Size of nipple areolar complex

Amount of skin excess and skin quality

The skin envelope plays a significant role in determining which will be the preferred approach. As outlined in Table-2 and Table-3, Dr. Rohrich modification of the original Simon classification serves as a guide for treatment. In cases with minimal skin excess and good skin quality a minimally invasive approach should suffice. This includes liposuction and perhaps limited skin incisions such as periareolar, intra-areolar, transaxilary, and edoscopic for excision of breast tissue. When the skin envelope is enlarged and/or stretched such as in postbariatric population, or in moderate to severe cases of gynecomastia, a larger excision should be planned.

The position of the nipple areolar complex (NAC) is also an important factor and will determine if a minimally invasive approach will be sufficient, or a mastopexy, and even a free nipple graft, will be required.

The different methods to address a significant skin excess and ptosis include crescentic excision, periareolar mastopexy, vertical mastopexy, Wise pattern mastopexy and inframammary fold scar. Crescentic mastopexy will allow for minimal mobilization up to 1 cm of the NAC in a cephalad direction. At the same time allows for access for direct excision of the breast tissue. This method is reserved for cases with mild to moderate ptosis and good skin quality. Periareolar mastopexy can be utilized also when a mild amount of excess skin is to be excised allowing for better access to excision of breast tissue. Vertical mastopexy can address cases of moderate ptosis allowing a comfortable access for removal of breast tissue. This method could be used for moderate to severe cases where skin excision and NAC repositioning form 1 to 5 cm is required. Wise pattern mastopexy is usually reserved for cases where a significant amount of excess tissue is to be removed. This approach also allows for an open access for removal of breast tissue and at the same time allows for easy repositioning of the NAC. The scars resulting from this procedure are usually the limiting factor as patients prefer a less invasive approach. The inframammary fold scar allows a large resection of excess tissue with a transverse scar along the inframammary fold but often requires free nipple graft for transposition of the NAC.

Adipose component

The amount of adipose tissue plays an important role on the method required to address the gynecomastia. The main line of treatment for adipose tissue is suction assisted liposuction (SAL). Some patients may present with dense fibrous septi within the adipose tissue. In these cases ultrasound assisted liposuction (UAL) or power assisted liposuction (PAL) in combination with SAL delivers the best result. If the adipose component is the main cause of gynecomastia, liposuction alone or combined with a minimal access excision should be the preferred option.

Glandular component

If the glandular component of the breast is prevalent the fibrous architecture becomes the main concern. Liposuction techniques alone are often insufficient to completely address the issue and a direct excision of some kind is required. While SAL still play a significant role in addressing the adipose tissue and sculpting of the periphery, the central glandular component should be excised. Some authors advocate a minimally invasive approach either by performing minimal access incisions in the periphery of the NAC or using arthroscopic shavers as a mean to break down the fibrous capsule of the glandular component and retrieve it with conventional liposuction methods.[22] If skin excess is also a significant concern, direct excision becomes the method of choice as the access is granted by the larger skin incisions.

Size of the nipple areolar complex

In some cases the diameter of the NAC is too large and other times there is a significant asymmetry between the sizes of the NACs. In either of these circumstances a reduction of the NAC is required. A periareolar incision is performed and the excess tissue is removed reducing the diameter of the NAC. This procedure can also be performed in combinations with either of the mastopexy techniques described above.

Classification	Clinical Features	Treatment Options
Grade I	Breast fullness without ptosis	Excision plus liposuction
Grade II	Breast fullness with the nipple at the IMF	Excision, liposuction and nipple transposition
Grade III	Significant hypertrophy with the nipple below the IMF	Breast reduction with nipple transposition

Table 2. Classification of Gynecomastia

Classification	Clinical Features	Treatment Options
Grade I: Minimal hypertrophy, less than 250 g.	IA: Primarily fatty breast tissue IB: Primarily fibrous breast tissue	Suction assisted lipectomy (SAL) is highly successful Additional excision is often required
Grade II: Moderate hypertrophy, 250 to 500 g.	IIA: Primarily fatty breast tissue IIB: Primarily fibrous breast tissue with peripheral fat	SAL is highly effective Usually requires central excision with peripheral suction
Grade III: Severe hypertrophy, more than 500 g.	Severe hypertrophy with grade I ptosis	Requires resection with suction
Grade IV: Severe Hypertrophy with grade II or III ptosis	Severe hypertrophy with grade II or III ptosis	Requires resection with suction and possible nipple transposition.

Table 3. Rohrich Classification of Gynecomastia

7.2 Operative technique

Markings are made to outline the boundaries of treatment. The inframammary fold is also marked preoperatively with the patient standing. Further markings for NAC repositioning are performed with the patient in the upright position. All patients undergo general anesthesia and are positioned supine with the arms abducted. The entire chest wall and upper abdomen are included in the operative field. Appropriate antibiotic and deep venous thrombosis prophylaxis are used.

Liposuction

Suction assisted liposuction alone or in combination with UAL and PAL play an essential role in the treatment of pseudogynecomastia or those cases where mild gynecomastia is present with a predominant adipose component. Our preferred technique includes infiltration of the surgical area with superwet solution (1:1 ratio) with a solution containing 50 ml of 1% lidocaine, and one ampule of 1:1000 epinephrine in 1 liter of lactated Ringer's solution. A remote access at the anterior axilary line is used for a 3-4 mm liposuction canula.

Following the initial conventional SAL the UAL is used to address the areas of dense tissues. Ultrasound-assisted liposuction is first performed using the LySonix 3000 Ultrasonic Surgical Aspirator System (Byron Medical, Tucson, Ariz.). It is set on the pulse mode at amplitude of 90 percent. A plastic port is placed into the incision through which the ultrasound probe is passed. The endpoint for ultrasound application is loss of tissue resistance throughout the marked area (approximately 4 to 10 minutes per side). We do not perform PAL although it is a viable alternative. The skin flaps are thinned to a thickness of approximately 1.5 cm. Extra SAL is utilized if further refinements are necessary after UAL. Sequential pressure with a rolled gauze-sponge is applied at the end of the procedure to evacuate the excess of fluid through the access ports. The ports are sutured and a compression garment is applied.

Liposuction and endoscopic excision of breast tissue

Liposuction is usually performed as previously explained. The transaxilary approach is used for the excision of the breast tissue. Similarly to the approach for transaxilary breast augmentation, a tunnel is developed and the breast tissue including adipose and glandular tissue are excised under direct visualization using and endoscopic guidance. This technique is reserved for conditions where there is no need for repositioning of the NAC and good skin quality.

Liposuction with direct excision and repositioning of the nipple areola complex

Liposuction is performed as explained above and once completed the direct excision and NAC repositioning are undertaken following the preoperative markings. If no NAC repositioning is required a minimal access direct excision is performed through an inferior periareolar incision. The authors find that the morbidity of this approach is minimal and, at the same time, more efficient and cost effective than other minimally invasive techniques described. Case 1

Case 1

Grade II gynecomastia treated with periareolar approach with liposuction (SAL and UAL) followed by direct excision of breast tissue - Preop and 6 months follow up.

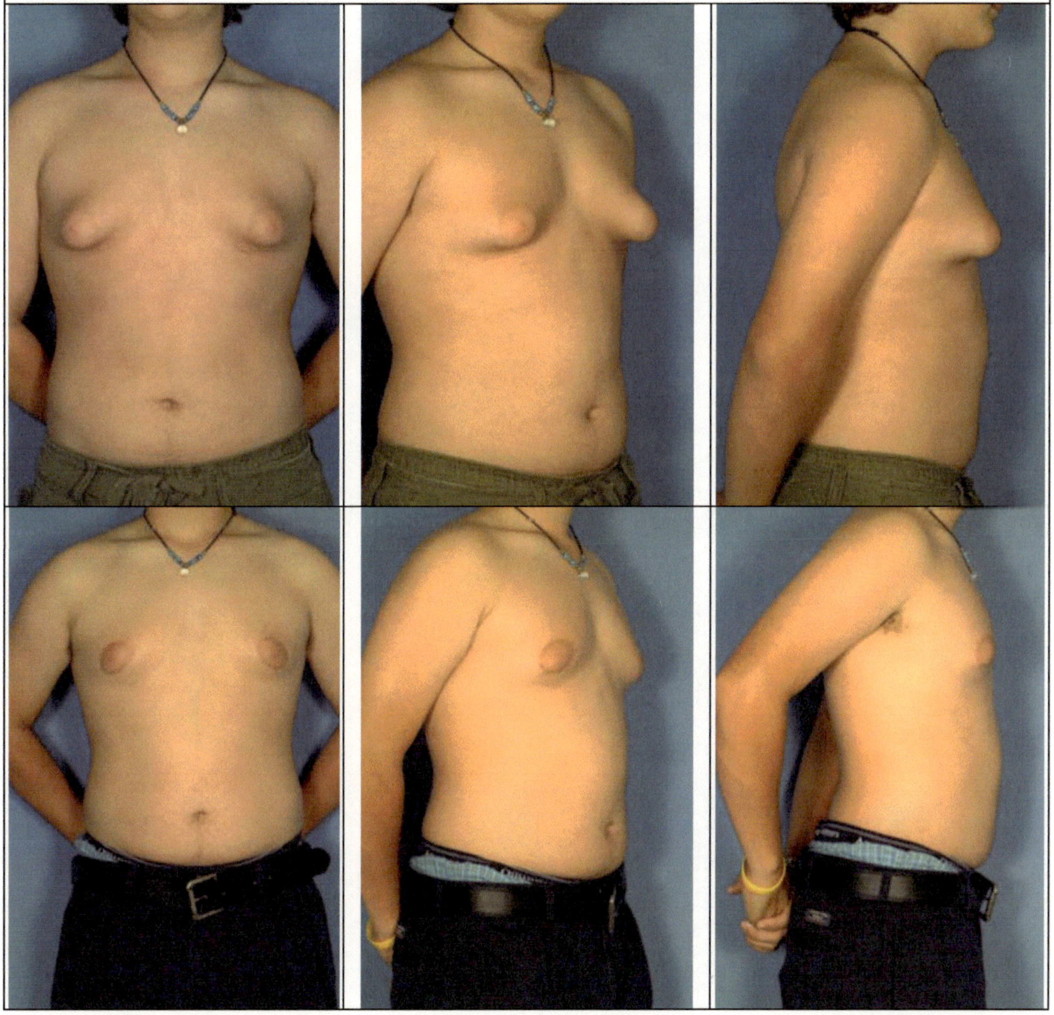

Wise pattern and inframammary approach with or without free nipple graft

This is the treatment of choice for the severe ptosis and the massive weight loss patient. In some cases a radical resection with free nipple grafting is necessary and delivers the best results to those patients with Grade III or severe gynecomastia. In these cases we favour an inframammary approach with resection of excess skin, subcutaneous and glandular tissue and repositioning of the NAC as a free NAC graft. The position of the new NAC is determined once the excision has been undertaken and the flaps approximated with staples. The new NAC position is deepithelialized and the free nipple graft sawn into position with a bolster dressing. Case 2

Case 2

Grade III gynecomastia on a massive weight loss patient. Treatment included inframmamary fold approach with direct excision of excess skin and breast tissue followed by free nipple graft. Preop and one month follow up.

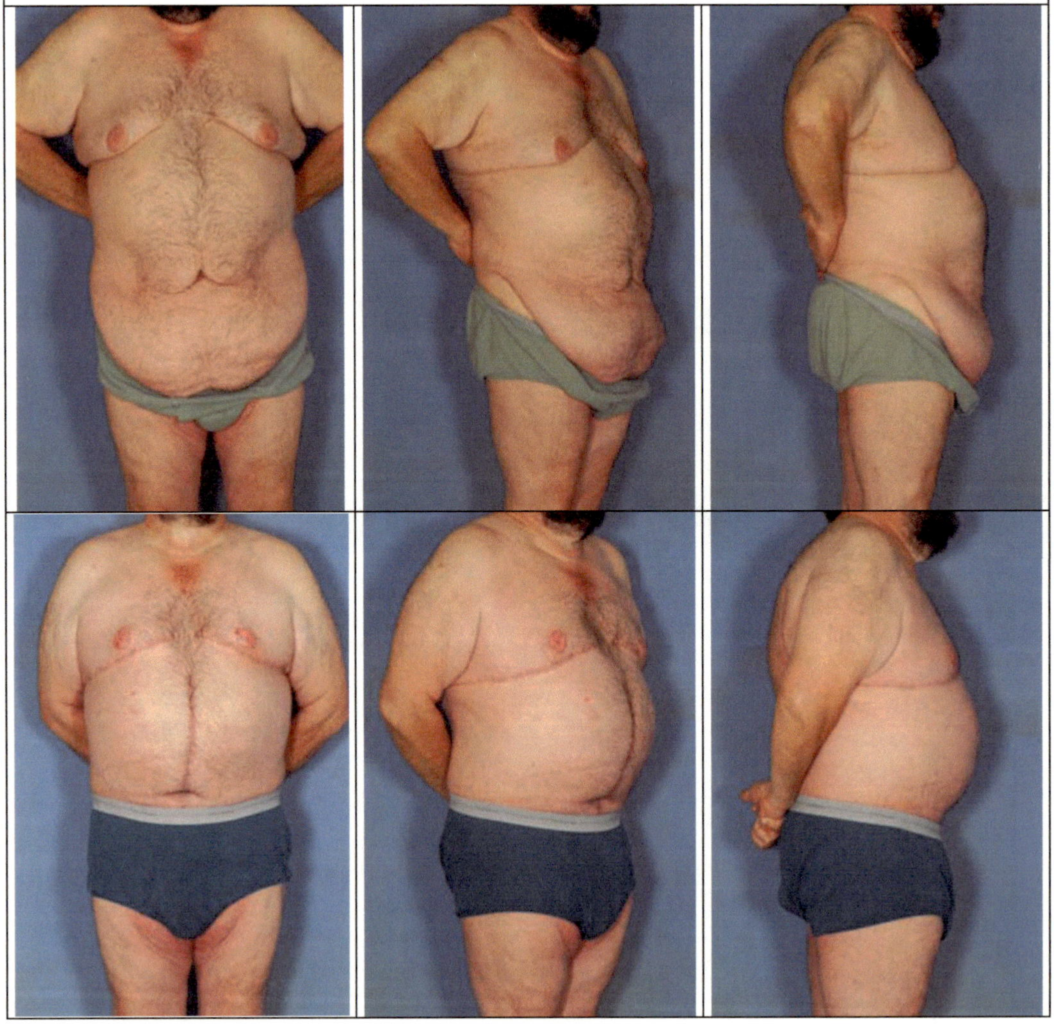

The algorithm on Figure 1 demonstrates our propose treatment plan for the different degrees of gynecomastia

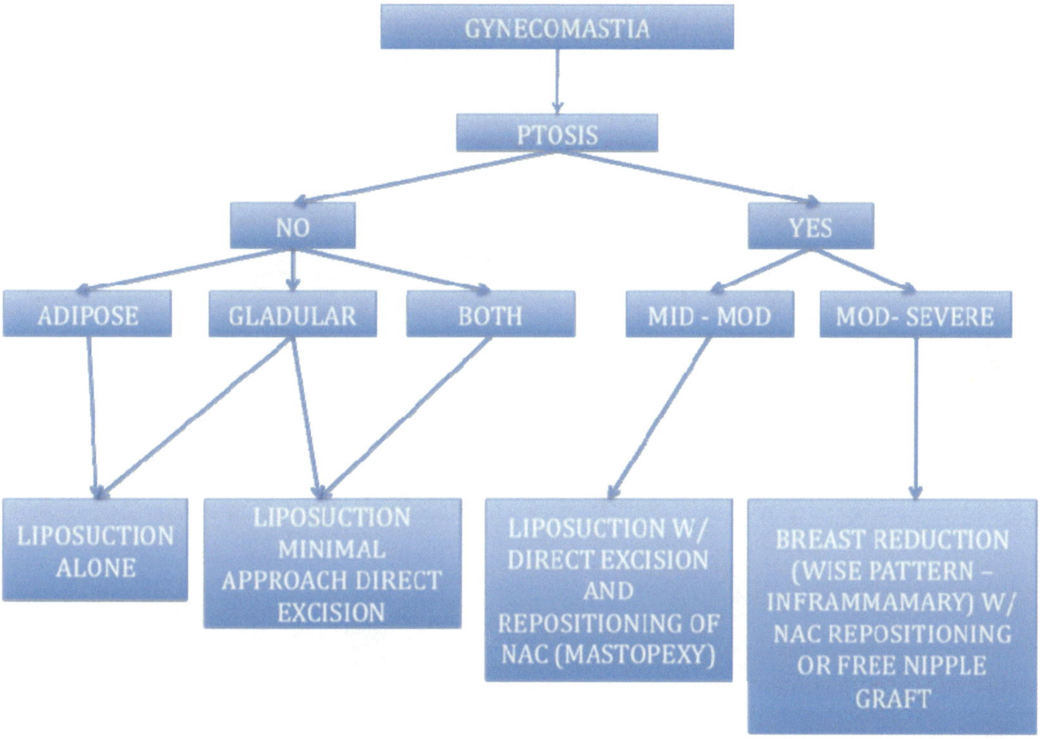

Fig. 1.

7.3 New developments

Laser assisted liposuction

Laser assisted liposuction has been described. The adjunct of laser therapy facilitates the lipolysis process without undue risk. [23, 24]

Dermoglandular repositioning for re-contouring of the masculine chest

Resection of breast an adipose tissue is not always the answer to gynecomastia. With the new developments and techniques in body contouring a new path for the treatment of gynecomastia has emerged. Some cases of gynecomastia require a reshaping procedure more than an ablative one. Although not yet published, we would like to present a case that illustrates this concept. Case 3. On a weight loss patient with gynecomastia a dermoglandular flap containing the NAC was fashioned and repositioned. The resulting shape of the chest contour shows restoration of the masculine contour of the anterior chest wall, where an ablative procedure would have resulted in a flat appearance.

Case 3

Grade I gynecomastia with caudal displacement of the NAC following weight loss. Treatment included dissection and repositioning of the NAC based on a dermoglandular flap. Preop intraop and post operative pictures are shown.

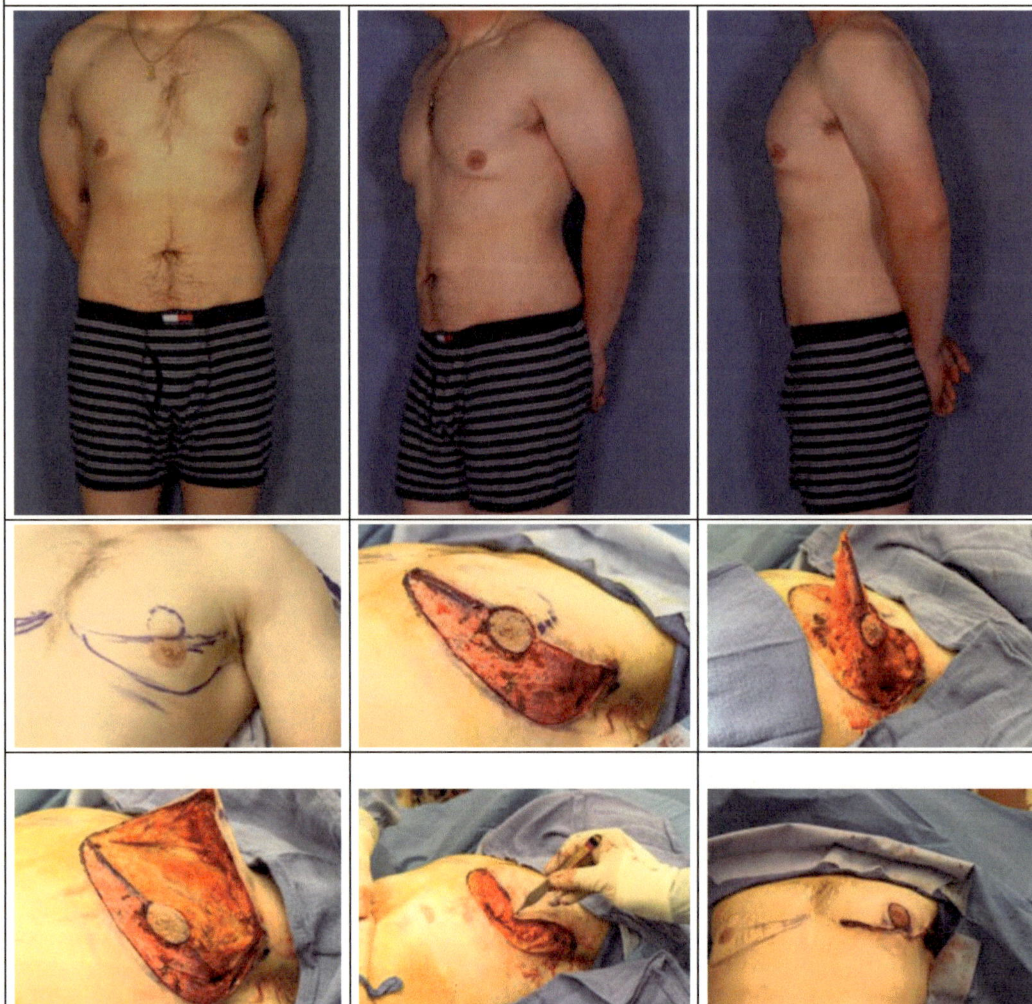

POSTOPT1	POSTOPT2	POSTOPT3

8. Postoperative care

All patients received compression garment treatment for six weeks to minimize the formation of seromas and avoid dead space. Those patients that undergo a large excision with wide undermining get drained for approximately 10 to 14 days. Patients are advised to refrain from strenuous activity for a period of 4 weeks with a recovery time of 7 to 10 days before returning to regular activities. We strongly believe a compliant postoperative course has a significant impact in speed of recovery and avoidance of complications.

9. Complications

The development of seromas is the number one complication. Often times and despite the rigorous measures to avoid seromas the dead space created by liposuction is prone to subsequent accumulation of fluid that needs to be drained during the follow up period. Hematomas are much less frequent with an incidence under 1%. Infection is uncommon but would healing complications can be a problem, especially in those cases with a large resection and free nipple grafting. The avoidance of undue tension and the use of drain and/or quilting sutures may help to decrease the common misadventures of the postoperative period. Skin necrosis and skin damage from aggressive liposuction, ultrasound liposuction, or arthroscopic shaver use have been reported. These complications are due to technical errors and should be avoided by the use of a consistent and careful technique.

10. Conclusion

Gynecomastia is a condition with increase prevalence and the advent of new developments and techniques require a dynamic update to deliver the best possible outcome. Several options are available today to address the different degrees of gynecomastia. The careful analysis of individual patients will permit the selection of the appropriate treatment method to deliver the best result. Psychological guidance plays an important role in the treatment of the condition.

11. References

[1] Georgiadis E, Papandreou L, Evangelopoulou C, Aliferis C, Lymberis C, Panitsa C, Batrinos M: Incidence of gynaecomastia in 954 young males and its relationship to somatometric parameters. *Ann Hum Biol* 1994, 21(6):579-587.

[2] Niewoehner CB, Nuttal FQ: Gynecomastia in a hospitalized male population. *Am J Med* 1984, 77(4):633-638.

[3] Nordt CA, DiVasta AD: Gynecomastia in adolescents. *Curr Opin Pediatr* 2008, 20(4):375-382.

[4] Nydick M, Bustos J, Dale JH, Jr., Rawson RW: Gynecomastia in adolescent boys. *JAMA* 1961, 178:449-454.

[5] Carlson HE: Gynecomastia. *N Engl J Med* 1980, 303(14):795-799.

[6] Hands LJ, Greenall MJ: Gynaecomastia. *Br J Surg* 1991, 78(8):907-911.

[7] Hanavadi S, Banerjee D, Monypenny IJ, Mansel RE: The role of tamoxifen in the management of gynaecomastia. *Breast* 2006, 15(2):276-280.

[8] Al-Allak A, Govindarajulu S, Shere M, Ibrahim N, Sahu AK, Cawthorn SJ: Gynaecomastia: A decade of experience. *Surgeon* 2011, 9(5):255-258.

[9] Laron Z, Dickerman Z: Clomiphene in pubertal-adolescent gynecomastia. *J Pediatr* 1978, 92(1):169.

[10] LeRoith D, Sobel R, Glick SM: The effect of clomiphene citrate on pubertal gynaecomastia. *Acta Endocrinol (Copenh)* 1980, 95(2):177-180.

[11] Stepanas AV, Burnet RB, Harding PE, Wise PH: Clomiphene in the treatment of pubertal-adolescent gynecomastia: a preliminary report. *J Pediatr* 1977, 90(4):651-653.

[12] Beck W, Stubbe P: [Excessive gynecomastia in boys. Effective medical treatment using danazol (Winobanin)]. *Monatsschr Kinderheilkd* 1984, 132(1):32-37.

[13] Beck W, Stubbe P: Endocrinological studies of the hypothalamo-pituitary gonadal axis during danazol treatment in pubertal boys with marked gynecomastia. *Horm Metab Res* 1982, 14(12):653-657.

[14] Swoboda W, Bohrn E: [Steroid treatment of adolescent gynecomastia with danazol (author's transl)]. *Wien Med Wochenschr* 1981, 131(5):127-132.

[15] Ting AC, Chow LW, Leung YF: Comparison of tamoxifen with danazol in the management of idiopathic gynecomastia. *Am Surg* 2000, 66(1):38-40.

[16] Derman O, Kanbur N, Kilic I, Kutluk T: Long-term follow-up of tamoxifen treatment in adolescents with gynecomastia. *J Pediatr Endocrinol Metab* 2008, 21(5):449-454.

[17] Devoto CE, Madariaga AM, Lioi CX, Mardones N: [Influence of size and duration of gynecomastia on its response to treatment with tamoxifen]. *Rev Med Chil* 2007, 135(12):1558-1565.

[18] Webster JP: Mastectomy for Gynecomastia Through a Semicircular Intra-areolar Incision. *Ann Surg* 1946, 124(3):557-575.

[19] Simon BE, Hoffman S, Kahn S: Classification and surgical correction of gynecomastia. *Plast Reconstr Surg* 1973, 51(1):48-52.

[20] Teimourian B, Perlman R: Surgery for gynecomastia. *Aesthetic Plast Surg* 1983, 7(3):155-157.

[21] Rohrich RJ, Ha RY, Kenkel JM, Adams WP, Jr.: Classification and management of gynecomastia: defining the role of ultrasound-assisted liposuction. *Plast Reconstr Surg* 2003, 111(2):909-923; discussion 924-905.

[22] Petty PM, Solomon M, Buchel EW, Tran NV: Gynecomastia: evolving paradigm of management and comparison of techniques. *Plast Reconstr Surg* 2010, 125(5):1301-1308.

[23] Wollina U, Goldman A: Minimally invasive esthetic procedures of the male breast. *J Cosmet Dermatol* 2011, 10(2):150-155.

[24] Rho YK, Kim BJ, Kim MN, Kang KS, Han HJ: Laser lipolysis with pulsed 1064 nm Nd:YAG laser for the treatment of gynecomastia. *Int J Dermatol* 2009, 48(12):1353-1359.

Part 4

Research and Microsurgery

10

Autologous Fat Grafting – Factors of Influence on the Therapeutic Results

Regina Khater[1] and Pepa Atanassova[2]
[1]*Division of Plastic and Craniofacial Surgery, St. George University Hospital, Medical University of Plovdiv*
[2]*Department of Anatomy, Histology and Embryology, Medical University of Plovdiv*
Bulgaria

1. Introduction

The correction of soft tissue defects has always been a challenge for plastic surgery. In the different stages of its historical development these problems has been solved by a variety of complicated techniques or filler materials some of which proved in time not only to be ineffective but even harmful for the human body. The ideal filler should be physically and chemically stable, long lasting and immobile in body, nonimmunogenic, noninfectious, nonpyogenic and nonallergic, should not require pretesting and should be cheap and easily stored. Some of these characteristics has been defined back in 1953 (Scales, 1953) but still there is no consensus regarding the perfect injectable material. Nowadays, despite of the growing number of alloproducts, the autologous fat grafting is recognized as one of the basic methods for soft tissue defects correction. It represents a three staged procedure of aspiration, purification and reimplantation of fat cells (Mojallal et al, 2004). The considerable presence of adipose tissue in the body and its autogenous origin guarantying advantages as biocompatibility, structure stability and polyvalent usage are reasons for the growing popularity of this intervention and its broading spectrum of indications. Nevertheless there are still a lot of controversies and unsolved questions regarding the autologous fat grafting. Its efficiency is still often doubted due to the variable resorption rates and the unpredictability of the post operative outcomes. In attempts of optimizing the results many surgical techniques have been created (Billings at al., 1989; Mojallal, Foyatier, 2004). The new concepts were built on attempts to avoid excessive pressure changes during harvesting and reimplantation, improving the means of purification from potential local inflammation promotors, and application in a fashion that assures sufficient nutritional sources (Mojallal, Foyatier, 2004; Shiffman, Mirrafati, 2001). Though none of the newly invented techniques is considered optimal a consensus has been reached on some stages of the technical implementation of autologous fat grafting such as manual syringe lipoaspiration and three-dimensional reimplantation (Niechajev, Sevcuk, 1994; Coleman, 2001; Jauffret et al., 1994; Lalikos et al., 1997; Moore et al., 1995; Novaes et al., 1995). To date the optimal method of transplant purification still remains unclear as well as the impact on the therapeutic results of factors as combination with other interventions, intraoperative extent of correction and the need of numerous transplantations as methods counteracting the postoperative resorption. At the same time the growing knowledge on adipose tissue and the revealed importance of the preadipocytes for transplant survival set questions about the influence of factors as age and gender, indications (esthetic or reconstructive), recipient site, etc. These and other issues will be discussed in this chapter as the profound knowledge on the existing techniques, the characteristics of the transplant and the influence of certain factors on therapeutic results could contribute to one's outcomes or technique refinement.

2. Surgical characteristics of adipose tissue

Adipose tissue is a particular sort of connective tissue existing in three different in morphology and function types. These are: white, brown and medullar adipose tissue which under the influence of various stimuli could turn into one another (Ashjilian et al., 2002; Casteilla et al., 2004; Mojallal, 2003; Jauffret, 1998).

The white adipose tissue is of greatest surgical importance. In people with normal body mass index it constitutes 15%-20% of the mass in males and 25%-30% in females (Ryan at al., 1989). It is scattered or distributed in depots localized in various anatomical regions according to age, gender and different nutritional and hormonal stimuli.

Morphologically white adipose tissue consists of stromovascular fraction and lipid inclusions containing mature adipose cells called adipocytes. Adipocytes together with hondrocytes and miocytes originate and differentiate from a multipotent cell of a mesodermal type (Ashjilian et al., 2002; Mojallal, 2003; Jauffret, 1998). The mature adipose cells have a roundish form and a diameter varying between 10μm and 120 μm. They are known as unilocular fat cells as their lipid inclusions are organized in one big lipid drop occupying almost the entire cell and pushing the nucleus and cytoplasm to the periphery. In the adipose tissue they are structured in lobules divided by connective tissue fibers.

The stromovascular compartment of adipose tissue contains nerves, capillary vessels, connective tissue fibers, fibroblasts, macrophages and endothelial cells localized in the interadipocytary spaces and immature multilocular fat cells called preadipocytes. Single preadipocytes could be found in the fat lobules among adipocytes as well. The immature adipose cells strongly resemble the fibroblasts' morphology. In comparison with adipocytes they are smaller with centrally placed nucleus and a great number of little lipid droplets. Unlike the mature adipose cells, preadipocytes have the ability to divide and proliferate into adipocytes and thus are realizing the process of adipogenesis, now recognized to extend throughout life (Atanassova, 2000; Dugail, Ferre, 2002; Casteilla et al., 2004)

Nowadays, the growing knowledge on the complexity of adipose structure and functions revealed great potentials of influence on surgical results. Though fat tissue was initially accepted as passive energy storage, it is now clear that it is a major endocrine and paracrine organ producing a variety of hormones and signalling molecules, generally referred to as adipokines (Mohamed-Ali et al., 1998; Fruhbeck et al., 2001; Chaldakov et al., 2006; Tore at al., 2007). Leptin is recognized as a hormone of great importance for the process of auto regulation, assimilation of nutritional sources, puberty and fertility (Zhang et al., 1994, Montague et al., 1997; Lafontan, Bouloumie, 1999). It is synthesized mainly in adipocytes and in very small quantities in preadipocytes. This makes it an original marker for identification of mature and immature fat cells (Markman, 1989; Atanassova, 1996; Lafontan, Bouloumie, 1999; Atanassova, Popova, 2000; Ashjilian et al., 2002). Of greatest importance for the autologous fat transplantation is the participation of leptin in the process of angiogenesis. The hormone exerts a strong stimulating effect on endothelial cells and consequently on graft microvascularization and fat tissue de novo synthesis.

The considerable presence of adipose tissue in the human body is a great advantage for autologous fat grafting. Its distribution in the anatomical regions is very specific and it strongly influences the choice of donor sites (Ryan, Curri, 1989; Jauffret, 1998). Adipocytes' number and size vary according to their localization due to the differences in blood supply and the response to neuroendocrine factors (Hudson et al., 1990; Dugail, Ferre, 2002; Casteilla et al., 2004). Y. J. Illouz describes two types of adipose tissue: an "ordinary" - which chemical homeostasis is constant and its volume varies and a "fat tissue of reserve" which almost never disappears except in cases of malnutrition and physiological insufficiency (Markman, 1989). The existing of those two types is determined by metabolic and biochemical differences resulting from the non identical distribution of the β-1 and α-2 receptors which are responsible for fat tissue sensibility to lipolysis stimuli. For example the α-2 receptors suppress lipolysis in the pelveotrochanteric region which is exactly the reason for the sometimes observed inability for weight loss in these zones. The latter is also valid for the intraorbital, plantar, palmar and Bichat bulle fat. All those variations in distribution and stability of adipose tissue are of great importance for the therapeutic strategies in autologous fat surgery and will be later thoroughly discussed (5. Factors of influence on the therapeutic results).

3. Evolution of autologous fat grafting – Historical overview

The use of fat tissue as a material for soft tissue defects correction or augmentation dates back from the end of 19th century. In 1989 E. Billings and J. May (Billings, May, 1989) published a historical overview of autologous fat grafting and in 2004 A. Mojallal divided it into three periods (Mojallal et al., 2004):

- First period - before the invention of lipoaspiration called an "open surgery" period (from 1889 to 1977)
- Second period - after the invention of lipoaspiration called "non refined", "traumatic" (from 1977 to 1994)
- Third period - after the popularization of S.R. Coleman's lipostructure called "refined" (from 1994 to nowadays)

The "open surgery" period represents the en block transplantation of fat tissue without any changes of its structure. The first report on autologous fat grafting was published by G. Neuber in 1893. He described implanting of small quantities of adipose tissue for filling of cicatrix depressions. Neuber reported good postoperative results though he encountered considerable rates of graft resorption in cases of big volumes transplantation (Neuber, 1893).

In the first half of the 20th century the method gained a lot of popularity and it was applied in almost all surgical specialties (Billings, May, 1989; Mojallal, Foyatier, 2004). Of course, the technique was widely used in plastic and aesthetic surgery for breast reconstructions and augmentations (Czerny, 1895; Bames, 1953; Schrocher, 1957), deep wrinkles corrections, cheek-bones area augmentation (Lexer, 1910), corrective rhinoplasties (Brunning, 1919) and etc. All authors reported good immediate results and different resorption rates in the late postoperative period which led to a creation of many technical modifications pretending for improving of transplant stability.

The second period is associated with the invention of liposuction in 1977 (Illouz, 1986, 1986, 1988). Initially created to eliminate the unharmonious adipose accumulations the technique turned out an ideal supplier of fat tissue without causing any unnecessary cicatrices. This led to new horizons for autologous fat transplantation. The first one used the unpurified product of liposuction as a transplant was Y. Illouz (Illouz, 1986, 1986, 1988). Later, in 1989 P. Fournier proposed a technique for reinjection of the aspirated fat called liposculpture (lipofilling) but the quoted necessity of hypercorrection and the instability of the results prevented its recognition (Fournier, 1996). In this period, however, many surgeons were applying autologous fat grafting in their practice. This led to a new wave of negative publications, modifications and even an attempt for reviving the idea of the en block transplantation (Ellenbongen, 1986). On the other hand many authors in Europe and USA reported big series of patients with successful application of autologous fat tissue harvested by liposuction and each one of them suggested a personal technique of processing and reinjection of the graft (Asken, 1987; Bircoll, 1987; Bircoll, Novack, 1987; Carraway, Mellow,1990; Chajhir et al., 1990; Ersek et al., 1998; Illouz, 1986; Fournier, 1996). One of them is S.R. Coleman, with the popularization of whose work starts the third period called "nontraumatic", "refined" (Mojallal et al, 2004). After a profound analysis he summarized the methods and the results of his predecessors and created a new surgical protocol changing utterly the philosophy of the known by this time autologous fat grafting from free transfer of intact adipose tissue to free fat cells transplantation. The method was published in 1994 and called Lipostructure® (Coleman, 1994; 1995; 2001). It is a three staged procedure consisting of:

1. manual lipoaspiration under low pressure
2. three minutes of centrifugation at 3400rpm eliminating the blood, oil and detergents and
3. reinjection in three-dimensional plan

In creating this technique S.R. Coleman pays great attention to the atraumatic handling of adipose tissue which is of paramount importance for autologous fat grafting results improvement. The method was presented and popularized in Europe in 1994. Afterwards, many authors published series of good results after applying Coleman's technique and summarized its advantages and disadvantages (Amar, 1999; Jaufret et al., 2001; Trepsat, 2001; Mojallal, 2003; Laurent et al., 2006). In comparison with the existing fillers the autologous fat transplanted by this technique is an ideal substitute material because of its quantity, autogenous origin and the ability of full integration with the surrounding tissue (fig.1, 2). It is not palpable and the results seem quite natural. The technique is easily applied under general and local anesthesia, more productive than the other methods stated and not harmful for the adipose tissue. According to that, nowadays, lipostructure® is the officially recognized method of autologous fat grafting. Nevertheless one could still find lots of co-existing techniques pretending for equally good results (Ellenbongen, 1986; Teimourian 1986; Guerrerosantos, 1996; 2000; Toledo, 1996). Their technical modifications act in a different way on graft's biology which creates a variety of factors of influence on the postoperative effect. Thus, even though there are irrefutable proofs for the advantages of autologous fat grafting, still there are some controversies regarding its technical implementation.

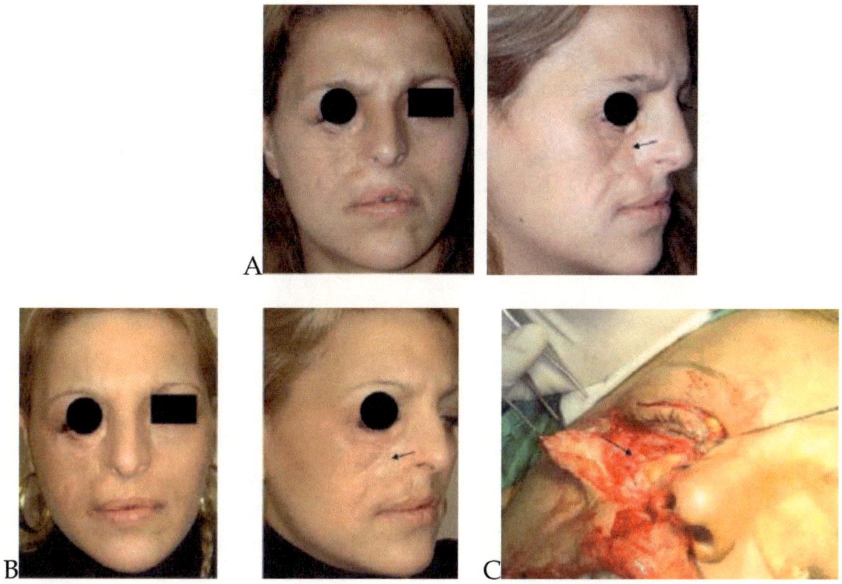

Fig. 1. A patient with cleft №4 according to Tessier classification: A - preoperatively; B - 14,5 months after autologous fat grafting of 3cc in the upper lip and 10cc in right and 7cc in left suborbital region; C - fat tissue found intraoperatively in the recipient site 2 years after the fat grafting

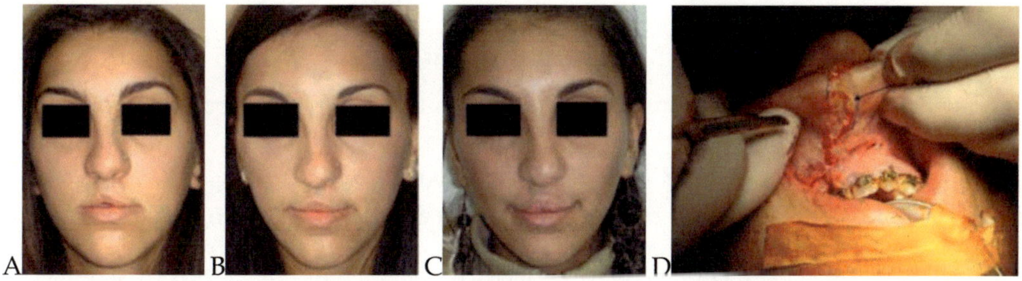

Fig. 2. A patient with bilateral cleft lip and palate, operated according protocol earlier: A - preoperatively; B - 10,5 months after autologous fat grafting of 6cc in the upper lip; C - 12 months after second grafting of 4cc; D - fat tissue found intraoperatively in the recipient site 1 year after the second fat grafting

4. Surgical technique

Nowadays the universal method of autologous fat transplantation is Coleman's technique "lipostructure" with some variations of its technical implementation. In general it consists of three stages: fat harvesting, specific processing of the aspirate and reimplantation performed in sterile conditions with respect to the fragility of adipocytes.

In our practice fat harvesting is done by deep manual lipoaspiration of the donor site using different in length 2,6mm-inner-diameter blunt cannulas, allowing the free passing of fat cells, attached to a 10-cc syringes of a Luer-lock type. The so described vacuum system is brought in through a miniature incision placed in the natural creases. The donor site could be any of the subcutaneous depots with or without excessive fat accumulation but we always choose the pelveotrochanteric region for the more appropriate size of the fat cells and their higher activity of lipoprotein lipase (Hudson et al., 1990; Niechajev, Sevcuk, 1994; Fulton et al., 1998). Lipoaspiration is performed under manual regulation of the negative pressure not exceeding 2cc. In the cases operated under general anesthesia no local infiltration is used. For local anesthesia or in the cases of neurosedation between 40cc and 80cc of modified Klein's solution (500ml NaCl, 150mg Lidocain®, 0,5mg Epinephrine®) are applied. Until processing the harvested material is kept in the syringes used for aspiration obturated with sterile caps preventing the harmful contact with air.

The harvested quantity and the choice of anesthesia are individual and depending on patient's character and indications.

The processing of the graft could be done by various methods: centrifugation at different revolutions per minute and durations; decantation; serum washing and so on. In our practice we use centrifugation at 3400 rpm for 3 minutes and serum lavage but we recommend the second method for reasons that will be later discussed.

The graft is centrifuged in the same 10-cc syringes in which it is harvested. The pistons are being removed and the obturated syringes are placed in the centrifuge in sterile metal flasks ensuring sterility. Centrifugation results in sedimentation of material and formation of three layers:

- at the top - an oily layer which is an effect of adipocytes disintegration
- in the middle - the adipose graft
- at the bottom - mainly serum and blood products

This method of processing is considered done when the serum at the bottom and the oil at the top are removed.

The advised by us technique of serum lavage is realized by transferring of the harvested material from the 10-cc syringe in which it was obtained to 20-cc syringe and washing by additionally drawn 10cc of physiological serum. To obtain a fat graft free of oil and blood the saline solution is changed one or two times. The removal of the washing material could be done in two ways according to surgical time: 1) after a short stay in vertical position the saline precipitates at the bottom of the syringe and it is gently pushed by the piston or 2) by pulling up the piston which results in saline leak.

For the next stage the so processed grafts are transferred into 1cc-syringes. Reinjection is done by 1,2mm or 1mm-inner-diameter blunt cannulas which allow structure-safe passing of fat cells and in the same time creates tunnels which diameter do not exceed the critical one for revascularization (1,5±0,5mm). The combination of cannulas and syringes of these sizes is optimal as they exert very low pressure on the fragile graft and in the same time they are easy for managing. The cannulas are introduced in the recipient site by lots of miniature incisions placed in a manner reassuring the creation of a three-dimensional trellis of grafted tunnels. For prevention of possible embolism reinjection is done while gently pulling backwards the cannula.

Grafted quantities and intraoperative extent of correction is individual and should be planned after a thorough discussion with patients explaining the advantages and disadvantages of the method, the discomfort of the hypercorrection and the expected resorption. However we do recommend the realization of a slight overcorrection for better results.

The incisions are sutured with Prolene® 6/0 - 7/0. At the end of the operation a light modulating massage of the recipient site and application of epithelotonic unguents is advised. According to localization a bandage or ice compresses in regular basis could be placed for the first 24 hours. At the donor site the wearing of a compressive bandage or garment for a period of 7 days is advised.

5. Factors of influence on the therapeutic results

Fat tissue is very fragile and requires a delicate handling. In view of that every stage of the contemporary surgical protocol as well as all related factors have been subjected in time to various investigations aiming an establishment of potential agents of influence on the postoperative results. Hereby we represent a summary on the existing information in literature and our personal contribution by a survey on 148 protocols of autologous fat transplantation realized for a period of 3 years in the Division of plastic and craniofacial surgery, St. George University Hospital, Plovdiv, Bulgaria. The comparison of the investigated factors was realized by application of the described below methods of outcomes assessing (6.Methods of outcomes assessing).

5.1 Local anesthetics

There are various reports and different preferences on the optimal type of anesthesia based on quite controversial data on the impact of local anesthetics (Ellenbongen, 1986; Chajhir, Benzaquen, 1989; Ersek, 1998; Har-Shai, 1998; Amar, 1999; Coleman, 2001). In 1995 Jr. Moore published the results of a profound analysis stating no negative influence of the adrenalin on fat cells survival (Moore, 1995). On the contrary, lidocain leaded to inhibition of glucose transport, lipolysis and growth of adipocytes but the effect was irreversible after cease of contact. Later on, in 2003 the latter was confirmed by J. MacRae's histomorphological research. It found no significant differences between most of the known anesthetics according to their influence on graft viability.

In our practice we always choose local anesthesia when possible - for grafting small quantities or working in limited locations. For the donor site we apply 0,5% lidocain for anesthetizing the place of incision and a tumescent type of infiltration of modified Klein solution (500ml NaCl, 150mg Lidocain®, 0,5mg Epinephrine®) for the rest of the zone. In these cases we prefer a subsequent processing by serum lavage for better purification of the graft. For the recipient site we tend to apply local blocks as the terminal type of local anesthesia leads to tissue edema perplexing the exact planning of the transplant quantity.

In cases with general anesthesia no local infiltration is advised.

5.2 Donor site

Any of the subcutaneous adipose tissue depots could be used as a donor site. More frequently these are the places of excessive fat accumulation such as the pelveotrohanteric region (thighs), abdomen, knees, ankles or even chin and hands. According to needed quantity numerous sites could be used. Nevertheless for treatment of mirror zones (nasolabial folds, cheeks, etc) we advise application of grafts harvested from one place as fat tissue differs according to cells size and activity in different locations (Hudson et al., 1990; Dugail, Ferre, 2002; Casteilla et al, 2004). For example D. Hudson at al. found out that the adipocytes in pelveotrohanteric region are bigger and with higher activity of the lipoprotein lipase. Later on J. Fulton and I. Niechajev proclaimed as optimal for fat harvesting the pelveotrohanteric zone, followed by the abdomen and face region (Hudson et al., 1990; Niechajev, Sevcuk, 1994; Fulton et al., 1998). Many other statements of preferences could be found in literature but we always choose the pelveotrochanteric zone when possible especially in female patients.

5.3 Fat harvesting

According to the optimal method of fat harvesting there are many investigations in favor of the manual lipoaspiration (liposuction). This technique combines the advantages of machine liposuction and surgical excision and in the same time it does not have the burden of their disadvantages - respectively adipocytes destruction due to the high negative pressure and disfiguring cicatrices (Novaes et al., 1998; MacRae et al., 2003; Mojallal, Foyatier, 2004). Manual lipoaspiration is noninvasive and as atraumatic towards adipose cells as surgical excision (Moore et al., 1995; Lalikos et al., 1997) which makes it an optimal method for fat harvesting.

5.4 Graft processing

The product obtained by fat harvesting consists not only of morphologically preserved adipose structures but also of products of tissue disintegration which sets the need of subsequent specific purification. This stage of the surgical technique is still disputed and there are several known methods of its realization - decantation, filtration, centrifugation and washing with saline solution (Mojallal, Foyatier, 2004; Khater, 2010). Filtration has already been denied for its traumatizing mechanical impact on fat cells and the too long exposition to air (Ersek, 1991; Niechajev, Sevcuk, 1994). The method of decantation is also not preferred for its duration which prolongs surgical time.

Nowadays the techniques of choice for most surgeons are centrifugation and washing with saline solution. 0,9% NaCl is experimentaly proved to be not harmful for fat cells viability which makes the method of serum lavage preferable for many authors (Ersek, 1991; 1998; Horl et al., 1991; Marques et al., 1994; Fulton, 1998; Har-Shai, 1999; MacRae et al., 2003; Smith at al., 2006; Khater et al., 2008). The method of centrifugation is applied in 3000-3400 rpm for 3 minutes. Though there have been many controversial researches concerning its safety, optimal rpm and duration, the technique is proved to be atrauamatical (Jauffret, 1998; MacRae et al., 2003; Smith at al., 2006; Khater et al., 2008).

To investigate the potential influence of the two techniques on surgical outcomes we compared results assessments (subjective and expert) and changes in quantity and morphology of aspirates after their application. From 148 cases of autologous fat transplantation 80,4% were operated with centrifugation of the graft at 3400rpm for 3min. and 19,6%with the already described (4.Surgical technique) technique of serum lavage. At the end of the follow up period the subjective and expert analysis found out considerably better results in the group with non centrifuged fat grafts ($p<0,01$ (fig.3)). The latter proved a dependency of the postoperative effect on the technique of purification in favor of serum lavage (fig.4, 5).

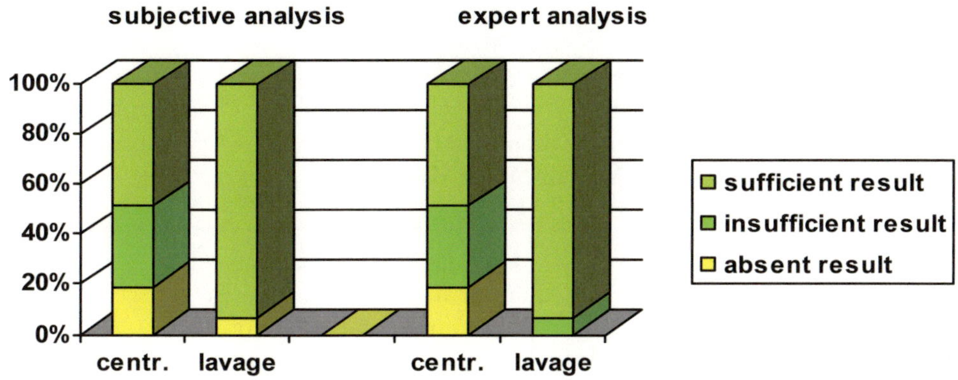

Fig. 3. Assessment of patients and expert jury according to the method of purification: centrifugation (centr.) and serum lavage (lavage).

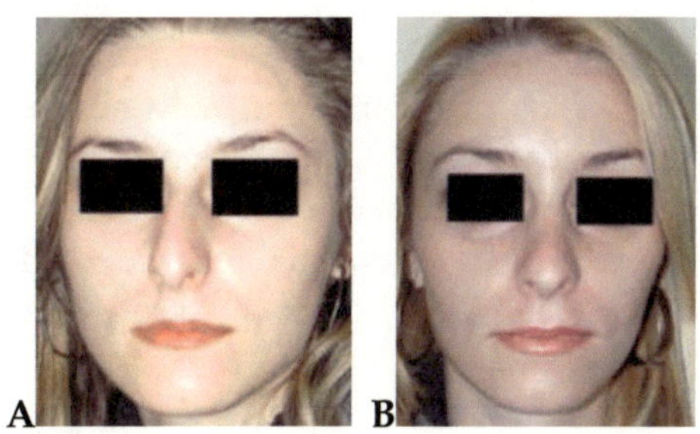

Fig. 4. 26-years old patient with transplantation of 4cc centrifuged autologous fat graft in the upper lip region. A - preoperatively; B – 12 months postoperatively

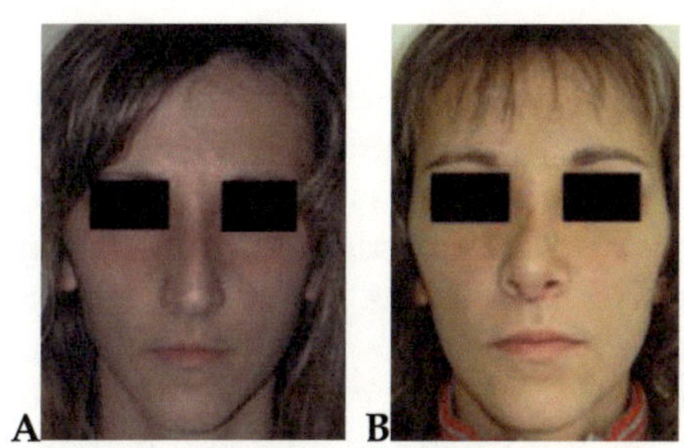

Fig. 5. 24-years old patient with transplantation of 4cc purified by the technique of serum lavage autologous fat graft in the upper lip region. A - preoperatively; B – 12 months postoperatively

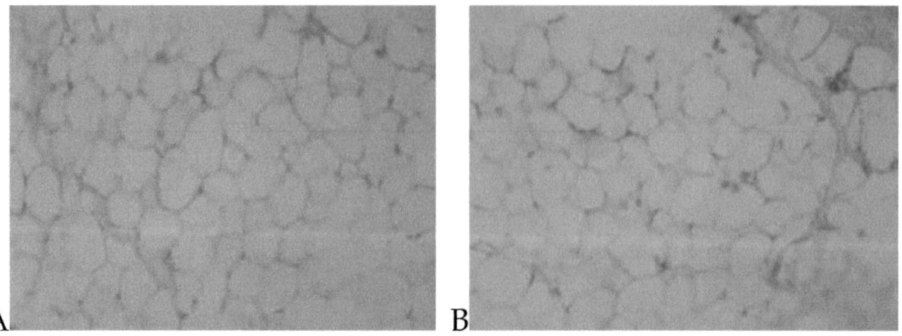

Fig. 6. Syringe aspirated adipose tissue processed by centrifugation (A) and serum lavage (B). Hematoxylin -Eosin staining. Magnification: x200.

Parameters / processing type	Average amount before processing	Average amount after processing	Average difference in quantity	T	P
Centrifugation	31,74cc	22,24cc	9,50cc	3,27	<0,01*
Serum lavage	50,72cc	31,75cc	18,98cc		

Table 1. Average difference in aspirate quantity before and after centrifugation and washing with saline solution. *The difference is statistically significant

Histological analysis found out more preserved tissue elements in the non centrifuged samples (fig.6). Of greatest importance among them was the presence of more immature adipose cells (preadipocytes) which in comparison with adipocytes are more resistant to ischemia, easier for revascularization and capable of proliferation and differentiation. The observed differences in preadipocytes preservation makes the technique of serum lavage more favorable for postoperative outcomes especially in view of recent assumptions that the primary flow of previous techniques was selecting the wrong component of adipose tissue – adipocytes (Scholler et al., 2001).

The quantative analysis found out that in comparison with saline washing the method of centrifugation preserves two times bigger amount of the harvested material (tabl.1). In view of the worse results and the presence of less tissue elements, the latter makes us think that the method of centrifugation is imperfect according to graft purification by detergents.

The influence of the two methods on grafts viability was studied in vitro in floating tissue cultures and diffusion chambers (Khater et al., 2008). After 7 days of cultivation the morphological analysis again found greater presence of preadipocytes in the non centrifuged samples (fig.7). Among the grafts cultivated in diffusion chambers these results were additionally confirmed (fig.8) by investigation of the immunohistochemical expression of leptin (Alexis Biochemicals; dilution 1:5000) which is a significant marker of adipose cells (Klein et al., 1996; Cinti et al., 1997; Atanassova, Popova, 2000). By analogy, in view of the fact that adipocytes do not have the ability to divide, the immunohistochemical expression of Cyclin D1 (DACO corp.; dilution 1:200) - an universal marker of proliferation (Klein et al., 1996; Cinti et al., 1997) showed higher proliferative activity in the non centrifuged grafts (fig.9). The latter spurs the notion of greater possibility of de novo fat formation in the recipient site after transplantation of adipose tissue processed by serum lavage. This idea was also supported by the results observed after cultivation in floating tissue cultures (fig.10). In centrifuged grafts weak manifestation of proliferation and differentiation was observed. In comparison, in the non centrifuged grafts could be seen a vast proliferative zone and a zone of distant cell migration containing differentiating preadipocytes.

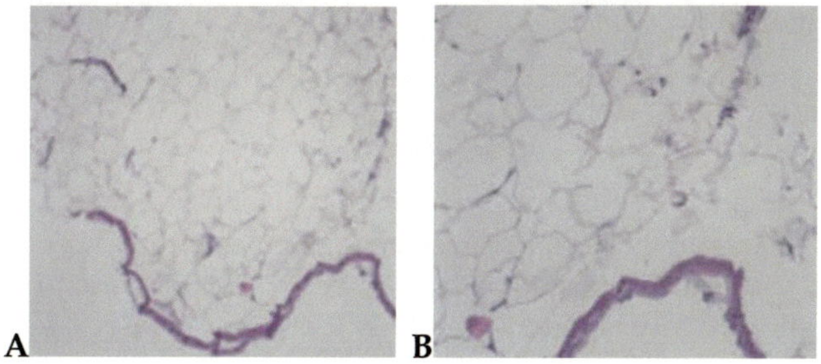

Fig. 7. Diffusion chamber tissue culture, hematoxylin - eosin staining. Magnification x200: A - centrifuged adipose graft culture: presence of adipocytes and a small amount of preadipocytes among them. B – non centrifuged graft culture: presence of adipocytes, preadipocytes and connective tissue fragments containing preadipocytes.

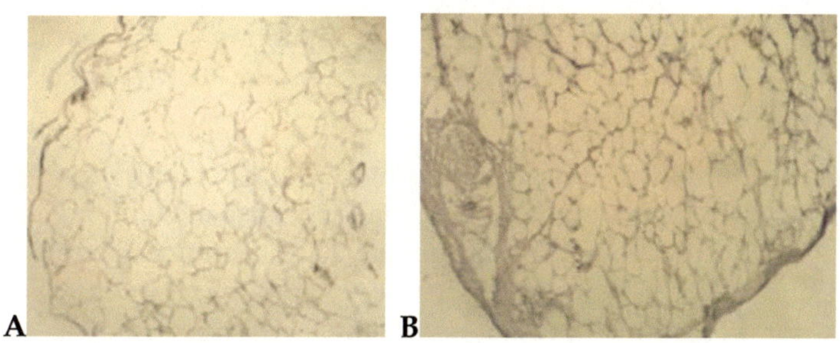

Fig. 8. Immunohistochemical expression of leptin in adipocytes and preadipocytes. Diffusion tissue chambers, magnification – x200. A - centrifuged adipose graft culture - expression of leptin in adipocytes and in small amount of preadipocytes among them. B – non centrifuged graft culture - expression of leptin in adipocytes and in the preadipocytes among them and within the connective tissue fragments.

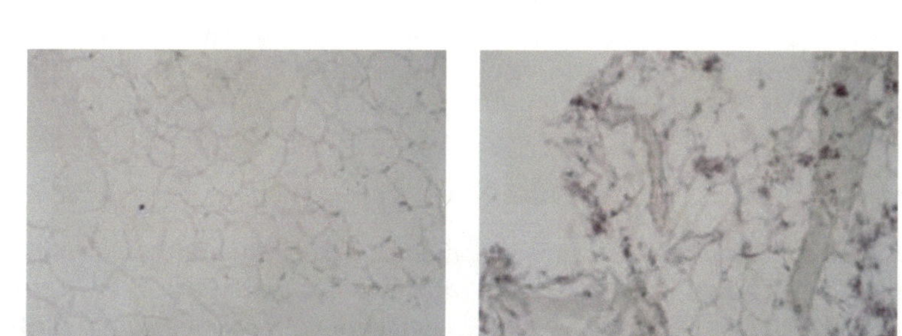

Fig. 9. Immunohistochemical expression of Cyclin D1 in preadipocytes. Diffusion tissue chambers, magnification – x200. A - centrifuged adipose graft culture; B – non centrifuged graft culture

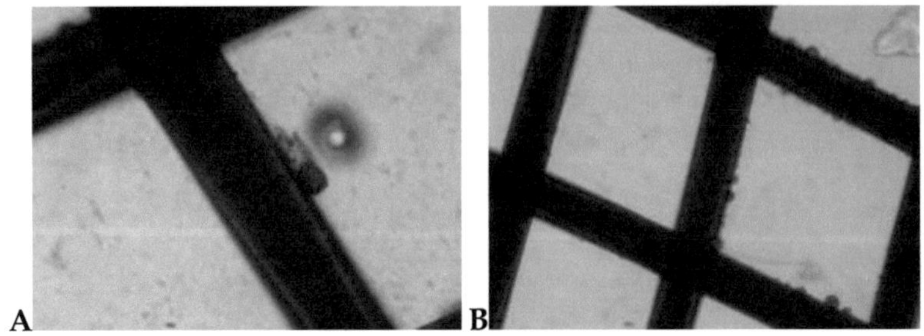

Fig. 10. Floating tissue cultures. Sudan III – hematoxylin staining, magnification x200.
A - centrifuged adipose graft culture: primary zone of cultivation and proliferative zone;
B – non centrifuged graft culture: primary zone of cultivation, proliferative zone and a zone of distant cell migration.

5.5 Recipient site

The quality of the recipient site is of great importance for transplant survival. The optimal conditions are to have anatomically and physiologically undamaged tissue structures with good blood supply. It is proved that fat grafting in zones of fibrosis is done under pressure which leads to structure changes in cells and diminishes the chances of survival (Har-Shai, 1999). For optimal results in these cases a certain repetition of the method is needed and after a few applications a considerable improvement of such a zone quality could be observed (Mojallal, Foyatier, 2004).

As good vascularization is of utmost importance for successful transplantation many authors consider the muscle optimal for graft intake because of its blood supply (Nguyen et al., 1990; Niechajev, Sevcuk, 1994; Guerrerosantos, 2000). Though this recipient site still has its supporters (Colic, 1999; Jackson, 2001; Stampos, Xepoulias, 2001) it was proved that it is of a much risk for hematoma formation and fat cells lysis (Mojallal, Foyatier, 2004). Nowadays there is not a unified opinion for the optimal anatomical structure but it is experimentally proved that fat grafting in zones without fat tissue by nature is unsuccessful (Van, Roncari, 1977; 1982).

We investigated the potential influence of recipient site anatomical location on the therapeutic results (Khater, 2010). The comparison of outcomes assessments after grafting in head and neck region, limbs and body found more favorable results with statistical significance ($p<0,05$) in the head and neck region (fig.11). We attribute the latter to the higher blood supply of this region.

5.6 Indications

The method of autologous fat grafting is suitable for soft tissue defects correction or volume augmentation. It is widely used for esthetic indications – esthetic surgery of the face, aging hands corrections etc. There are still some controversies on applying the method for breast augmentation. Though many surgeons think that the technique impedes breast cancer diagnosis by formation of micro calcifications and cicatrices it works quite well in the hands of others if the fat is not directly injected into the gland (Gradinger 1987; Hartrampf 1987; Ousterhout 1987; Khouri et al., 2000; Delay 2009).

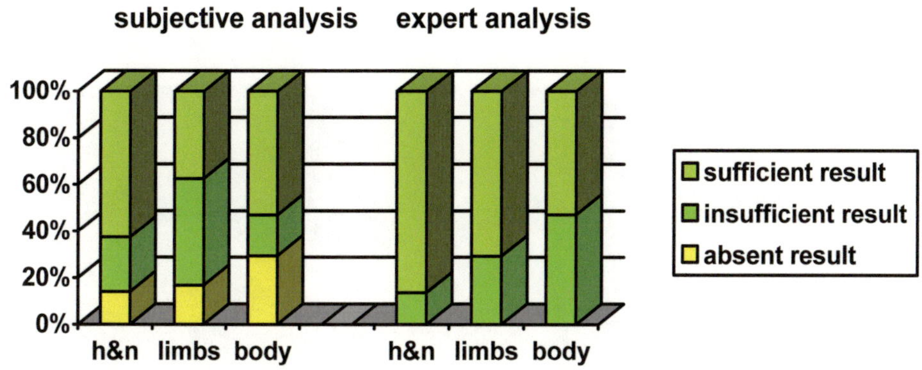

Fig. 11. Assessment of patients and expert jury according to recipient zone location: head and neck (h&n), limbs, body

Initially designed to fulfill the esthetic surgery needs nowadays the method has a broad spectrum of reconstructive indications though there is still a certain lack of distinctness which defect or condition is appropriate for such a surgical solution. Back in 2000 J. Guerrerosantos published a classification of soft tissue defects dividing them into four stages (Guerrerosantos, 2000). The first two groups affect only the subcutaneous tissue and could be treated successfully only by autologous fat transplantation. For the other two stages a combination with other surgical techniques is needed as the defects affect underlying structures in partial or full depth. This classification is very popular and advised for therapeutic strategies creation.

In our practice we compared the results assessments after autologous fat transplantation for esthetic and reconstructive indications and found considerably better results in the esthetic group (p<0, 0001 (fig.12)) probably due to the better qualities and blood supply of recipient sites. In view of that when treating cases with reconstructive indications a planning of multiple applications is advised.

Hereby we represent few cases of example from our practice (fig. 13 - 21).

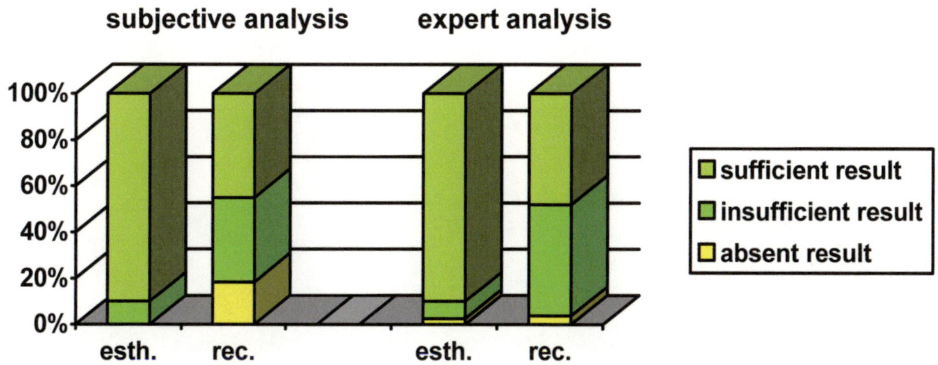

Fig. 12. Assessment of patients and expert jury according to indications: esthetic (esth.) and reconstructive (rec.)

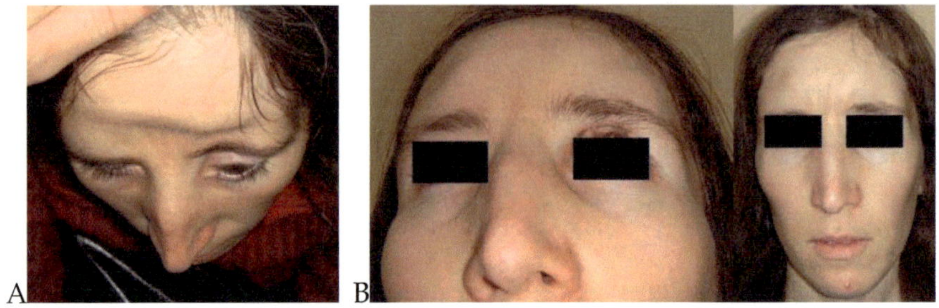

Fig. 13. A 27-year old patient with a forehead contour defect consequence of cranioplasty. A - preoperatively; B - 12 months after transplantation of 25cc purified by the technique of serum lavage autologous fat graft in the forehead region.

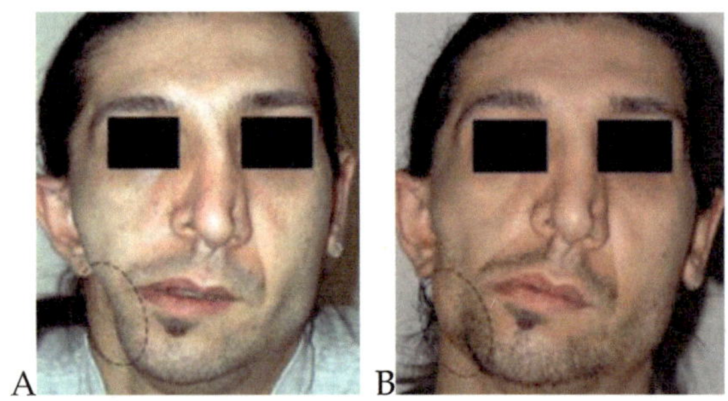

Fig. 14. A 35-year old patient with otomandibular syndrome in the right. A - preoperatively; B - one month after distraction and transplantation of 20cc centrifuged autologous fat graft in right mandibular area.

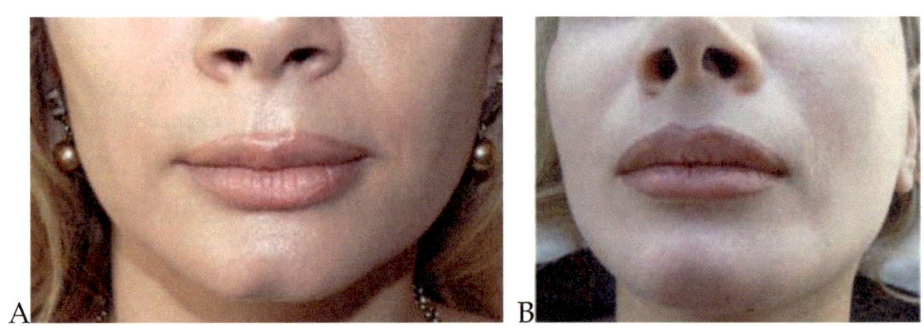

Fig. 15. A 33-year old patient with contour defect after mentoplasty. A - preoperatively; B - 9 months after 3 applications in 3 months of 16cc non centrifuged autologous fat graft in the chin area.

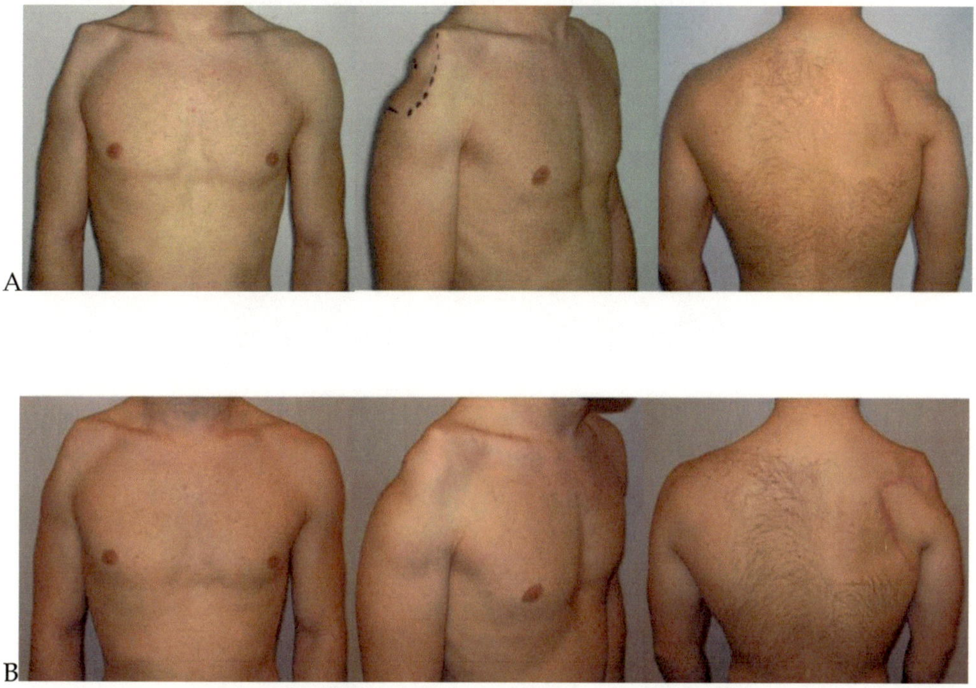

Fig. 16. A 23-year old patient with contour defect after operation for scapular fibrosarcoma 5 years ago. A - preoperatively; B - 3 months after transplantation of 51cc non centrifuged graft in scapular region.

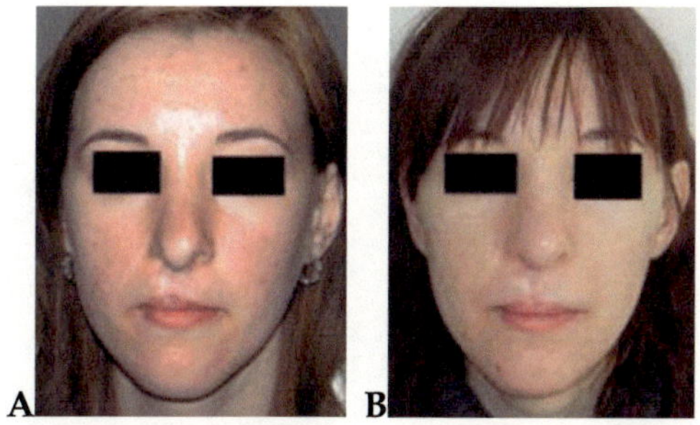

Fig. 17. A 28-year old patient with cleft lip and palate in the right operated in childhood. A- preoperatively; B - 18 months after rhynoplasty and transplantation of 4cc non centrifuged fat graft in the upper lip.

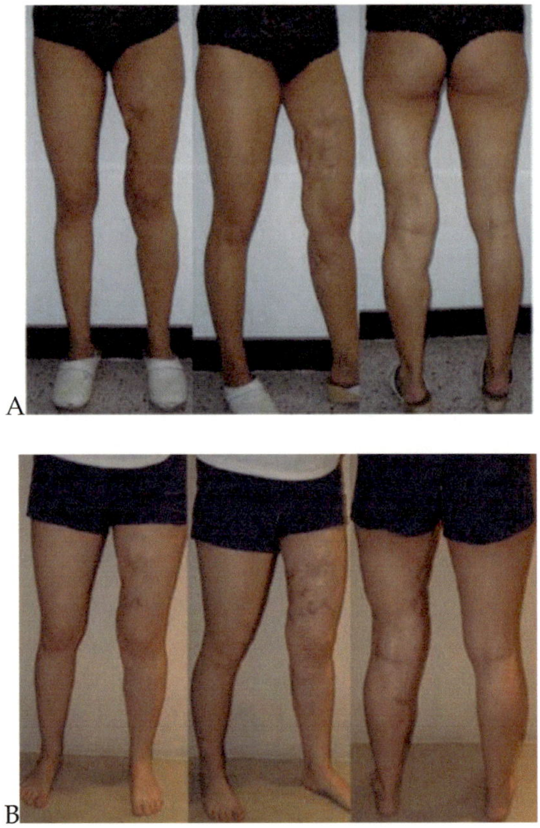

Fig. 18. A 29-year old patient with contour defects of the left leg sequence of clostridial myonecrosis in childhood. A – preoperatively; B – 16 months after transplantation of 100 cc centrifuged fat graft in the different regions.

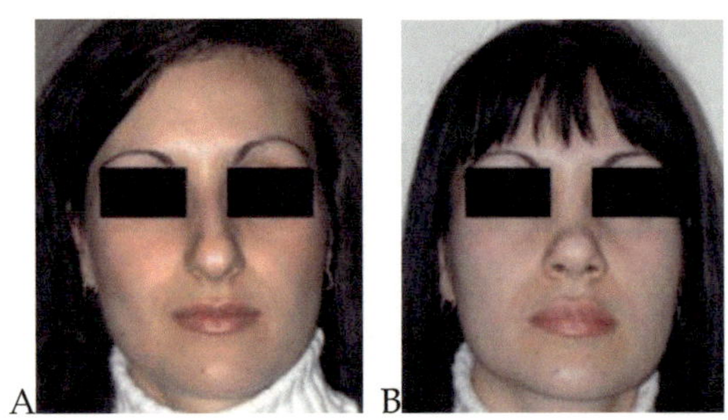

Fig. 19. A 24-year old patient with lip augmentation and rhynoplasty. A – preoperatively; B – 24 months after 2 applications in 6 months of centrifuged fat graft: 2x2,5cc in the upper and 2x2,5 in the lower lip.

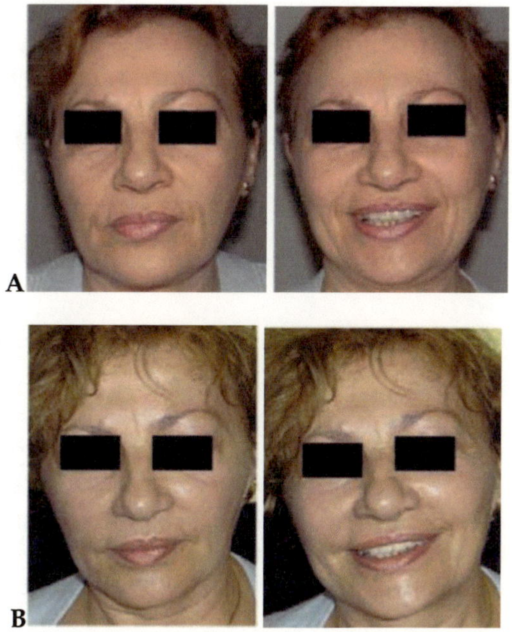

Fig. 20. A 56-year old woman with autologous fat grafting in the nasolabial folds. A - preoperatively; B - 12 months after transplantation of 10cc non centrifuged graft in each fold.

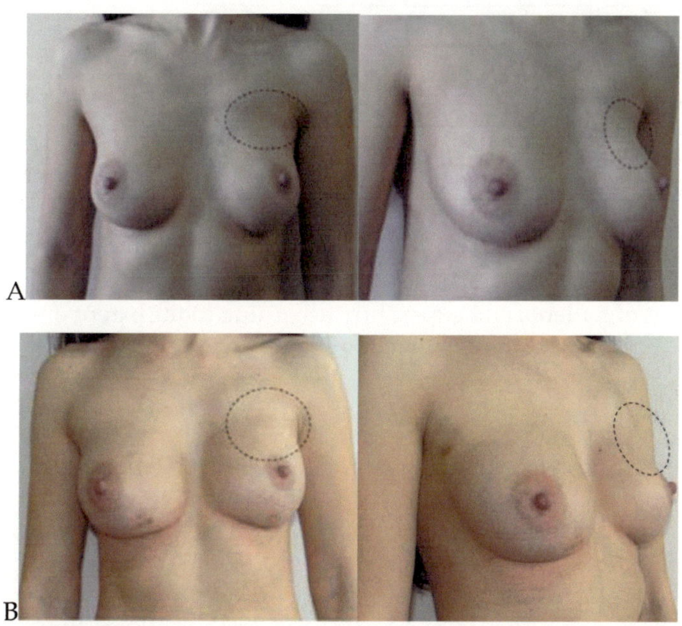

Fig. 21. A 33-year old patient with Poland Syndrome treated with breast augmentation 8 years ago (160cc round prosthesis). A - preoperatively; B - 2 weeks after operative change of prosthesis (180cc round prosthesis) and application of 18cc of non centrifuged fat graft.

5.7 Reimplantation

Although there are many stated preferences and created surgical instruments (Chajhir, Benzaquen 1990; Niechajev, Sevcuk, 1994; Toledo 1994; Amar 1999), nowadays the method of choice for fat grafts application is the three-dimensional technique of Coleman (Coleman, 2001). Most of the surgeons use the proceeded material immediately after fat grafting but in literature could be found examples for graft freezing and subsequent use (Coleman WP 1999; Fulton et al., 1998; Bertossi et al., 2000) or graft enrichment with growth factors and other substances increasing the chances of graft survival (Pinski et al., 1992; Scholler et al., 2001).

5.8 Intraoperative extent of correction – normo- and hypercorrection

The stated in literature graft survival varies but it is rarely 100%. There is always a certain percentage of transplant resorption. For optimization of postoperative outcomes many authors advise a hypercorrection of the treated zone (Niechajev, Sevcuk, 1994; Amar 1999; Coleman 2001) or three and more applications in the recipient site at regular basis - between 3 and 6 months (Bircoll 1987; Boschert et al., 2002). In our practice the comparison of surgical outcomes assessments showed more favorable results after hypercorrection of the treated zones (p<0, 0001 (fig.22)). There were no statistical differences between multiple and single graft applications.

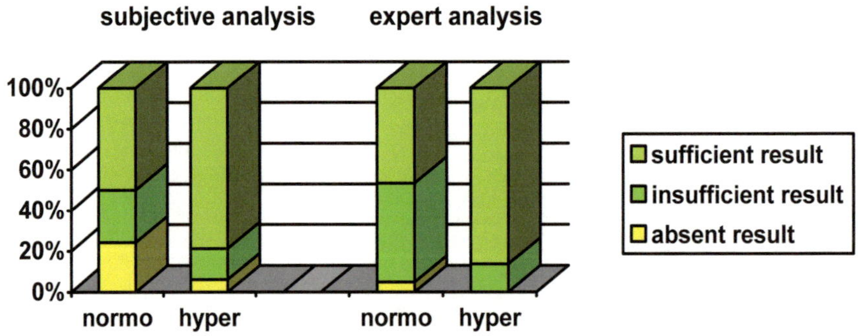

Fig. 22. Assessment of patients and expert jury according to the extent of surgical correction: normocorrection (normo) and hypercorrection (hyper)

5.9 Combinations with other interventions

The need of combinations with other surgical interventions is individual and it depends on the treated defect. Nevertheless an immediate combination with another surgical technique in the recipient site is not advised for increasing the chances of traumatism and graft lysis. On the other hand autologous fat grafting with execution of other interventions in adjacent regions such as augmentation of gluteus region with liposuction of thighs or lip augmentation with rhinoplasty was highly assessed by the patients (p<0,0001 (Fig.23)). The expert analysis showed no significant difference between the groups. These data are not informative for the efficiency of autologous fat transplantation as a surgical method but show that its combination sometimes could improve subjective results apprehension.

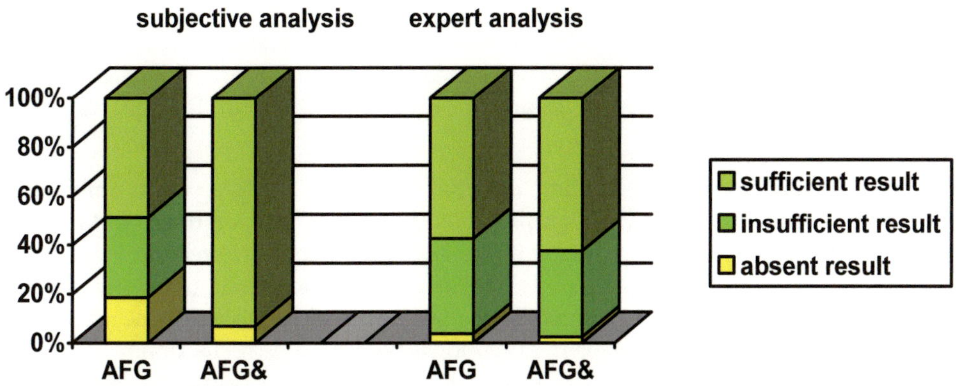

Fig. 23. Assessment of patients and expert jury according to the type of operation: autologous fat grafting (AFG) and autologous fat grafting in combination with other techniques in adjacent areas (AFG&)

6. Methods of outcomes assessing

The assessment of the postoperative results is closely related and dependent on the extent of graft survival. In general there are two theories about what happens in the recipient site after fat grafting: the theory of entire cell replacement by the host and the theory of adipocytes survival (Mojallal, 2003). According to the first one, which still has some followers, the induced volume augmentation in the recipient site is due to an entire phagocytosis of grafted cells and accumulation of phagocytes (Chajhir et al., 1990; Nguyen et al., 1990; Eremia, Newman, 2000; Sadick, Hudgins, 2001). The second theory states that the transplanted adipocytes survive and continue their development in the recipient site. Nowadays there are many researches in favor of this statement but the first and the most important one was published back in 1950 by L. Peer (Peer, 1956). The author described an autologous fat transplantation of grafts with different sizes in the rectus abdominis muscle area of 26 patients. The subsequent histological analysis discovered a periphery neovascularization starting at the fourth postoperative day and up to 50% of resorption to the end of the first year, more intensely expressed in the cases with bigger fragments transplantation. These findings were later supported by many experimental, biochemical and histological researches based on biopsies (Carpaneda, Ribeiro, 1993; 1994; Niechajev, Sevcuk, 1994; Jauffret, 1998; Moitra et al.,1998; Gavrilova et al., 2000; Rieck, Schlaak, 2003)

Unfortunately, since then there are not much more means of graft survival or results assessment. After the biopsy of the graft the most informative methods are the magnetic resonance imaging and the 3-D tomodensitometry of the recipient site pre and postoperatively but they are too expensive and not suitable for routine clinical practice (Horl et al., 1991; Liang et al, 1991; Har-Shai, 1999). Echography is not informative. Up to date the only approachable assessment method remains the standardized photo documentation.

After we summarized the experience of other authors we offer a protocol of results evaluation combining all known uninvasive methods. We suggest postoperative outcomes follow up in three stages:

- immediate - to the end of the first week,
- intermediate - between the 3d and 6th month, in which the results are still unstable and
- final - after the 9th month, after which according to literature the graft is steadily integrated (Horl et al., 1991; Carpaneda, Ribeiro, 1993) and further resorption is unexpected.

The follow up includes standardized photo documentation and filling up of specially designed protocols and patients' inquiries. Photographs should be taken preoperatively and in the three postoperative stages in same and as many as possible projections. We recommend a distance of 1 meter for the face and 2 meters for other regions. The protocols should be filled in by the operating surgeon and should record: personal data, indications, consecution of the intervention, combinations with other interventions, type of anesthesia, donor and recipient site, method of processing, harvested and grafted quantities, intraoperative extent of correction and complications as these two should be as well followed in the 3 postoperative periods. The patients' inquiries are not obligatory but very helpful for evaluating the subjective view of the postoperative period: donor or recipient site pain; any difficulties in social integration due to edema and ecchymoses and most importantly personal assessment of the results as sufficient, insufficient or absent. To avoid the subjectivity some surgeons are proposing a creation of an alternative jury for double blind assessing of the results.

7. Complications and disadvantages

Our practice showed that there are rarely any complications after application of autologous fat grafting (fig.24, 25). Among investigated cases complications in donor site were dependant on the aspirated quantity which sets the need for multiple donor sites planning if bigger amount of fat is needed.

Our investigation found out that the postoperative period is not painful in most cases and if it is there is a prevalence of the low intensity rates - 3,95±0,29 in recipient and 4,22±0,26 in donor site according to subjective pain assessment from 1 to 10.

Usually after autologous fat transplantation edema and ecchymoses of donor and recipient sites are observed. As the latter are almost always present they are considered as method's disadvantages. In the investigated cases edema was observed in 65,54% and ecchymoses in 20,95%. According to our patients the disadvantages were present for about one week and in most cases they did not interrupt their habits and social activity (fig.26).

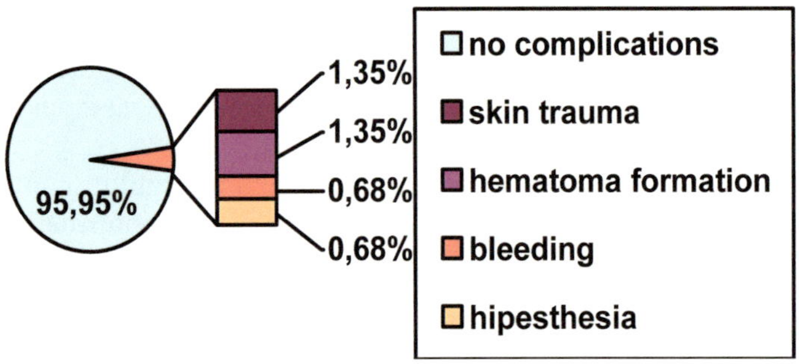

Fig. 24. Postoperative complications in donor site

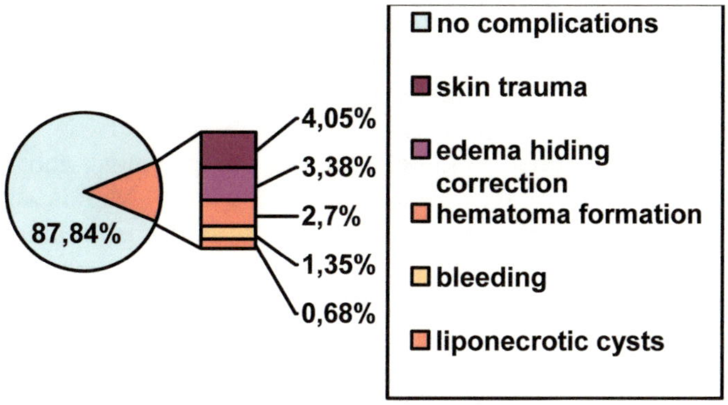

Fig. 25. Postoperative complications in recipient site

In conclusion we could say that the intervention is not painful and rarely leads to complications. It is well accepted by patients and does not require a long period of rehabilitation.

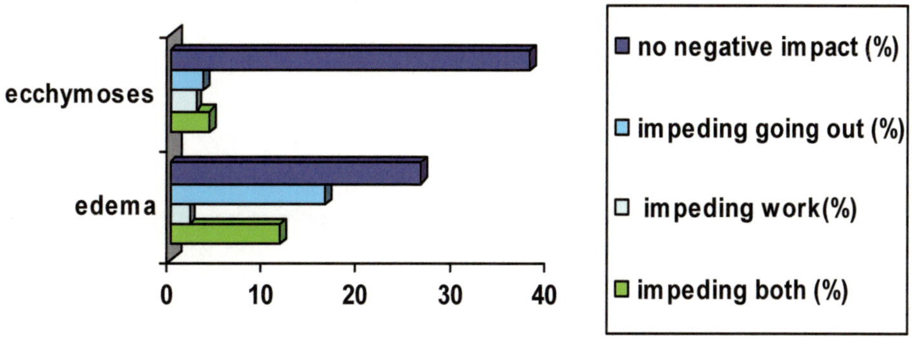

Fig. 26. Edema and ecchymoses impact on social activities. Data by patients' inquiry

Nevertheless there could be some complications due to a bad surgical technique such as:

- Graft migration - when applying big quantities in a cavity or in a manner different from the three-dimensional technique
- Skin irregularities or even necrosis in the cases of too superficial applications
- Liponecrotic cysts formation - when injecting big quantities unable of revascularization
- Infections
- Embolism after fat injection into vessels and so on

8. Perspectives

Nowadays, the growing knowledge on the complexity of adipose structure and functions revealed great potentials of influence on the therapeutic results. The contemporary strategies in autologous fat grafting improvement are concentrated on gaining presence of particular tissue structures in the graft (preadipocytes, etc), provoking different substances secretion or creation of methods for transplant enriching and thus improving the chances of its survival and integration.

It is now clear that fat tissue is a major endocrine and paracrine organ producing a variety of hormones and signalling molecules, generally referred to as adipokines (Mohamed-Ali et al., 1998; Fruhbeck et al., 2001; Chaldakov et al., 2003; Trayhurn, Wood, 2004). Among those is the nerve growth factor (NGF), recently proved to be synthesized in the main white adipose tissue depots by the stromo-vascular cell compartment and mature adipocytes (Peeraully et al., 2004; Ryan et al., 2008; Sornelli et al., 2009). NGF is a pentameric protein complex which neutrophic activities are mediated by the tyrosine kinase A (trkA) - high affinity receptor, specific for NGF and p75 - non-specific, low affinity receptor. Its expression in adipocytes is associated with wound healing and plasticity (Tore at al., 2007) and it exerts metabotrophic effect on glucose, lipid and energy homeostasis as well as antilipolytic, lipogenic and angiogenic effects (Emanueli et al., 2002; Hansen-Algensteadt et al., 2006). Moreover, NGF has an indirect effect on fat cells viability, proliferation and differentiation (Peeraully et al., 2004).

In our practice the expression and cellular localization of nerve growth factor and its' receptors - trkA and p75 was investigated in non centrifuged adipose grafts in view of potential possibilities for influence on outcomes. Immunohistochemical investigations demonstrated a moderate positive expression of NGF in both types of adipose cells (mature and immature) and a much stronger expression of the trkA receptor with higher intensity in the preadipocytes (fig.27 - A, B). No expression of p75 was detected.

In future these findings could influence upon the strategies of outcomes improvement as the mechanisms of NGF expression and secretion regulation are already known.

Our investigations also pose some questions on postoperative graft intake. For example, it would be interesting to know to what extent the neutrophin is involved with postoperative swelling after autologous fat grafting. In 1995 Amman et al. proved that local injection of NGF in rat's paw causes oedema and hyperalgesia (Amman et al., 1995). In the same time the widely used in clinical practice low temperature and glucocorticoids for their anti-edematous effects are known to decrease the neutrophin's release. Another question which answers would also need further investigations is related to the expected postoperative outcomes after autologous fat grafting in patients with altered levels of NGF as in obesity or type 2 diabetes.

The determination of all those issues could bring to a new era for fat grafting strategies

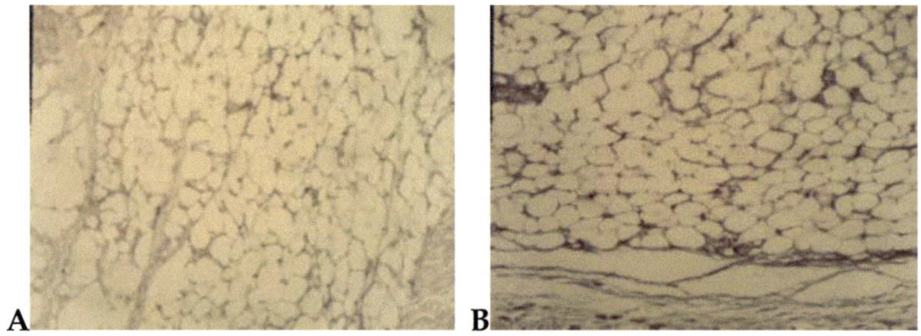

Fig. 27. Immunohistochemical analysis of NGF (A) and trkA (B) in non centruged fat grafts - ABC method with primary antibodies (Santa Cruz, USA) in dilution 1:200: A -moderate positive expression of NGF in both types of adipose cells (mature and immature); B - A much stronger expression of the trkA receptor with higher intensity in the preadipocytes

9. References

Amann R, Schuligoi R, Herzeg G, Donnerer J (1995) Intraplantar injection of nerve growth factor into the rat hind paw: local edema and effects on thermal nociceptive threshold. *Pain* 64: 323-329

Amar R.E. (1999) Microinfiltration adipocytaire (MIA) au niveau de la face, ou restructuration tissulaire par greffe de tissu adipeux. *Ann. Chir. Plast. Esthét* 44(6): 593-608

Ashjilian P.H, De Ugarte D.A, Katz A.J, Hedrick M.H. (2002) Lipoplasty: From body countouring to tissue engineering. *Aesthetic Surg J* 22: 121-127

Asken S. (1987) Autologous fat transplantation: micro and macro techniques. *Am J. Cosm. Surg.*, 4: 111-121

Atanassova P, Popova E (2000) Leptin expression during the differentiation of subcutaneous adipose cells of human embryos in situ. *Cells Tissue Organs 166: 15-19*

Atanassova P. (1996) Immunohistochemical expressionof the protein of the ob-gene, leptin, during early human embryogenesis. *Annals of anatomy. Supplementheft zum 183. Band des Anatomischen Anzeiger.*: 74

Atanassova Pepa (2000) Hystiogenesis and differentiation of subcutaneous adipose cells in human early embriogenesis in situ. Thesis for conferring a PhD title in medicine, Medical University of Plovdiv, Bulgaria

Bames HO. (1953) Augmentation mammaplasty by lipotransplant *Plast Recons Surg*; 11: 404

Bertossi D, Kharouf S, D'Agostino A, Fior A, Bedogni A, Zancanaro C. (2000) Facial localize cosmetic filling by multiple injections of fat stored at –30 degrees C. Techniques clinical follow-up of 99 patients and histological examination of ten patients. *Ann Chir Plast Estet*, 45: 548 - 555

Billings E Jr, May JW Jr (1989) Historical review and present status of free fat graft autotransplantation in plastic and reconstructive surgery. *Plast Reconstr Surg* 83:368–381

Billings E Jr, May JW Jr. (1989) Historical review and present status of free fat graft autotransplantation in plastic and reconstructive surgery. *Plast Reconstr Surg*; 83: 368-81

Bircoll M. (1987) Cosmetic Beast Augmentation Utilizing Autologous fat and liposuction techniques *Plast Reconst. Surg*. 79: 267-271

Bircoll M., Novack B.H. (1987) Autologous fat transplantation with liposuction techniques. *Ann of Plast. Surg*. 18(4): 361-2

Boschert MT, Beckert BW, Puckett CL, Concannon MJ. (2002) Analysis of lipocyte viability after liposuction. *Plast Reconstr Surg* 109: 761 -6

Brunning P. (1919) Contribution à l'étude des greffes adipeuses. *BullMémAcadRMéd Belg*; 28: 440

Carpaneda CA, Ribeiro MT. (1994) Percentage of graft viability versus injected volume in adipose autotransplants. *Aesthetic Plast Surg* 18: 17-19

Carpaneda CA, Ribeiro MT. (1993) Study of the histologic alterations and viability of the adipose graft in humans. *Aesthetic Plast Surg* 17: 43-47

Carraway J.H., Mellow C.G. (1990) Syringe aspiration and fat concentration: a simple technique for autologous fat injection. *Ann. Plast. Surg*. 24: 293-296

Casteilla L, Charriere G, Laharrague P, Cousin B, Planat-Benard V, Pericaud L, Chavoin J.P. (2004) Adipose tissue, plastic and reconstructive surgery: come back to sources *Ann Chir Plast Esthet* 49: 409-418

Chajhir A., Benzaquen I. (1989) Fat grafting injection for soft tissue augmentation. *Plast. Reconst. Surg* 84(6): 921-934

Chajhir A., Benzaquen I., Wexler E., Arellano A. (1990) Fat injection. *Aesth. Plast. Surg.* 14: 127-316

Chaldakov G, Stankulov I, Hristova M, and Ghenev P (2003) Adipobiology of disease: adipokines and adipokine-targeted pharmacology. *Curr Pharm Des* 9: 1023–1031

Chaldakov G, Tonchev A, Tunsel N, Atanassova P, Aloe L. (2006) dipose tissue and mast cells. Adipokines as yin-yang modulators of inflammation. Nutrition and health: Adipose tissue and adipokines in health and disease, edited by G. Fantuzzi and T. Mazzoni, *Humana Press Inc., Totowa, NJ* (12): 147-154

Cinti S, Frederich RC, Zingaretti MC, De Matteis R, Flier JS, Lowell BB. (1997) Immunohistochemical localization of leptin and uncoupling protein in white and brown adipose tissue. *Endocrinology* 138: 797-804

Coleman S.R. (1994) Lipoinfiltration in the upper lip white roll. *Aesth. Surg.* 14: 231-234

Coleman S.R. (1995) Long term survival of fat transplants: Controlled Demonstrations. *Aesth. Plast. Surg.* 19: 421-425

Coleman S.R. (2001) Structural fat grafts: the ideal filler? *Clin. Plast. Surg.*, 28: 111-119

Coleman WP. (1999) Fat transplantation. *Dermatol Clin* 17:891-898

Colic M. (1999) Lip and Perioral Enhancement by Direct Intramuscular Fat Autografting *Aesth. Plast. Surg.* 23: 36–40

Czerny V. (1895) Plasticher Ersatz der Brustdrüse durch ein lipom. *Zentralb Chir* 27: 72

Delay E., Garson S, Toussoun G, Sinna R. (2009) Fat injection to the breast: technique, results, and indications based on 880 procedures over 10 years. *Aesth Surg Journal* 29: 360-76.

Dugail I, Ferre P. (2002) Développement du tissu adipeux. *Encycl Méd Chir 2002; (Elsevier SAS, Paris), Endocrinologie- Nutrition*, 10-506-A-10, 8

Ellenbongen R. (1986) Free autologous pearl fat graft in the face - a preliminary report of a rediscovered technique. *Ann. Plast. Surg.* 16: 179-194

Emanueli C, Salis M, Pinna A, Graiani G, Manni L, Madeddu P (2002) Nerve Growth Factor Promotes Angiogenesis and Arteriogenesis in Ischemic Hindlimbs. *Circulation* 106 (17): 2257-2262

Eremia S, Newman N. (2000) Long term follow-up after autologous fat grafting: analysis of results from 116 patients followed at least 12 months after receiving the last of a minimum of two treatments. *Dermatol. Surg* 26: 1150-1158

Ersek R.A. (1991) Transplantation of purified autologous fat: a 3-year follow-up is disappointing. *Plast. Reconst. Surg.* 87: 219-228

Ersek R.A., Chang P., Salisbury M.A. (1998) Lipo layering of autologous fat: an improved technique with promising results. *Plast. Reconst. Surg.*, 101(3): 820-826

Fournier P. (1996) Liposculpture: *Ma technique. (2eme edition) Paris, Arnette*

Fruhbeck G, Gomez-Ambrosi J, Muruzabal FJ, and Burrell MA (2001) The adipocyte: a model for integration of endocrine and metabolic signaling in energy metabolism regulation. *Am J Physiol Endocrinol Metab* 280: 827–847

Fulton JE, Suarez M, Silverton K, Barnes T. (1998) Small volume fat transfer *Dermatol Surg* 24:857-865

Gavrilova O, Marcus-Samuels B, Graham D, Kim JK, Shulman GI, Castle AL (2000) Surgical implantation of adipose tissue reverses diabetes in lipoatrophic mice. *J Clin Invest;* 105: 271-278

Gradinger G.P. (1987) Breast augmentation by autologous fat injection (correspondence). *Plast. Reconst. Surg* 80(6): 868

Guerrerosantos J. (1996) Autologous fat grafting for body contouring. *Clin. Plast. Surg* 23: 619-631.

Guerrerosantos J. (2000) Long-term outcome of autologous fat transplantation in aesthetic facial recontouring: sixteen years of experiencewith 1936 cases. *Clin Plast Surg* 27:515-544

Hansen-Algensteadt N, Algensteadt P, Schaefer C, Hamann A, Wolfram L, Cingoz G, Kilic N, Schwarzloh B, Schroeder M, Joescheck C, Wiesner L, Ruther W, Ergun S (2006) Neural driven angiogenesis by overexpression of nerve growth factor *Histochem Cell Biol* 125: 637-649

Har-Shai Y. (1999) An integrated approach for increasing the survival of autologous fat grafts in the treatment of contour defects. *Plast. Reconstr. Surg* 104: 945-954

Hartrampf C.R., Bennett G.K. (1987) Autologous fat from liposuction for breast augmentation (correspondence). *Plast. Reconst. Surg* 80(4): 646

Horl HW, Feller AM, Biemer E. (1991)Technique for liposuction fat reimplantation and long-term volume evaluation by magnetic resonance imaging. *Ann Plast Surg* 26:248-258

Hudson DA, Lambert EV, Bloch CE. (1990) Site selection for fat autotransplantation: some observation. *Aesth Plast Surg* 14:195-197

Illouz Y.G. (1988) Present results of fat injection. *Aesth. Plast. Surg* 12: 175-181

Illouz Y.G. (1986) The fat cell graft: a new technique to fill depressions. *Plast. Reconstr. Surg* 78: 122-123

Illouz Y.G. (1985) Utilisation de la graisse aspire pour combler les defects cutanes. Revue de chirurgie esthetique de langue francaise. 40(10): 13-20

Jackson I. (2001) A successful long-term method of fat grafting: Recontouring of a large subcutaneous postradiation thigh defect with autologous fat transplantation. *Aesth Plast Surg* 25: 165-169

Jauffret J.L. (1998) Utilisation de la graisse autologue en chirurgie plastique et esthétique : la technique de S.R. Coleman. Thèse de Doctorat d'Etat en Médecine, Universite de la Mediterrannee, Faculte de Medecine de Marseille, Marseille

Jauffret JL, Champsaur P, Robaglia-Schlupp A, Andrac-Meyer L,Magalon G (2001) Arguments in favor of adipocyte grafts with the S.R. Coleman technique. *Ann Chir Plast Esthe´t* 46:31–38; in French

Khater R, Atanassova P, Anastassov Y, Pellerin P, Martinot-Duquennoy V (2008). Clinical and experimental study of autologous fat grafting after processing by centrifugation and serum lavage *Aesth Plast Surg* 33: 37-43 (1)

Khater R. (2010) Autologous fat transplantation - clinical and experimental researches. Thesis for conferring a PhD title in medicine, Medical University of Plovdiv, Bulgaria

Khouri, RK, Schlenz, I, Murphy, BJ, Baker, TJ. (2000) Nonsurgical breast enlargement using an external soft tissue expansion system. *Plast Reconstr Surg* 105: 2500-2514

Klein S, Coppack SW, Mohamed-Ali V, Landt M. (1996) Adipose tissue leptin production and plasma leptin kineticks in humans. *Diabetes* 45: 984-987

Lafontan M, Bouloumie A. (1999) Angiogenèse : une implication physiologique de plus pour la leptine. *Méd/Sci* 15: 382-1185

Lalikos JF, Li YQ, Roth TP, Doyle JW, Matory WE, Lawrence WT (1997) Biochemical assessment of cellular damage after adipocyte harvest. *J Surg Res* 70:95–100

Laurent F., Capon-Dégardin N., Martinot-Duquennoy V., Dhellèmmes P., Pellerin P. (2006) Intérêt du lipofilling dans le traitement des séquellesde chirurgie des craniosténoses *Ann. Chir. Plast. Esthét.* 23-28

Lexer E. (1910) Freie Fett transplantation. *Dtsch Med.Wochenschr*; 36: 640

Liang MD, Narayanan K, Davis PL, Futrell JW. (1991) Evaluation of facial fat distribution using magnetic resonance imaging. *Aesthetic Plast Surg* 15: 313-319

MacRae J.W., Tholpady S.S., Katz A.J., Gampper T.G., Drake D.B., Ogle R.C., Morgan R.F. (2003) Human adipocyte viability testing: a new assay *Aesth. Surg. J* 23:265-269

Markman B. (1989) Anatomy and physiology of adipose tissue. *Clin Plast Surg*; 16: 235-241

Marques A, Brenda E, Saldiva PH, Amarante MT, Ferreire MC. (1994) Autologous fat grafts. A quantitative and morphometric study in rats. *Scand J Plast Reconstr Surg Hand Surg* 28:241-247

Mohamed-Ali V, Pinkney JH, and Coppack SW. (1998). Adipose tissue as an endocrine and paracrine organ. *Int J Obes* 22: 1145–1158

Moitra J, Mason MM, Olive M, Krylov D, Gavrilova O, Marcus-Samuels B et al. (1998) Life without white fat: a transgenic mouse. *Genes Dev* 12: 3168-3172

Mojallal A, Breton P, Delay E, Foyatier J-L (2004) Greffe d'adipocytes: applications en chirurgie plastique et esthetique. Encyclopedie Medico-Chirurgicale: Techniques chirurgicales, 1st edn. Elsevier SAS, Amsterdam

Mojallal A, Foyatier JL (2004) The effect of different factors on the survival of transplanted adipocytes. *Ann Chir Plast Esthe´t* 49:426–436; in French

Mojallal A. (2003) Greffe d'adipocytes. Interet dans la restauration des volumes de la face – a propos de 100 cas. Thèse de Doctorat d'Etat en Médecine, Universite Claude Bernard Lyon I, Faculte de Medecine Lyon-Sud, Lyon

Mojallal A., Foyatier J.L (2004) Historique de l'utilisation du tissu adipeux comme produit de comblement en chirurgie plastique. *Ann chir plast esthet* 49: 419-425

Montague CT, Farooqi IS, Whitehead JP, Soos MA, Rau H, Wareham NJ (1997) Congenital leptin deficiency is associated with severe early-onset obesity in humans. *Nature*; 387: 903-907

Moore JH Jr, Kolaczynski JW, Morales LM, Considine RV, Pietrzkowski Z, Noto PF (1995) Viability of fat obtained by syringe suction lipectomy: effects of local anesthesia with lidocaine. *Aesthetic Plast Surg* 19: 335–339

Neuber GA (1893) Fettransplantation. Chir Kongr Verhandl Dtsch Gesellsch Chir 22:66

Nguyen A, Pasyk KA, Bouvier TN, Hassett CA, Argenta LC. (1990) Comparative study of survival of autologous adipose tissue taken and transplanted by different techniques. *Plast Reconstr Surg* 85: 378-387

Niechajev I, Sevcuk O (1994) Long-term results of fat transplantation: clinical and histologic studies. *Plast Reconstr Surg* 94: 496–506

Novaes F, Reis N, Baroudi R (1998) Counting method of live fat cells used in lipoinjection procedures. *Aesthetic Plast Surg* 22:12–15

Ousterhout D.K. (1987) Breast augmentation by autologous fat injection (correspondence). *Plast. Reconst. Surg.* 80(6): 868

Peer L.A. (1956) The neglected free fat graft *Plast Reconstr. Surg* 18: 234-250

Peeraully M.R, Jenkins J.R, Trayhurn P (2004). NGF gene expression and secretion in white adipose tissue: regulation in 3T3-L1 adipocytes by hormones and inflammatory cytokines. *Am J Physiol Endocrinol Metab* 287: 331-339

Pinski KS, Roenigk HH. (1992) Autologous fat transplantation: long tern follow-up. *J Dermatol Surg Oncol* 18:179-184

Rieck B, Schlaak S. (2003) Measurement in vivo of the survival rate in autologous adipocyte transplantation. *Plast Reconstr Surg* 111 (7): 2315-2323

Ryan TJ, Curri SB. (1989) The cutaneous adipose tissue. *Clin Dermatol* 7: 37-47

Ryan V.H, German A.J, Wood I.S, Morris P, Trayhurn P (2008) NGF gene expression and secretion by canine adipocytes in primary culture: upregulation by the inflammatory mediators LPS and TNF-α. *Horm Metab Res* 40:1-8

Sadick NS, Hudgins LC. (2001) Fatty acid analysis of transplanted adipose tissue. *Arch Dermatol*; 137: 723-727

Scholler T, Lille S, Wechselberger G, Otto A, Mowlawi A, Pizza-Katzer H. (2001) Histomorphologic and volumetric analysis of implanted autologous preadipocyte cultures suspended in fibrin glue: A potential new source for tissue augmentation. *Aesth Plast Surg*, 25: 57-63

Schrocher F. (1957) Fettgewebsverpflanzung bei zu kleiner Brust. *Munschen Med Wochenschr*; 99: 489

Shiffman MA, Mirrafati S (2001) Fat transfer techniques: the effect of harvest and transfer methods on adipocyte viability and review of the literature. *Dermatol Surg* 27:819–826

Smith P, Adams W.P, Lipschits A.H, Chau B, Sorokin E, Rohrich R.J, Brown S.A. (2006) Autologous human fat grafting: effect of harvesting and preparation techniques on adipocyte graft survival *Plast. Reconstr. Surg* 117: 1836-1844

Sornelli F, Fiore M, Chaldakov G, Aloe L (2009). Adipose tissue-derived nerve growth factor and brain-derived neutrophic factor: results from experimental stress and diabetes. *Gen. Physiol. Biophys* 28: 179-183

Stampos M., Xepoulias P. (2001) Fat Transplantation for Soft Tissue Augmentation in the Lower Limbs. *Aesth. Plast. Surg.* 25: 256–261

Teimourian B. (1986) Repair of soft-tissue contour deficit by means of semiliquid fat graft. *Plast. Reconstr. Surg* 78: 123-124

Toledo L. S. (1991) Syringe liposculpture: A 2 year experience. *Aesth. Plast. Surg* 15: 321-326

Tore F, Tonchev A.B, Fiore M, Tuncel N, Atanassova P, Aloe L, Chaldakov G.N. (2007) From adipose tissue protein secretion to adipopharmacology of disease. *Immun., Endoc. & Metab. Agents in Med. Chem., Bentham Science Publishers Ltd.* (7): 1871-5222

Trayhurn P and Wood S (2004) Adipokines: inflammation and the pleiotropic role of white adipose tissue. *Br J. Nutr* 92: 347-355

Trepsat F. (2001) Volumetric face lifting. *Plast. Reconstr. Surg* 108: 1358-1371

Van RL, Roncari DA. (1982) Complete differentiation in vivo of implanted cultured adipocyte precursors from adult rats. *Cell Tissue Res* 225: 557

Van RL, Roncari DA. (1977) Isolation of fat cell precursors from adult rat adipose tissue. *Cell Tissue Res* 181:197-201

Zhang Y, Proenca R, Maffei M, Barone M, Leopold L, Friedman (1994) Positional cloning of the mouse obese gene and its human homologue *J.M. Nature*, 372-425

11

Importance of Anatomical Landmarks on Axillary Neurovascular Territories for Surgery

Nuket Gocmen Mas[1], Hamit Selim Karabekir[2],
Mete Edizer[1] and Orhan Magden[1]
[1]*Department of Anatomy, Faculty of Medicine, Dokuz Eylul University, Izmir,*
[2]*Department of Neurosurgery, Faculty of Medicine, Afyon Kocatepe University, Afyonkarahisar, Turkey*

1. Introduction

The anatomy of axillary neurovascular architechture is very important for neurosurgeon, plastic and cardiovascular surgeons, and also radiologists to aid in diagnosis, treatment and planning surgical procedure. Walsh and Willar were firstly described brachial plexus (BP) anatomy in details from 1877 (Akboru et al, 2010). After rapid development of microsurgical approaches, variations and injuries of the plexus, their diagnosis and treatment were searched by many authors. Inspite of the belief that BP malformations together with the vascular malformations, variations of BP may be encountered without arterial or venous abnormalities. Variations of axillary vessels and BP are of importance for clinicians either the diagnostic interventions or the surgical applications. The knowledge of the anatomical variations of the vascular and BP can help to give explanation when encountering incomprehensible and extraordinary clinical signs. While planning flap surgery, the surface landmarks on axillary skin area and variations of the neurovasculatures are of significance for surgeons. Iatrogenic BP injuries have been reported during infraclavicular and transaxillary biopsy, general anesthesia and resection of space occupying lesions in axillary region. Cause of iatrogenic injuries include needle trauma and haematoma during central venous catheterization due to neural ischaemia may be encountered. The vein catheterization is more likely with multiple needle passes and generally affects BP (Zhang et al, 2011).

Anatomical knowledge on peripheric nerves position of cords of BP is also important in order to prevent an iatrogenic nerve injury during traumatic lesions of humerus, postoperatively. In literature, limited cadaveric data revealed a close relationship between inserted screws which are used in fractures of the humerus and anatomical nerves direction is present (Ligsters et al 2008). The diagnosis and advanced surgical methods were described as neurolysis, nerve transfers and vascularized or non-vascularized nerve grafts combined with local and free muscle transfers for reanimation of the upper extremity and the axillary region in plexopathy cases with regaining functional outcomes.

2. Anatomy of axillary region

Anatomically, the axilla is a space between the medial side of the upper extremity and the lateral aspect of the chest wall. Many major neurovascular structures pass between the thorax and upper limb via the space (Standring et al., 2005, Moore & Dalley 1999). The usual anatomy of the axilla is clearly well-known to all operators, hovewer, anatomical variations of the region are not well defined, though they are neither uncommon nor few. Classically, the axilla covers the lateral branches of some intercostal nerves, the neurovascular structures such as axillary vein, artery and their branches, the infraclavicular part of BP and its pheripheric branches, loose adipose areolar connective tissue, some lymph nodes and vessels, and sometimes the axillary tail of the breast (Natsis et al, 2010).

Its appearance is such like a pyramid. Its obtused apex runs into the root of the neck which is called cervico-axillary canal (Standring et al, 2005). The apex is circumscribed by the first rib, the scapula and the clavicle. The anterior wall limits the pectoralis major and minor muscles. The posterior wall overlies the subscapular muscles. The margin of the medial wall is the serratus anterior muscle. The lateral wall is narrow and formed by the intertubercular groove. The base overlies fascia of the axillary fossa and the skin. The posterior borders are the latissimus dorsi and subscapularis muscles, the medial boundry is the serratus anterior muscle and the anterior border is the pectoralis major and also lateral boundries are the fascia of the axilla, chest wall and humerus. In literature there are some anomalies on the axillary components. The most encountered variation on the axillary region is localization anomaly of axillary arch. For instance, as a variant, the arch may originate from lateral margin of the latissimus dorsi, lying across the axilla, and inserting into tendon of the pectoralis major muscle nearby its humeral insertion point. Occasionally, variations are also defined in the literature (McWhirter & Malyon 2008). In classical anatomy texts described on the axillary arches inserting into the long head of the triceps muscle or the medial intramuscular septum of the arm. The axillary arch does not show large significance in clinically. When removing an axillary node, the presence of an axillary arch may confuse the normal anatomical structure. As a mistake the arch for the free margin of the latissimus dorsi muscle can give rise to the operator to dissect along the arch rather than the muscle in a more proximal manner instead of usual application (Bartlett et al, 1981). The major risk of unwitting injury to the BP and axillary vein may also cause an incomplete removing of nodes, so the surgeons might be more superordinate in the axilla. If an axillary arch is represented during a breast reconstructive surgery using a latissimus dorsi flap, it may need to be seperated in the axilla because of causing a compression of the vascular pedicle leading to failure of the flap (Kayvan et al, 2008; Bartlett et al, 1981).

The axilla includes many neurovasculature and important structures of the region. The axillary artery which is begin as a continuation of the subclavian artery, when it pass under the first rib's outer margin, ending point is nominally at the inferior border of the teres major where it is called as the brachial artery (Fig 1). It placed on deep to infraclavicular part of the BP. During dissection, the axillary vein takes place approximately 1 cm cranial direction from the lateral margin of the latissimus dorsi muscle. The inferolateral part of the clavipectoral fascia at the upper extent of the area is readily represented. When it is removed and the underlying fat gently send away, the blue hue of the axillary vein can be seen easily. Mostly, two axillary veins are identified (Ung et al, 2006).

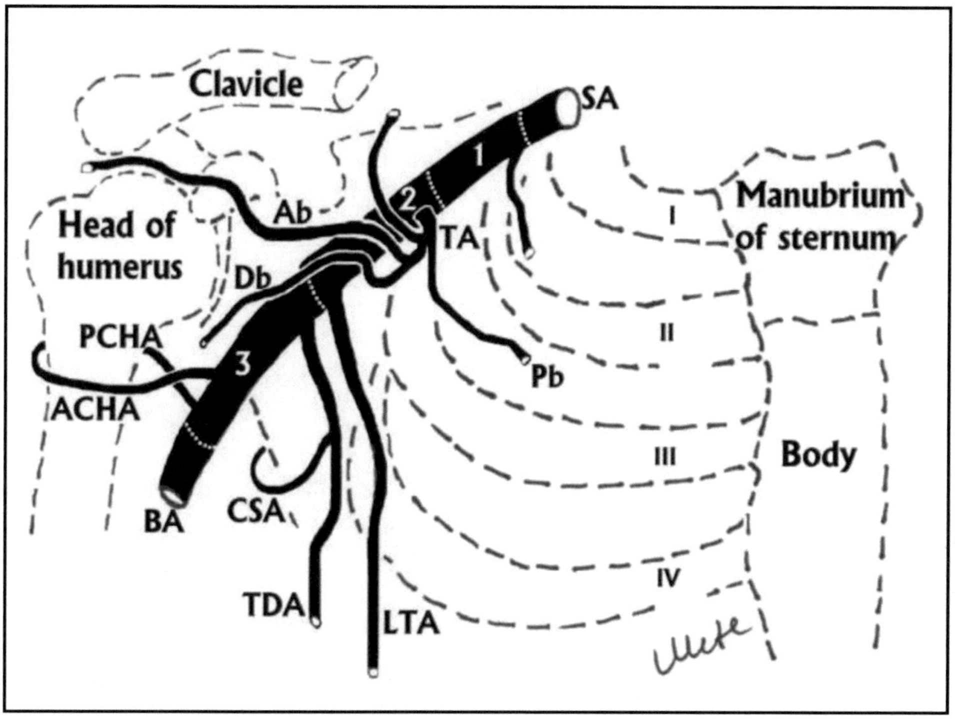

Fig. 1. The subclavian artery and its branches have been demonstrated. (SA: Subclavian artery, STA: Superior thoracic artery, TA: Thoracoacromial artery, PB: Pectoral branch of thoracoacromial artery, AB: Acromial branch of thoracoacromial artery, DB: Deltoid branch of thoracoacromial artery, LTA: Lateral thoracic artery, TDA: Thoracodorsal artery, CSA: Circumflex humeral artery, BA: Brachial artery, ACHA: Anterior circumflex humeral artery PCHA: Posterior circumflex humeral artery, 1: First part of axillary artery, 2: Second part of axillary artery, 3: Third part of axillary artery, I, I, III, IV have been indicated the first, the second, the third and the fourth costae) [Illustrated by Asc.Prof.Edizer M.].

A typical brief definition of the BP is usually found in classical anatomy textbooks as follows: The BP composed of the anterior primary rami of C4 through T1 spinal nerves. Each root which innervates a particular myotome and dermatome represent the anterior primary rami of the spinal nerve. The roots placed between the anterior and middle scalene muscles. The roots are come together and then form the trunks in the posterior cervical triangle. As posteriorly and anteriorly divisions are formed by bifurcation of the trunks deep to the clavicle. Primitive posterior musculature like extensor muscles are innervated by the posterior divisions of the trunks. The primitive anterior musculature like the flexor muscles are also innervated by the anterior divisions. The anterior or the posterior divisions come together and form cords. The cords placed on the axillary region beneath the pectoralis minor muscle and neighbouring of the axillary artery. The lateral cord which derived C4-C7, is composed of the joining of the anterior divisions of the upper and middle trunks and is called for its localization according to the axillary artery. The lateral pectoral nerve (C5-C7), the musculocutaneous nerve (C4-C6) and lateral cord of the median nerve (C5-C7) derive from the lateral cord of BP. The medial cord (C8-T1) is continuation as anterior division of the lower trunk and is called for its localization according to the axillary artery. The medial pectoral nerve (C8-T1), the medial cord of the median nerve (C6-C8), the ulnar nerve (C8-T1), the medial antebrachial cutaneous nerve (C8-T1) and the medial brachial cutaneous nerve (T1) are derived from the medial cord of BP. The posterior cord which is composed of the fusion of the posterior divisions of the upper, middle and lower trunks, is also called for its localization according to the axillary artery. The upper subscapular (C5-C6), the middle subscapular (thoracodorsal) (C6-C8), the lower subscapular (C5-C6), the axillary (C5-C6) and the radial (C5-T1) nerves come from the posterior trunk of BP (Fig 2).

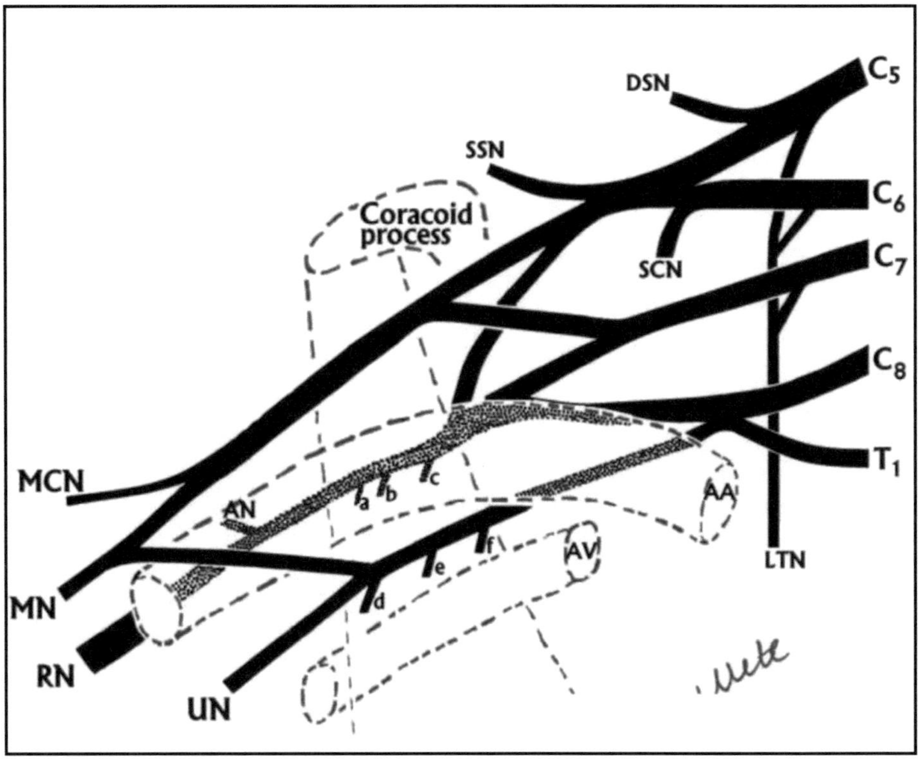

Fig. 2. The brachial plexus and the peripheral nerves have been demonstrated (The pectoralis minor muscle which is originated from the coracoid process has been shown as projection by dotted line. AA: Axillary artery, AV: Axillary vein, DSN: Dorsal scapular nerve, SSN: Suprascapular nerve, SCN: Subclavius nerve, MCN: Musculocutaneous nerve, MN: Median nerve, RN: Radial nerve, AN: Axillary nerve, UN: Ulnar nerve, LTN: Long thoracic nerve, a: Inferior subscapular nerve, b: Thoracodorsal nerve, c: Superior subscapular nerve, d: Medial cutaneous nerve of forearm, e: Medial cutaneous nerve of arm, f: Superior subscapular nerve) [Illustrated by Asc.Prof. Edizer M.].

Infraclavicular part of BP has complex structure in axillary region. There are many investigations on some variations in nerve contributions to the BP and vasculature of the axillary region in literature (Loukas et al, 2010; Shaw et al, 1995). Understanding the variations in the nerve distributions of the BP may assist both anatomists and surgeons for analysis of normal anatomy, diagnosis and application of clinical conditions that involve the BP (Fig 3).

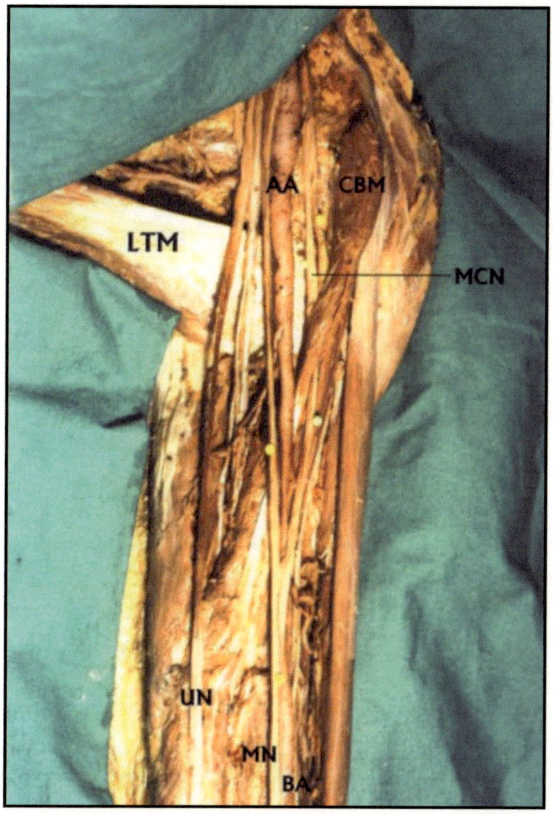

Fig. 3. The axillary region and the peripheral nerves which are originated from the brachial plexus have been shown on a cadaver (LTM: Latissimus dorsi muscle, AA: Axillary artery, BA: Brachial artery, UN: Ulnar nerve, MN: Median nerve, MCN: Musculocutaneous nerve, CBM: Coracobrachialis muscle) [From the archive records of Prof. Magden O].

Relations with BP and the adjacent structures of the axillary region are also important for clinicians. Many diagnostic and therapeutic invasive application like angiographic procedures on the axillary artery and vein, ligation of traumatic vessels and repairing damaged nerves due to trauma, and also surgical or radiological interventions on aneurysms and/or arteriovenous malformations are applied on the axillary region. It is also significant to avoid potential BP or vascular injuries during flap surgery (Shaw et al, 1995). Critical and usual architecture should represent in axillary region, and their relations with various anatomical landmarks should identify for safety surgical interventions. Many flaps which are named external mammary, thoracodorsal, superficial thoracic, lateral thoracic and axillary flaps, have been practically displayed from the axillary region and the lateral chest wall. They divide into mainly two groups. The first groups are predicated on the lateral thoracic and superficial thoracic arteries. The second groups are also based on a cutaneous branch of the thoracodorsal artery (Fig 4). Evidently potential flaps which include both vessels and flaps compose varying parts of latissimus dorsi muscle and its overlying skin based on the thoracodorsal artery, particularly perforators of the musculocutaneous. The blood source of the pectoralis major muscle is the branches of the superficial thoracic and the lateral thoracic arteries (Kim et al, 2011).

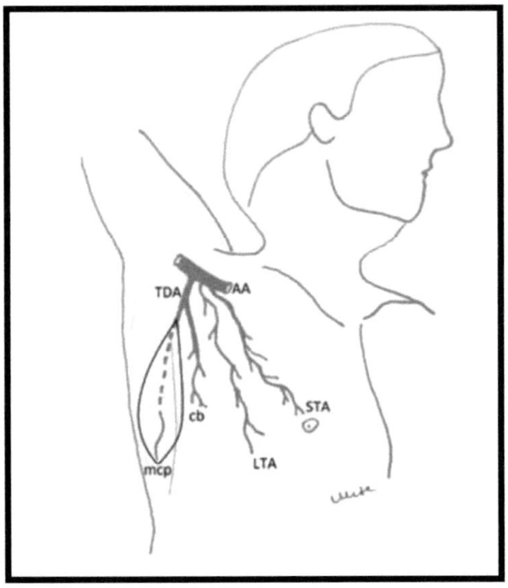

Fig. 4. Vascular anatomy of axillary flap. A schematic representation of the blood supply to the axilla and lateral chest wall in which all the possible vessels which may supply skin in this area are known. AA: Axillary artery, TDA: Thoracodorsal artery, mcp: musculocutaneous perforators of thoracodorsal artery, cb: cutaneous branch , LTA: Lateral thoracic artery, STA: Superficial thoracic artery [Illustrated by Asc.Prof.Edizer M].

3. Variation of vascular and neural territories on axillary region

Variations of BP have been displayed either in cadaver dissections or in clinical cases. Studies on the BP anatomy was firstly described by Walsh (1877), Willar (1888), Franz (1889) and Harris (1904). After developments on microsurgical techniques, BP variations, injuries, their diagnosis and treatment were well-described by the authors. In the light of these developments inspite of the belief that BP malformations together with the arterial and venous malformations, variations of BP can be seen without vascular abnormalities. Variations are commonly seen as attaching or detaching of contributional complements.

Several studies try to clarify the spatial relations of BP with its adjacent structures such as nerves, bones, arteries and veins and to find out the best way of surgery without complications (Akboru et al, 2010).

Variations in the architecture of the BP have often been displayed, and terms such as supraclavicular and infraclavicular, high and low, or prefixed and postfixed have been used to refer on the nerve composition of the BP (Kerr, 1918). The anatomy of the BP can create confusion, particularly due to common variations in length and size of each of its elements (Leinberry et al, 2004).

The branching pattern of the BP shows significant variations. Bilateral variations in the structure and branching of the BP are immensely uncommon (Aggarwal et al, 2009; Goyal et al, 2005). Variant BP architecture with two trunks and two cords is also rare. A unilateral variation in the formation of the BP accompanied by unusual positional relationship with the axillary artery was well defined in literature. Second part of axillary artery was determined lying inferomedial to the BP instead of passing between medial and lateral cords. In literature there was some authors observed branching pattern of the subscapular, lateral thoracic, and posterior circumflex humeral arteries, as well as those branches' topographic relationships to the two terminal branches of the posterior cord of the BP (Olinger & Benninger, 2010).

Generally, the variations in formation, location, and courses of cords of the BP are defined in literature. These variations are divided into three groups. The first group is abnormal location of the cords. The second group is absence of the posterior cord. The third group is abnormal formation and course of the median nerve. As a variation, Pandey et al (2007) declarated absence of the posterior cord in their series and they defined the lateral cord and the medial root of the median nerve had received communicating branches from the posterior cord. However, as a rare variation, absence of the musculocutaneous nerve can be encountered (Song et al, 2003; Gumusburun et al, 2000). A rare constellation of multiple upper limb anomalies were declerated by Wadhwa et al in 2008. Variations in the branching pattern of the posterior cord are clinically important. This knowledge may help the anesthesiologists and the surgeons during operation. It is also significant for avoiding unexpanded injury of the nerves and the axillary artery during blocks, interpreting effects of nervous compressions, while repairing of the plexus injuries and other surgical procedures (Aggarwal et al, 2010; Muthoka et al, 2011; Johnson et al, 2010).

Iatrogenic BP damages have been shown during infraclavicular and transaxillary biopsy, general anesthesia and resection of tumours in axillary region. An ulnar nerve pressure palsy which is the most frequent positioning damage under general anaesthesia, may occure because of malpositioning of the patient. Cause of the damage may include needle trauma and haematoma during central venous catheterization due to neural ischaemia. The vein catheterization with multiple needle passes generally affects BP. Some damages, such as those correlated with uncommon variations, may not be preventable. However, many if not most cases are preventable by the way of a detailed anatomical knowledge on axillary region and displaying of situations in which peripheral nerves are primarily under risk (Zhang et al, 2011; Minville et al, 2006).

Injuries of the BP may affect in the axillary region due to blunt or penetrating traumas. Axillary artery injury might be accompanied with brachial plexus injury because of haematoma (Murata et al, 2008). Although the supraclavicular strecth injuries are more common than infraclavicular stretch injury lesions, the infraclavicular lesions can be treated technically more difficult than the supraclavicular. Because the infraclavicular injuries are related with a higher incidence of vascular and dislocation or fraction damages (Kim et al, 2004).

The variations have also value because a large range of diagnostic or therapeutic invasive procedures are carried out on the axillary artery or its branches (Reid et al, 1984; Mas et al, 2006). Previously, the variations in origins of the lateral thoracic, the superficial thoracic, the thoracodorsal, the axillary arteries were also described by many authors in details (Taylor et al, 1975; Harii et al, 1978; Rowsell et al, 1984; Anson et al, 1939; Ricbourg et al, 1975; Ricbourg 1975; Conink et al, 1976; Bhattacharya et al, 1990; Chandra et al, 1988; De Coninck et al, 1975; Baudet et al, 1976; Irigaray et al, 1979; Cabanié et al, 1980; Yang et al, 1983).

The axillary artery is a continuation of the subclavian artery, originates at the outer margin of the first rib, ending at the distal border of the teres major muscle. The pectoralis minor muscle crosses it and divides it into three parts as the first (proximal), the second (posterior) and the third (distal). The first part of the axillary artery is lie between the first rib and the upper margin of the pectoralis minor muscle. The first branch of the first part is the superior thoracic artery which harvests the first and second intercostal space and the upper part of the serratus anterior muscle. It anastomoses with the intercostal arteries. There were many variations on superior thoracic artery in literature. Pandley and Shukla implied that the superior thoracic artery arose from the thoracoacromial trunk in 16.8% cases of the right and 6.1% of the left axilla and the lateral thoracic artery in 39.8% cases of the right and 29.3% of the left axilla. Magden et al (2007) claimed that the superior thoracic artery was found out of the position as a variation. Differ from the knowledge of the classical textbook, it was originated from the first part of the axillary artery as the second branch. Instead of the superior thoracic artery, an aberrant independent origin of the serratus anterior branch as the first branch which originated directly from the first part of the axillary artery was presented in the case (Magden et al, 2007).

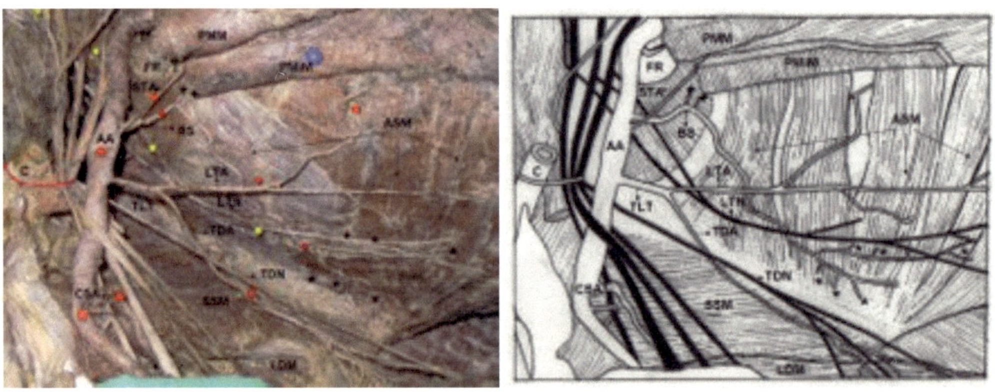

A B

Fig. 5. A-B: Anomalous axillary artery tree has been presented.The serratus anterior vascular branch (BS) as the first branch (newly reported anomaly), the lateral thoracic-thoracodorsal common trunk (TLT) and the circumflex scapular artery arise directly from the axillary artery (CSA). The branches which supply the first external intercostal muscle are indicated by plus signs, the common slip arteries which arise from the serratus branch are indicated by asteriks. AA: Axillary Artery, BS: Branch to Serratus Anterior Muscle, STA: Superior Thoracic Artery, TLT: Lateral Thoracic-Thoracodorsal Trunk, LTA: Lateral Thoracic Artery, TDA: Thoracodorsal Artery, CSA: Circumflex Scapular Artery, LTN: Long Thoracic Nerve, TDN: Thoracodorsal Nerve, ASM: Anterior Serratus Muscle, PMM: Pectoralis Major Muscle, PMiM: Pectoralis Minor Muscle, LDM: Latissimus Dorsi Muscle, SSM: Subscapular Muscle, FR: First Rib, C: Clavicle. [A: From the archive records of Prof. Magden O, the case was published in International Journal of Morphology at 2007, B: Illustrated by Prof.Magden O].

The second part of the axillary artery locates deep to the pectoralis minor muscle. The lateral cord of the BP places on laterally to the artery, the medial cord is medial to it, and the posterior cord is also posterior to it. The second part of the axillary artery has two branches as the thoracoacromial and the lateral thoracic arteries. Generally, the long thoracic artery which is originates directly from the second part of the axillary artery courses along the thoracic wall superficially to the serratus anterior muscle and branches of the blood supply to the muscle (Moore & Dalley, 1999; Magden et al, 2007). Magden et al defined a common trunk containing the lateral thoracic artery and the thoracodorsal arteries that originate together from the second third of the axillary artery. They suggested to call the arteries "a lateral thoracic- thoracodorsal" common trunk. In literature, the thoracodorsal artery was described different origin and percentage as a branch of the subscapular artery in 97% of the cases by Goldberg et al (1990) and 94% of the cases by Roswell et al or a branch of the lateral thoracic artery in 1% of the cases (Magden et al. 2007). Roswell et al found that in 24% of dissections, the thoracodorsal artery gave two branches to the serratus anterior muscle; one of them was 1 mm in diameter and the other one was on average 2 mm in diameter (Roswell et al. 1984). According to Magden et al all of the branches which harvested to the serratus anterior muscle had diameter of more than 1.0 mm and each had average diameters large enough for anastomosis, so they considered that these branches were safe to use as the pedicles of flaps.

The third part of the axillary artery has three branches which are called as the subscapular, the anterior circumflex humeral and the posterior circumflex humeral arteries. The subscapular artery is the largest branch of the axillary artery which ends as the circumflex scapular and thoracodorsal arteries (Moore & Dalley, 1999). In literature many variations were defined on subscapular arterial tree (Fig 6).

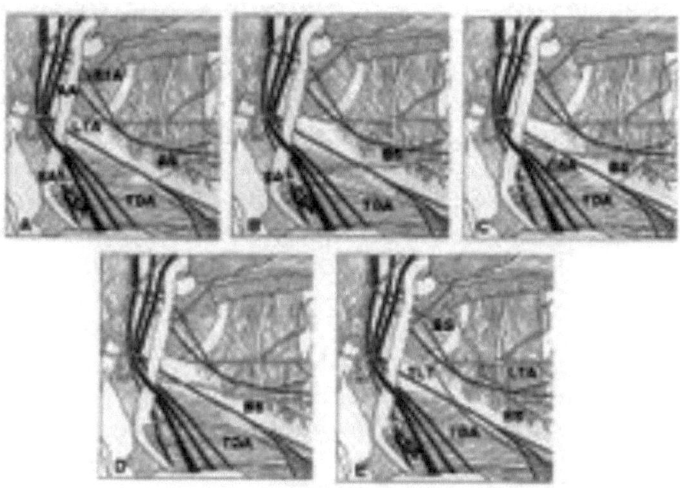

Fig. 6. Patterns of subscapular vascular tree have been illustrated. (A) The subscapular artery gives off the circumflex scapular and the thoracodorsal arteries. The subscapular artery sends one to three branches to the serratus anterior muscle. (B) The thoracodorsal artery which arises from the subscapular artery, sends the branches to the serratus anterior muscle. (C) The thoracodorsal and the serratus anterior branches originate separetely from the subscapular artery. (D) The subscapular artery gives off the serratus anterior branches. The thoracodorsal artery arises directly from the axillary artery. The circumflex scapular artery not visualized. (E) The serratus anterior vascular branch (BS) as the first branch, the lateral thoracic-thoracodorsal trunk (TLT) and the circumflex scapular artery arise directly from the axillary artery (Magden et al, 2007, Illustrated by Prof.Magden O). AA: Axillary Artery, SA: Subscapular Artery, CSA: Circumflex Scapular Artery, TDA: Thoracodorsal Artery, BS: Branch to Serratus Anterior Muscle, LTA: Lateral Thoracic Artery, STA: Superior Thoracic Artery, TLT: Lateral Thoracic-Thoracodorsal Trunk.

The blood supply to the serratus anterior muscle typically originates as the branches from the lateral thoracic artery (Moore & Dalley, 1999). The lateral thoracic artery originates in 40% of cases from the second part of the axillary artery. The artery is also arises from the subscapular or the the thoraco-acromial arteries in 60% of cases. It lies on the lateral border of the pectoralis minor to the chest wall. The blood supply to the pectoralis major, the pectoralis minor, the serratus anterior, the subscapular muscles and the skin are by the artery. Firstly, Taylor and Daniel were tried to represent the artery and were not find the artery in three out of twenty cadaveric dissections in 1975 (Taylor & Daniel). Similarly Harii et al (1978) failed to identify the vessel in two out of eleven clinical cases. The lateral thoracic artery generally lies no further than the fifth interspace and distributes various branches to the skin which pass through the lateral border of pectoralis major and mainly contribute blood supply of the female breast as rami mammarii laterales. There is clearly classical description on the artery, numerous variations are reckoned on this theme. The lateral perforating branches of the intercostals may replace the lateral thoracic artery. The artery becomes a major cutaneous branch when it pierces the deep fascia on 4th rib level. The cutaneous branch runs anteroinferiorly at oblique direction, and then it may anastomose with a cutaneous branch of the thoracodorsal artery. Due to anomalies correlated with axillary variations; the vascular anatomy of the muscle might be inconstant (Magden et al, 2007). Barlett et al (1981) found that in 100% of dissections, one or more branches from the subscapular-thoracodorsal arterial vasculature to the serratus anterior muscle. In 99% of dissections this artery was branch of the thoracodorsal artery itself. In 96% dissections one (72%) or two (24%) branches were exist from the thoracodorsal artery to the serratus anterior muscle. Goldberg et al (1990) found an anomalous serratus anterior pedicle which arose directly from the subscapular pedicle from the first part of the axillary artery and the thoracodorsal originated separately from the third part of the axillary artery. Valnicek et al (2004) ascerted that, three major arterial branching patterns of the subscapular artery were displayed with one, two and three major branches to the serratus anterior in 60%, 29% and 9% of cases, respectively. The serratus anterior pedicle originated from the thoracodorsal pedicle in 100% of cases by Takayanagi et al (1988). The authors implied that, the arterial supply to the serratus anterior muscle clasically arose as branches from the thoracodorsal artery which originated from the subscapular artery in 97% of cases and only 3% of them originated outright from the axillary artery. Former studies declerated that the serratus anterior branch originated from the thoracodorsal artery in 99% of cases or 100% of cases (Rowswl et al, 1975; Takayagani et al, 1982).

Daraemaecker et al (1988) and Kawamura et al (2005) defined that the angular branch which originated from the thoracodorsal artery, supplied the serratus anterior muscle. According to their data, the thoracodorsal artery was finally divided into the branches to the serratus anterior muscle and the latissimus dorsi muscle. The average diameter of the branch to serratus anterior muscle at its origin was 1.6 mm. The mean diameter its origin was 1.5 mm (Daraemaecker et al, 1988; Kawamura et al, 2005). Roswell et al (1984) and Kawamura et al (2005) also defined the multiple branches of the serratus anterior muscle, the branches which were preffered flap surgery had to show a consistent existence and safely diameter of more than 1.0 mm. Goldberg et al (1990) claimed that the serratus anterior branch and lateral thoracic artery were the vessels of suitable size and potentially a good feeding for microvascular free flaps or rotation pedicle flaps which moved from the serratus anterior muscle. Magden et al (2007) represented the origin point of the branches, distance between the branches and the surgical reference points, the diameters, the courses, and supplying pattern of the serratus anterior muscle in the case report. Five through nine slips were harvested by one (40%), two (50%), or three (10%) branches from the thoracodorsal artery (Cuadros et al, 1995). Godat et al (2004) defined a different arterial architecture to the lower part of the serratus muscle. Basically, a single serratus artery which was the terminal branch of the thoracodorsal artery had multiply branches, each lying between two neighbourhood serratus slips. Differ from the knowledge of the classical textbook; Magden et al (2007) found an aberrant independent origin of the serratus branch which arose directly from the first part of the axillary artery was presented as a first branch. The inferior part of the serratus anterior muscle was also harvested by the serratus anterior branch. They also defined that the superior and middle part of the serratus anterior muscle which was supplied by the lateral thoracic artery as "a lateral thoracic-thoracodorsal common trunk", arose from the axillary artery (Magden et al, 2007).

In classical textbook, the subscapular artery, about 4 cm from its origin, it gives off the circumflex scapular artery, usually larger than continuation of the subscapular artery (Moore & Dalley, 1999; Williams & Warwick, 1989). Sometimes, the circumflex scapular artery may originate directly from the axillary artery in 14.7% of cases (Valnicek et al, 2004). Goldberg et al (1990) noted that the serratus anterior branch arose directly from subscapular artery from the proximal third of the axillary artery and the thoracodorsal artery originated separately from the distal third of the axillary artery as variations.

Several authors declerated that a branch or branches to the serratus anterior muscle arose from the thoracodorsal artery which originated from the subscapular artery in all of the cases (Tobin et al, 1990; Barlett et al, 19981). Magden et al (2007) declerated that they could not encountered the subscapular artery in their case as a variation.

The data on the variations is of anatomical and surgical interest. The results on axillary tree confirm the anatomical safety of the serratus anterior flaps to eradicate ambiguity due to variations of the axillary artery. Detailed knowledge on variations of axillary architecture can prevent damage on the branches of the axillary artery during elevating serratus anterior flaps. It is also important to understand anatomic characteristics on neigbourhood area of axillary region (Magden et al, 2007). Magden et al offered to great care should be taken during flap surgery for moving the axillary artery and its branches as completely. The superficial thoracic artery which is placed on in front of the lateral part of pectoralis major, is a cutaneous artery of anterolateral thoracic wall. Adachi and Manchot both firstly defined it (Anson et al, 1939). Anson et al (1939) called it as the accessory lateral thoracic artery but its course was not same from that of the lateral thoracic in that it was a direct cutaneous artery purely supplying the skin and run on apex of the lateral part of pectoralis major muscle. It originated from the proximal part of the brachial artery or distal part of the axillary arter in the 5 cm segment associated to the lower border of insertion of the tendo pectoralis major muscle. It might lie down to 6th intercostal space and 26 cm down the anterior thoracic wall. Rowsell et al described the cutaneous branches which was originating from directly the axillary artery in 7% of cases in 1984. Salmon (1936) also defined it originating from the lateral thoracic or the subscapular arteries, but did not see to detect in excess of 8 cm in length. Harii et al (1978) also described the artery as giving off a cutaneous branch to the medial side of the upper extremity and the upper lateral quadrant of the breast.

In the literature many authors defined importance of the anatomical landmarks for describing relationship of the BP with the glenoid labrum because the procedures for stabilizing the shoulder and to success the placement of the sutures to the glenoid rim either through the bone or with suture hinges.

According to these cadaveric studies, the musculocutaneous, axillary, and subscapular nerves locate on inferior and lateral to the coracoid process. The musculocutaneous nerve is especially at risk while using the arthroscopy on the shoulder. This nerve originates from the lateral cord of the brachial plexus and pierces the coracobrachialis four to five centimeters inferior to the coracoid process. Lateral and inferior to the coracoid process, the superior and inferior subscapular nerves innervate the subscapularis and the teres major muscles. The brachial plexus and the axillary vessels, placed medial to the coracoid process, have no risk as long as the surgical approach is made lateral to the coracoid process.

Pedicled serratus anterior muscle flap wrapping around the brachial plexus is also used as a treatment for severe axillary neuropathic pain and distress due to neuroma formation. Many surgeons tried to find new techniques with good results for the treatment of the severe neuropathic pain syndromes arise from the brachial plexus. For the brachial plexus reconstruction microneurolysis, interposition nerve grafts, direct end to end repair or vascularized grafting required. In the light of the authors' experimental studies the techniques to repair injured nerves like neurolysis, nerve grafting, nerve transfer, nerve coaptation, direct muscle neurotization, fascicular transfer and end to side neuroraphy are discussed.

The BP injuries commonly are seen with multisystem trauma. The main mechanism of the BP injury is extreme traction of the nerves or direct impact. Upward traction results generally in the lesion of the lower cervical nerve roots like C8 and T1 whereas the downward traction results in the lesion of the upper cervical nerve roots. Paralysis of the shoulder, arm, and/or hand with parasthesias and altered sensation were the common symptoms of the BP injuries. The temperature and color of the limb may be changed because of the autonomic nervous system damage. The main opinion of the BP injuries treatment depends on the mechanism and the time of the trauma. Acute BP trauma in the axillary region with vascular trauma is a great challenge for the surgeon for restoring the upper extremity function. For these cases interdisciplinary operative and postoperative approach is essential to obtain the best results.

For the diagnostic interventions and surgical procedures variation of the axillary nerves and vessels are also significant for surgeons and clinicians. With varying frequency iatrogenic axillary neurovasculatory injuries during surgical interventions on the shoulder have been described previously. These complications may involve axillary vessels, axillary nerve, median nerve, ulnar nerve, radial nerve and or musculocutaneous nerve.

4. Pedicled flap elevation

Clinically, the branches of the axillary artery used in pedicled flap transferred applications. The lateral thoracic artery originates from the second part of the axillary artery, revert the lateral border of the tendo pectoralis minor muscle and runs the lateral margin of the muscle for nearly 4-5 cm before extend along under of the pectoralis major muscle. Therein, it associated with the pectoral branch of the thoraco-acromial artery and by perforators which traverse round the lateral margin of pectoralis major muscle and harvest to the lateral part of the breast in female. It may lie along the community between the pectoral branch and the lateral thoracic artery. A pedicled flap from the lateral thoracic wall was well defined and named the lateral thoracic region flap by Bhattacharya (1990). The flap is based on more than just the lateral thoracic artery. There may also be a supply from the acromio-thoracic axis by its pectoral margin of pectoral branch which gives off terminal branches around the lateral margin of pectoralis major to over the superficial fascia and which also association with the lateral thoracic artery.

The surface landmarks of the ventral margin of the flap are of importance. The surgeon should start at the 3rd intercostal space and continue throughout a line dropped vertically downwards from the coracoid process, crossing the infero-lateral margin of the pectoralis major and passing over the serratus anterior and external oblique muscles to a point not more than 3 cm below the costal border. The dorsal incision should be at the 3rd interspace again, at a point 2 cm medial to the lateral margin of latissimus dorsi and runs vertically downwards crossing infero-lateral margin of the muscle and lies to not more than 3 cm below the costal border. The ventral and dorsal borders may be converged by a curve such that the end of the flap follows nearly 5 cm below the costal border in the mid-axillary line.

During elevating the flap special attention is represented the fascia and vessels for up to 1 cm from beneath the infero-lateral margin of pectoralis major muscle.

The subaxillary flap which is named the smaller pedicled flap is used for reconstruction of the opposite hand. The flap is based on a single artery and measures up to 7 cm x 20 cm (Chandra et al, 1988).

The intercostal arteries give off lateral cutaneous branches and posterior branches. Their anterior branches are given off either before or after the lateral branch crosses the deep fascia and lie antero-inferiorly, for a distance of 2-4 cm, along the the fibres of external oblique muscle together with the lateral cutaneous nerves and then distribute under skin. Generally, great variation on the branch is normally seen. The lateral cutaneous branch itself is intensive and is often replaced by many large musculocutaneous perforators. In the 3th, 4th and 5th interspaces the artery are so small as to be not significant. In the lower spaces the perforators are larger but one or more may be absent in which case the perforator in the directly neighbourhood space above or below compensates for the insufficiency. There are also three or four musculocutaneous perforators through external oblique muscle originating from intercostal, subcostal and lumbal arteries.

The thoracoacromial artery originates from the second part of the axillary artery, run round the medial border of tendo pectoralis minor muscle, pierces the claviopectoral fascia. Then it divides into four branches as acromial, clavicular, deltoid and pectoral. The branches supply the ventral part of deltoid muscle, pectoralis major muscle, and the cutaneous tissue in the region over the claviopectoral fascia. The pectoral branch is the largest branch and gives off a small artery to pectoralis minor muscle before run on the deep of pectoralis major muscle after piercing the muscle. In there, it comminicates with branches of the perforators of the internal thoracic artery where have run through the medial ends of the intercostal spaces. Musculocutaneous perforators are sent which supply overlying skin. The acromial or deltoid branches of the thoraco-acromial artery which send a major direct cutaneous branch which supplies out in the underskin fat tissue for an uncertain distance and rarely more than 10 cm traverse the thoracic wall and 7.5 cm below the clavicle. The branches of the artery which comminicates with those of the 2nd and 3rd intercostal perforators from the internal thoracic artery were encountered in up to nearly 60% of cases. Variations on the branching pattern of the thoracoacromial artery were studied by Reid & Taylor (1984) in over 100 cadaveric specimens. Classically, the subscapular artery originates from the third part of the axillar artery and lie down behind the axillary vein occasionally sends the posterior of circumflex artery. At a level between 0.5 and 5 cm under its origin locus it bifurcates as the circumflex scapular artery and the thoracodorsal artery. The thoracodorsal artery sends a cutaneous branch in nearly 75% of cases, before it pierces and supplies the latissimus dorsi muscle. The cutaneous branch originates between approximately 0.5-2 cm beyond the bifurcation of the subscapular artery. Hence, the utmost feasible length of the vascular pedicle is supplied by the subscapular and thoracodorsal arteries as variable between 1 and 7 cm. A further content to the vascularized pedicle is founded by the cutaneous branch itself, which is either of a long type or a short type, making the total length of the anastomosable vascular trunk between nearly 3-10 cm long with a mean of 6 cm (Olinger & Benninger, 2010; Magden et al, 2007; Valnicek et al, 2004, Reid & Taylor, 1984).

The thoracodorsal artery sends a cutaneous branch which may be used as a feasible flap from the lateral thoracic wall. The termed thoracodorsal axillary flap is developed from both the arterial supply and the topographical site, but flaps based on the artery occasionally termed another name in the literature. The feasibility of harvesting a flap based on the artery was first studied morphologically by De Conick et al (1975) and Taylor & Daniel (1975). Free flaps transfer was firstly defined by Baudet et al (1976) and Irigary et al (1979). The latter case was performed in a child where the authors defined the feasible flap for microvascular transfer of the large size of the thoracodorsal artery.

The subaxillary pedicled flap was found by Cabanie et al (1980). Chandra et al (1988) was firstly standardized the design of a convienent pedicled flap based on the artery. A wider and longer version of the pedicled flap, based on the cutaneous branch of the thoracodorsal artery together with any of the other artery may be present on the lateral thoracic wall. Chandra et al (1988) described that the artery pierces to the deep fascia at the level of the 4th intercostal space in the posterior axillary line; thereafter becoming more superficial as it lies downward nearly 1 cm ventral and parallel to free margin of the latissimus dorsi muscle.

The venous drainage of the flap is by a small cutaneous vein which drains into the two venae comicantes accompaning with the thoracodorsal artery. The nerve innervation of the flap is the lateral cutaneous branches of the 3rd and 4th intercostal nerves. The thoracodorsal nerve which is the motor nerve to latissimus dorsi lies ventral to the thoracodorsal artery (Chandra et al, 1988; Cabanie et al, 1980).

5. Planning surgical procedure

According to surgeons, in planning the axillary pedicled flap, the operator may use the horizontal continuation of a line drawn through the nipples to surface mark the base of the flap. Then, the long axis of the flap has its centre line 1 cm ventral and parallel to the margin of the latissimus dorsi muscle. The largest flap described by Chandra was 7 x 20 cm and all donor sites enable of direct closure (1988).

Due to variation of the site of the cutaneous branch which may even be not present, it is best to dissect the axilla first and restore the anatomy. If the cutaneous branch is too small or totally absent, then the muscle branch together with a piece of the margin of latissimus dorsi muscle might be needed to support the flap and outline of the flap may be in the dorsal of the positions with a strong cutaneous branch the flap may be positioned more ventrally.

For the cutaneous branch flap, the structure is surrounded by the margin of pectoralis major muscle ventrally, by a line 2 cm medial to the margin of latissimus dorsi muscle dorsally, and by the 8th intercostal space caudally (Chandra et al, 1988; Silverberg et al, 2003).

6. Surgery

There's different approaches to the axillary region for different pathologies of these area. The main approaches those use at the literature and we use in our daily practice were summerized at this section. After patient placed supine to operating table donor side elevated 45^0 and patient's arm abducted 130^0 for preparing free skin flap. For exposure of the axillary vessels a mid axillary incision is done. The incision slightly ventrally forms axilla downward along the outerside of the pectoralis major muscle and flap's anterior border incison follows a line slopping inferiorly and obliqually. The anterior board of the flap lies from the 3rd intercostal space and dropped vertically downwards from coracoid process and then after crossing the inferolateral border of the pectoralis major muscle and reached over the serratus anterior muscle at a point which is not more then 3 cm below the costal margin. At the distal end of the flap the incison curves round and passes up over the edge of latissimus dorsi muscle. The posterior incision starts at a point 2 cm lateral border of latissimus dorsi muscle from the 3rd intercostal space level and passes vertically at a point not extends more then 3 cm below the costal border and downwards crossing the inferolateral border of the muscle. At the mid-axillary line 5 cm below the costal border the anterior and posterior borders of the curve of the flap may be jointed.

Pedicled flap is a different type of axillary flap which has a base at the level of 4th costa is marked by a line to nipples with the arm by the same side and the centre line of the flap is approximately 1 cm ventral to the free edge of the latissimus dorsi muscle.

For the breast cancer cases the axillary dissection elicites detailed information related with the nerves, vessels, nodal status and the topography of the muscles. Local control of the axillary disease and establishing of systemic adjuvant therapy are dependent on axillary surgery additionally. When lymph nodes are removed from the axial region in operations for primer mammary carsinoma or other pathologies like lymphadenopathy, lipoma, sabeceous cyst, lipodsytrophy, hidradenitis suppurativa, vascular malformations and metastatic carcinomas, the anatomical relationship of the vessels and nerves in the axilla are important, so the positions of major structures are significant for surgeons (De Cholnoky 1951, Silverberg et al, 2003). The favored recipient vessels for microvasculary breast reconstruction have differency from the thoracodorsal to internal mammary vessels because of the deep location and bad exposure of the vessels in the axilla and the other technical difficulties. Many authors generally used the same arm adduction maneuver during microvascular anastomoses in the axillary region and compared that with conventional abducted arm position regarding the exposure of the vessels, the operation time and the position of the surgeon and his assistant (Gravvanis et al, 2008).

Recently improved reconstructive and microsurgical outcomes of the cases with brachial vascular and plexus injuries related traumatic BP palsy, avulsion, rupture, haematomas or tumors on axillary region was mentioned in the literature.

Several anatomical studies and a few surgical studies are determined the anatomical variations of the anterior serratus, the pectoralis major and the latissimus dorsi muscles. During the axillary lymphadenectomy for breast cancer all of these muscle anomalies are significant clinically. If there's a muscle anomaly pass through the surgical field the surgery may be affected so the border of the surgery can be changed. There have been few studies discovering these anomalous muscles of the axillary region (Natsis et al, 2010).

During axillary lymph nodes dissections due to breast cancer the detailed defination of the anatomical landmarks of the axillary region is very important. Facilitating to access to the axillary fossa in the cases of the tumor, the patient is positioned as supine with a rolled towel under the ipsilateral scapula. For surgical approach there is no consensus for axillary lymph node dissection surgery. The main goal of the lymph node dissection of axillary region is remove all of the lymph node-bearing tissue. This contains all of the lymphatic bearing tissue posterior, anterior, inferior and superior to the axillary vessels. The dissection limits extend approximately at the level of the areola inferiorly from the level of the thoracodorsal nerve insertion to the latissimus dorsi muscle to superiorly the subclavius muscle. The medial limit of the dissection is medial to the edge of the pectoralis minor muscle (the level of rib), extending laterally to the margin of the latissimus dorsi muscle.

There are transverse (a), U-shaped (b) and extended S-shaped (c) incision choices; a; extending form the border of the latissimus dorsi muscle to the edge of the pectoralis major; b or c incisions following the contour of the pectoralis major into the axillary apex and down the border of the latissimus dorsi muscle. C type incision can be done from the behind of the pectoralis major muscle and start from the posterior under the level of the axillary hairline and then inferior of the anterior edge of the latissimus dorsi muscle (Dzwierzynski, 2010).

The dissection should cover the nodal tissue named Rotter node above the pectoralis major muscle, between the pectoralis major and minor muscles, and also between the pectoralis major and latissimus dorsi muscles. The fascia of the pectoralis muscles, the subaxillary fat

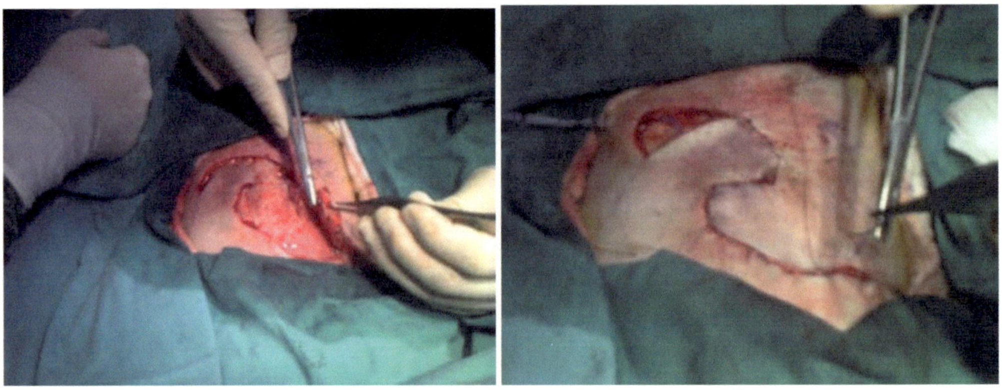

A B

Fig. 7. Elevation of the flap has been shown (A). S type of incision was shown (B). [From the archive records of Ass.Prof.Karabekir H.S., 2011].

pad, the interpectoral space, and lateral thoracic wall is also removed. The intercostal brachial nerves should be dissected, but the long thoracic and thoracodorsal nerves must be saved unless overly involved in tumor.

The axilla is frequently affected in severe burns that involve the body and the upper arm. Due to its unfavorable contour the acute treatment of the deep axillary burns still occured a difficult problem beacuse of a significant skin graft loss post-burn axillary contractures in the patients. The axillary disabilities deeply affect hand function because it affects the strategic positioning of the hand. Full hand motion is actually useless as the hand can not be positioned for the best function when significant contracture of this joint occurs. Because of the complex anatomy of the axilla which has been characterized as a unique three dimensional pyramid shape, the surgical correction of the axillary burn contracture has remained a forciable challenge. The restoration of the function of axilla is the goal of reconstructive surgery. The axillary surgery also may affect shoulder and hand surgery (Asuku et al, 2008; Larson et al, 1971; Robson & Smith, 1990; Yang, 2005; Hallock, 1993; Button et al, 2010).

Some cadaver studies have implied to define muscles of adjacent area of the axillary region. They also provide neurovasculary support in their usage as a flap for covering defects of the region. For flap survival recognition of any vascular and neural variation is very important to select the appropriate pedicle. In the literature the different type of surgical approach techniques are described for reaching axillary region. The best known type is curved upward incion, which is made just under the hairbearing region of the axilla. A diagonal incision made across the axilla and this incision extended for many centimeters in the space between the anterior and posterior axillary line, axillary fossa was represented by protecting neurovascular structures and lymph node of the axilla.

During axillary surgery a subclavicular mid-axillary incision may be performed then the skin and subcutaneous tissue are removed to present the axillary vessels and infraclavicular part of BP after clavipectoral fascia seperated, unilaterally. Dissection is carry on anteriorly and medially behind the anterior axillary fold until the lateral margin of pectoralis major is represented. The lateral border of the latter is easily represented as its muscle bundles lie upward to downward in relation to the horizontally lying fibres of serratus anterior. Although no surgical landmark represents the caudal extent of the dissection, lateral muscle boundry of the latissimus dorsi marks the lateral extent of the dissection. When the intercostobrachial nerve is represented as it crosses the lateral border of latissimus dorsi muscle, the surgeon should be aware that the axillary vein is approximately 1 cm to upward direction. Many times, double axillary veins are seen and the most inferior vessel indicates the limit of the dissection. The fat pad is retracted to inferior while axillar dissection dissected too far. The inferolateral part of the clavipectoral fascia at the upper extention of the dissection is easily seen. When clavipectoral fascia is seperated together with the axillary sheath, the axillary vessels and the brachial plexus are exposed. The musculocutaneous nerve is particularly at risk while arthroscopic approach to the shoulder. This nerve originates from the lateral cord of the brachial plexus and enters the coracobrachialis four to five centimeters distal to the coracoid process. Lateral and inferior to the coracoid process, the superior and inferior subscapular nerves innervate the subscapularis and the teres major muscles. The fragility of the axillary nerve has been well known to during shoulder arthroscopic and open surgical interventions. Iatrogenic injuries to the axillary nerve during surgical applications on the axillary region have been declerated previously with varying frequency (Lögters et al, 2008). Kulkarni et al (1992) have studied the course of the axillary nerve in the deltoid muscle. The nerve was found to extent 2.2–2.6 cm. above the midpoint on the vertical plane of the deltoid muscle, and parity was drawn to give the certain course of the nerve in this muscle (Kulkarni et al, 1992). Tubbs et al (2001) have described surgical landmarks for the proximal portion of the axillary nerve and defined an anatomical "triangle" within which the axillary nerve was recognized in all cadavers and evaluated the relationship of the axillary nerve with the musculocutaneous nerve. A triangle configuration of anatomic area that contains the axillary neurovascular bundle, containing the proximal part of the axillary nerve was recognized for the anterior approach. The coracoid process constituted the apex of this triangle while the medial rim of the coracobrachialis and the lateral border of the pectoralis minor were developing its lateral and medial margins, respectively.

A virtual horizontal line associating the superior margin of the tendon of the latissimus dorsi to the coracobrachialis constituted the floor of the triangle. According to result of a cadaveric study by Apaydin et al (2007), it was suggessted that the axillary nerve was an average of 3.7 cm. away from the coracoid (Apaydin et al, 2007). The result in concordance with the results of the study by Lo et al (2004), which defined this distance as mean, 30.3 mm, Tubbs et al (Tubbs et al, 2001; Apaydin et al, 2010; Apaydin et al, 2007). Surgeons should be taken care, during dissection, to evade injury of the axillary nerve, which pierces the deep surface of the deltoid approximately five centimeters lateral to the acromion.

The longest distance from the mid-acromion to the lower border of the axillary nerve was approximately 80-85 milimeters with the arm forward abduct. Some authors claimed that the distance of the axillary nerve to the mid-acromion in neutral and 90 degree vertical abduction, and found it to be 61 milimeters and 45 milimeters. Several authors examined the posterior deltoid splitting approach, and displayed the distance from the axillary nerve to the posterolateral corner of the acromion to be 65 milimeters in neutral and decreased to 51 milimeters in 90 degree vertical abduction and 46 milimeters in 30 degree extension. They also found the distances at 45 degree pronation and 45 degree supination to be 62 and 61 milimeters (Tubbs et al, 2001; Apaydin et al, 2010; Robinson et al, 2007; Zlotolow et al, 2006).

It must be noted that smaller branches of the axillary nerve may pierce to the deltoid as close approximately one or one and a half centimeter lateral to acromion. Also the axillary nerve is nearly six centimeters inferior to the apex of the humeral head. The nerve is placed high on the axilla, dorsal to the axillary artery and ventral to the subscapularis muscle. It presents the posterior cord at the level of the lower margin of the pectoralis minor muscle and travers lateral and dorsally. The axillary nerve is initially lateral to the radial nerve, dorsal to the axillary artery, and ventral to the subscapularis muscle; in the lower margin of this muscle, it curves backward and runs through the quadrangular space with the posterior circumflex humeral artery, where it bifurcates anterior and posterior branches.

Alternatively, a long deltopectoral incision may be made from the deltopectoral triangle to the axilla. Then, the skin may be elevated and laid down to both sides by making perpendicular incisions to the first incision. The pectoralis major and the clavicular part of the deltoid are displayed by cutting the deltopectoral fascia. Then the humeral insertion of the pectoralis major is cut and elevated medially. At this step, pectoralis minor and the axillary neurovascular bundle that is placed lateral to this muscle are exposed. Tendon of the pectoralis minor should be cared for disturbance. Then, the fascicles of the brachial plexus, the axillary vessels, and their branches are represented.

Skin and bony anatomical landmarks of the axillary region have crucial significance for the surgeons who interested in microsurgery and reconstructive surgery.

Our anatomical evaluations and representing objective criterias of the landmarks on the axillary region may support the literature for safety surgical approach.

7. Case report

A 22-year-old woman presented with severe rightsided pain affecting the shoulder, arm and neck. She also experienced numbness in her rightupper extremity. There was history of trauma before three months as traffic accident. The patient's complaints were not alleviated by analgesic treatment during three months. On physical examination the range of motion of the shoulder was limited and more painful in overhead movements. On palpation she had tenderness in the shoulder, axillary region, clavicle and neck. Shoulder and neck radiographs did not reveal any pathology. Generalized numbness and pain on the right extremity suggested a probable diagnosis of brachial plexus injury or cervical radiculopathy. The magnetic resonance imaging (MRI) studies of the shoulder, neck and cranium did not reveal any pathology, but we detected radicular hyperintensity at C7 and C8 levels on brachial plexus MRI (Fig 8).

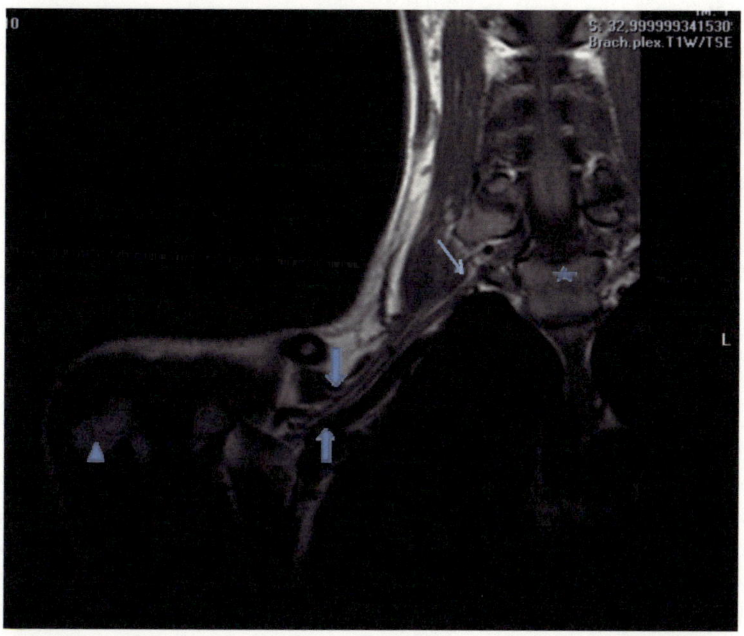

Fig. 8. Brachial plexus MRI of the patient were shown (Asterix showed the level of T1, thin arrow showed the hyperintensity of the radicule, thick arrows showed infraclavicular part of the BP, triangle showed the caput of the humerus) [From the archive records of Ass.Prof. Karabekir H.S., 2011].

The hyperintensity revealed as edema. EMG examination revealed as plexopathy. The pain of the patient diagnosed as neuropathic pain, because of persistant pain during three mounths. Analgesic, anti-inflammatory and antidepressant therapies were arranged with the combination of gabapentine. After two weeks medical treatment, the patient had still severe shoulder, arm and forearm persistant pain. So, operation was offered to the patient, but she did not accept the surgery. Activity limitation and a new analgesic management were rearranged.

8. References

Aggarwal, A., Harjeet, K., Sahni, D., Aggarwall, A. (2009). "Bilateral multiple complex variations in the formation and branching pattern of brachial plexus." *Surg Radiol Anat.* Nov; 31(9):723-31.

Aggarwal, A., Puri, N., Aggarwal, A.K., Harjeet, K., Sahni, D. (2010). "Anatomical variation in formation of brachial plexus and its branching." *Surg Radiol Anat.* Nov; 32(9):891-4.

Akboru, I.M., Solmaz, I., Secer, H.I., Izci, Y., Daneyemez, M. (2010). "The surgical anatomy of the brachial plexus." *Turkish Neurosurgery* Vol: 20, No: 2, 142-50.

Anson, B.J., Wright, R.R., Wolfer, J.A. (1939). "Blood supply of the mammary gland." *Surgery, Gynaecology and Obstetrics.* 69; 468-73.

Apaydin, N., Uz, A., Bozkurt, M., Elhan, A. (2007). "The anatomic relationships of the axillary nerve and surgical landmarks for its localization from the anterior aspect of the shoulder." *Clin Anat.* Apr;20(3):273-7.

Apaydin, N., Tubbs, R.S., Loukas, M., Duparc, F. (2010). "Review of the surgical anatomy of the axillary nerve and the anatomic basis of its iatrogenic and traumatic injury." *Surg Radiol Anat.* Mar; 32(3):193-201.

Asuku, M.E., Ibrahim, A., Ijekeye, F.O. (2008). "Post-burn axillary contractures in pediatric patients: a retrospective survey of management and outcome." *Burns.* Dec;34(8):1190-95.

Bartlett, S. P., May, J.W., Yaremchuk, M. J. (1981). "The latissimus dorsi muscle: Fresh cadaver study of the primary neurovascular pedicle." *Plast. Reconstr. Surg.* May; 67(5)631-6.

Baudet, J., Guimberteau, J.C., Nascimento, E. (1976). "Successful clinical transfer of two free thoraco-dorsal axillary flaps." *Plast Reconstr. Surg.* Dec; 58(6): 680-8.

Bhattacharya, S., Bhagia, S.P., Bhatnagar, S.K., Chandra, R. (1990). "The lateral thoracic region flap." *Br J Plast Surg.* Mar; 43(5): 162-8.

Button, J., Scott, J., Taghizadeh, R., Weiler-Mithoff, E., Hart, A.M. (2010). "Shoulder function following autologous latissimus dorsi breast reconstruction. A prospective three year observational study comparing quilting and non-quilting donor site techniques." *J Plast Reconstr Aesthet Surg.* Sep;63(9):1505-12.

Cabanié, H., Garbé, J.F., Guimberteau, J.C. (1980). "Anatomical basis of the thoracodorsal axillary flap with respect to its transfer by means of microvascular surgery". *Anatomia Clinica.* 2: 65-73.

Chandra, R., Kumar, P., Abdi, S.H.M. (1988). "The subaxillary pedicled flap." *British Journal of Plastic Surgery.* 41: 69-173.

Conink, A., Vanderlinden, E., Boecks, W. (1976). "The thoracodorsal skin flap: A possible donor site in distant transfer of island flaps by microvascular anastomosis." *Chir. Plastica* (Berlin); 3: 283-91.

Cuadros, C.L., Driscoll, C.L., Rothkopf, D.M. (1995). "The anatomy of the lower serratus anterior muscle: a fresh cadaver study." *Plast Reconstr Surg* Jan;95(1):93-7.

Daraemaecker, R., Thienen, C. V., Lejour, M., Dor, P. (1988). "The serratus anterior-scapular free flap: A new osteomuscular unit for reconstruction after radical head and neck surgery." In proceedings of the second international conference on head neck cancer, Boston. Mass, July 31-August 5.

De Cholnoky, T. (1951). "Accessory breast tissue in the axilla". *NY State J Med.* Oct;51(19):2245-48.

De Coninck, A., Boeckx, W., Vanderlinden, E., Claessen, G. (1975). Autocraft with vascular microsutures. Anatomy of donor site. *Ann. Chir. Plast* 20(2): 163-70.

Dzwierzynski, W.W. (2010). "Complete lymph node dissection for regional nodal metastasis." *Clin Plast Surg* Jan; 37(1):113-25.

Godat, D.M., Sanger, J.R., Lifchez, S.D., Recinos, R.F., Yan, J.G., Godat, M.R., Ramirez, C.E., Matloub, H.S. (2004). "Detailed neurovascular anatomy of the serratus anterior muscle: implications for a functional muscle flap with multiple independent force vectors." *Plast Reconstr Surg* Jul; 114(1):21-9; discussion 30-1.

Goldberg, J.A., Lineaweaver, W.C., Buncke, H.J. (1990). "An aberrant independent origin of the serratus anterior pedicle". *Ann Plast Surg* Dec; 25(6):487-90.

Goyal, N., Harjeet, Gupta, M. (2005). "Bilateral variant contributions in the formation of median nerve." *Surg Radiol Anat* Dec; 27(6):562-5.

Gravvanis, A., Caulfield, R.H., Ramakrishnan, V., Niranjan, N. (2008). "Recipient vessel exposure in the axilla during microvascular breast reconstruction." *J Reconstr Microsurg* Nov; 24(8):595-8.

Gumusburun, E., Adiguzel, E. (2000). "A variation of the brachial plexus characterized by the absence of the musculocutaneous nerve: a case report." *E.Surg Radiol Anat* 22(1):63-5.

Hallock, G.G. (1993). "A systematic approach to flap selection for the axillary burn contracture." *J Burn Care Rehabil* May-Jun; 14(3):343-7.

Harii, I., Torii, S., Sekiguchi, J. (1978). "The free lateral thoracic flap." *Plast Reconst Surg* Aug;62(2):212-22.

Irigaray, A., Roncagliolo, A., Fossati, G. (1979). "Transfer of a free lateral thoracic flap in a child: Case report." *Plast Reconst Surg* Aug; 64(2):259-63.

Johnson, E.O., Vekris, M., Demesticha, T., Soucacos, P.N. (2010). "Neuroanatomy of the brachial plexus: normal and variant anatomy of its formation". *Surg Radiol Anat* Mar; 32(3):291-7.

Kawamura, K., Yajima, H., Kobata, Y., Shigematsu, K., Takakura, Y. (2005). "Anatomy of Y-shaped configurations in the subscapular arterial system and clinical application to harvesting flow-through flaps". *Plast Reconstr Surg* Sep 15;116(4): 1082-89.

Kerr, A.T. (1918). "The brachial plexus of nerves in man, the variations in its formations and branches." *Am J Anat* 23:285-395.

Kim, J.T., Ng, SW., Naidu, S., Kim, J., Kim, Y.H. (2011). "Lateral thoracic perforator flap: Additional perforator flap option from the lateral thoracic region" *J Plast Reconst Aesthet Surg* Dec; 64(12): 1596-602.

Kim, D.H., Murovic, J.A., Tiel, R.L., Kline, D.G. (2004). "Infraclavicular brachial plexus stretch injury." *Neurosurg Focus* May 15;16(5):E4.

Kulkarni, R.R., Nandedkar, A.N., Mysorekar, V.R. (1992). "Position of the axillary nerve in the deltoid muscle." *Anat Rec* Feb; 232(2):316-7.

Larson, D.L., Abston, S., Evans, E.B., Dobrkovsky, M., Linares, H.A. (1971). "Techniques for decreasing scar formation and contractures in the burned patient." *J Trauma* Oct; 11(10):807-23.

Leinberry, C.F., Wehbé, M.A. (2004). "Brachial plexus anatomy." *Hand Clin* Feb; 20(1):1-5.

Lögters, T.T., Wild, M., Windolf, J., Linhart, W. (2008). "Axillary nerve palsy after retrograde humeral nailing: clinical confirmation of an anatomical fear." *Arch Orthop Trauma Surg* 128 (12):1431–1435.

Magden, O., Gocmen-Mas, N., Caglar, B. (2007). "Multiple Variations in the Axillary Arterial Tree Relevant to Plastic Surgery: A Case Report". *Int J. Morphol. 25(2)*:357-61.

McWhirter, D., Malyon, A. (2008). "The axillary arch: a rare but recognised variation in axillary anatomy." *J Plast Reconstr Aesthet Surg* Sep; 61(9):1124-6.

Minville, V., Fourcade, O., Idabouk, L., Claassen, J., Chassery, C., Nguyen, L., Pourrut, J.C., Benhamou, D. (2006). "Infraclavicular brachial plexus block versus humeral block in trauma patients: a comparison of patient comfort". *Anesth Analg* Mar; 102(3):912-5.

Moore, L.K., Dalley, A.F.(1999) *Anatomy* 4 th.ed. Lippincott Williams & Wilkins. 703.

Murata, K., Maeda, M., Yoshida, A., Yajima, H., Okuchi, K. (2008). "Axillary artery injury combined with delayed brachial plexus palsy due to compressive hematoma in a young patient: a case report". *Journal Brachial Plex Peripher Nerve Inj* Mar; 28; 3:9.

Muthoka, J.M., Sinkeet, S.R., Shahbal, S.H., Matakwa, L.C., Ogeng'o, J.A. (2011). "Variations in branching of the posterior cord of brachial plexus in a Kenyan population". *J Brachial Plex Peripher Nerve Inj* Jun 7; 6:1.

Natsis, K., Vlasis, K., Totlis, T., Paraskevas, G., Noussios, G., Skandalakis, P., Koebke, J. (2010). "Abnormal muscles that may affect axillary lymphadenectomy: surgical anatomy". *Breast Cancer Res Treat.* Feb; 120(1):77-82.

Mas, N., Pelin, C. Zagyapan, R., Bahar, H. (2006). "Unusual relation of the median nerve with the accessory head of the biceps brachii muscle: An original case report." *Int. J. Morphol* 24(4):561-64.

Olinger, A., Benninger, B. (2010). "Branching patterns of the lateral thoracic, subscapular, and posterior circumflex humeral arteries and their relationship to the posterior cord of the brachial plexus". *Clin Anat* May; 23(4):407-12.

Pandey, S.K., Shukla, V.K. (2007). "Anatomical variations of the cords of brachial plexus and the median nerve." *Clin Anat* Mar; 20(2):150-56.

Reid, C.D., Taylor, G.I. (1984). "The vascular territory of the acromiothoracic axis." *Br J Plast Surg* 37:194-212.

Ricbourg, B., Lassau, J.P., Violette, A.M., Merland, J.J. (1975). "A propos de l'artère mammaria externe. Origine, territoire et intérêt pour les transplants cutanés libres." *Archives d'Anatomie Pathologique* 23:317-22.

Ricbourg, B. (1975). "Un nouveau site donneur pour transplant cutanè: le territorie mammaria externe." *Lettre d'information du Groupe d'Advancement pour la Microchirurgie* 2: 1-9.

Robinson, C.M., Khan, L., Akhtar, A., Whittaker, R. (2007). "The extended deltoid-splitting approach to the proximal humerus" *J Orthop Trauma* 21:657-62

Robson, M.C., Smith, D.J. (1990). "Burned hand. In: Jurkiewicz MJ, Krizek TJ, Mathes SJ, Ariyan S, editors." *Plastic Surgery; principles and practice.* St. Louis: CV Mosby; 781-802.

Rowsell, A.R., Davies, D.M., Eisenberg, N., Taylor, G.I. (1984). "The anatomy of the subscapular-thoracodorsal arteries system: study of 100 cadavers dissections." *Br J Plast Surg* Oct; 37(4): 574-6.

Song, W.C., Jung, H.S., Kim, H.J., Shin, C., Lee, B.Y., Koh, K.S. (2003). "A variation of the musculocutaneous nerve absent." *Yonsei Med J* Dec 30;44(6):1110-3.

Silverberg, M.A., Rahman, M.Z. (2003). "Axillary breast tissue mistaken for suppurative hidradenitis: an avoidable error." *J Emerg Med* Jul; 25(1):51-5.

Standring, S., Ellis, H., Healy, J.C., Johnson, D., Williams, A., Collins, P. (2005). *Gray's Anatomy* (ed 39). London, Churchill Livingstone.

Taylor, G.I., Daniel, R.K. (1975). "The anatomy of several free flap donor sites." *Plast Reconst Surg* Sep; 56(3):243-53.

Takayanagi, S., Ohtsuka, M., Tsukie, T. (1988). "Use of the latissimus dorsi and the serratus anterior muscles as a combined flap." *Ann Plast Surg* Apr; 20(4):333-9.

Tobin, G. R., Moberg, A., Ringberg, A., Netscher, D. (1990). "Mandibular-facial reconstruction with segmentally split serratus anterior composite flaps." *Clin Plast Surg* Oct; 17(4): 633-72.

Tubbs, R.S., Oakes, W.J., Blount, J.P., Elton, S., Salter, G., Grabb, P.A. (2001). "Surgical landmarks for the proximal portion of the axillary nerve. *Neurosurg* Dec; 95(6):998-1000.

Ung, O., Tan, M., Chua, B., Barraclough, B. (2006). "Complete axillary dissection: a technique that still has relevance in contemporary management of breast cancer." *Anz J Surg* Jun; 76(6):518-21.

Valnicek, S.M., Mosher, M., Hopkins, J.K., Rockwell, W.B. (2004). "The subscapular arterial tree as a source of microvascular arterial grafts." *Plast Reconstr Surg* Jun; 113(7):2001-05.

Wadhwa, S., Vasudeva, N., Kaul, J.M. (2008). "A rare constellation of multiple upper limb anomalies." *Folia Morphol* (Warsz) Nov; 67(4):236-39.

Williams, P.L. Warwick, R. (1989). *Gray's Anatomy.* 37th ed. Churchill-Livingstone, London, England; 611.

Yang, J-Y. (2005). Reconstruction of axillary contracture. In: McCauley RL, editor. *Functional and aestheticreconstruction of burned patients.* New York: Taylor and Francis; 367-78.

Yang, Z.N., Shih, R., Chao, L., Shih, T.S. (1983). "Free transplantation of sub-axillary lateral thoracodorsal flap in burn surgery." *Burns Incl Therm Inj* Feb; 10(3):164-69.

Zhang, J., Moore, A.E., Stringer, M.D. (2011). "Iatrogenic upper limb nerve injuries: a systematic review." *ANZ J Surg* Apr; 81(4); 227-36.

Zlotolow, D.A., Catalano, L.W. 3rd., Barron, O.A., Glickel, S.Z. (2006). " Surgical exposures of the humerus." *J Am Acad Orthop Surg* Dec; 14(13):754-65.

12

Simulation in Plastic Surgery Training: Past, Present and Future

Phoebe Arbogast and Joseph Rosen
Dartmouth-Hitchcock Medical Center, Dept. of Surgery, Division of Plastic Surgery and Thayer School of Engineering USA

1. Introduction

The face of medicine is characterized by rapid and constant evolution. New procedures, new technology, and new solutions to clinical challenges are forever changing the field. However, medical education has been historically stagnant. From the advent of medicine until Abraham Flexner's landmark report on the state of medical education in 1910, the apprenticeship model reigned. Training was highly variable and largely dependent on one's supervisor. As a result, by the turn of the 20th century the quality of health care in the United States (US) was cause for concern. Flexner's report proposed several radical changes to medical education and in doing so, redefined the fundamental contract between physicians and society (Flexner, 1910).

Today, new challenges in medical education demand a revolution similar to that which Flexner enacted a century ago. Present undergraduate medical education is rooted in lectures, laboratories, standardized patients, and (in some cases) simulators. Problems with this system include limited integration of basic and clinical sciences; a biology-centric rather than patient-centric focus; and an emphasis on knowledge and discrete skill over critical thinking, decision-making, and teamwork. This last issue is especially problematic, as physicians are routinely faced with the complex tasks of diagnosis and treatment in chaotic environments, in which information is often inadequate, inaccurate, or not readily available. Success in this setting requires the integration and synthesis of information from many sources – a skill set not adequately addressed in current medical education.

In response to these observed shortcomings, two seemingly contradictory goals in education have been put forth as priorities. On the one hand, there is a push for further standardization of education. To this end, the Accreditation Council for Graduate Medical Education (ACGME) and the American Board of Medical Specialties have defined six core competencies required of all residents. Standardization aims to increase patient safety by reducing surgical errors and improving the quality of care, while at the same time maximizing hospital resources. On the other hand, the medical education model ought to allow for individualization to reflect the fact that people learn differently from one another. In this line of reasoning, there should be room for one student's path to differ from another's to best accommodate the student's learning style. Richard Satava, MD, (a professor of surgery at the University of Washington and member of the American College of Surgeons (ACS) committees on Emerging Technologies and Resident Education, and Informatics; http://depts.washington.edu/biointel/biograph.html) cites three concepts that will be key in revolutionizing medical education, which exemplify these dual priorities: 1) an increased efficiency of education by standardizing curriculum; 2) an individualization of education; and 3) a shift from time-based training to competency-based training (Satava, 2010). In competency-based training, students practice a skill until they can demonstrate proficiency, at which point they proceed to the next skill. In contrast, time-based training requires only a set amount of time practicing the skill before it is checked off as complete, regardless of the student's competence at the end of that time period. Satava's first two concepts echo the previously mentioned goals of standardization and individualization, and his third concept demonstrates how such goals can coexist. Standardization here refers to the material presented, while individualization refers to the delivery of that material. By shifting to competency-based rather than time-based requirements, the end point of training can be standardized, while the path to reach it remains flexible from individual to individual.

Simulation can fulfill all three of Satava's educational goals, allowing for standardization of curriculum, individualization of delivery, and a shift to competency-based training. Wide adoption of simulation technology will facilitate a needed shift in education and will fundamentally change how we deliver medicine, just as Flexner's report did in 1910. Simulation offers residents the chance to advance along a learning curve, without subjecting patients to a novice's initial practicing of a skill or procedure. Furthermore, practicing skills outside of the operating room may decrease the operating room (OR) time for a procedure, and thus its cost. In recognition of simulation's power as a training tool, the American College of Surgeons is pursuing a strategy to incorporate simulation into general surgery residency programs. Their plan comprises three phases: skills training, procedure training, and team training.

This paper discusses how plastic surgery might follow the example set by the ACS and adapt the ACS's simulation training strategy to the needs and challenges specific to plastic surgery. Since many of the skills required in plastic surgery are taught during general surgery residency, Phase 1 (skills training) would require few modifications. Phase 2 (procedure training), however, necessitates the development of procedure simulations particular to plastic surgery. The team training of Phase 3 will overlap considerably with general surgery requirements, as competencies in teamwork are similar across specialties. Simulators in Phase 3 (team training) would facilitate cooperation and communication within a diverse team in a variety of environments, from the operating room to the clinic to the emergency department. Incorporating simulation in plastic surgery training is only the beginning of the needed changes in medical education; we will conclude this paper by anticipating the future roles of simulation in settings ranging from medical school to point of care.

2. Surgical simulation: Definitions and history to present

2.1 Definitions

To proceed with a discussion of simulation, it is first necessary to establish definitions of key terms. Here, a *model* refers to "a physical, mathematical, or logical representation of a system, entity, phenomenon, or process" (Rosen *et al.*, 2009). Examples of models in medical simulation include mathematical representations of tissue deformation under pressure from surgical instruments or a three-dimensional visualization of a lung. A *simulation* is "a model implemented over time, from nanoseconds to centuries, displayed either in 'real time' or faster or slower than real time" (Rosen *et al.*, 2009). Such simulations can be used to condense 100 years' worth of glacial change to a few minutes, or, alternatively, to teach cellular metabolism with a significantly decelerated animation. Building on these definitions, a *simulator* is "a device that uses simulation to replace a real-world system or apparatus, allowing users to gain experience and to observe and interact with the simulation via realistic, visual, auditory, or tactile cues" (Rosen *et al.*, 2009).

2.2 History to present

Medical simulators, in one form or another, have been used for centuries to develop and practice surgical procedures without breaching the Hippocratic promise to do no harm to the patient. Around 600 BC in India, leaf and clay models were used in the first recorded surgical operation, a forehead flap nasal reconstruction (Limberg, 1984). More recently, simulators have taken the form of animals, cadavers, and bench models to allow trainees to practice various skills. Live animals have the advantage of providing a living anatomy; however, their downsides include availability, anatomical differences from humans, and ethical concerns. Human cadavers supply a high level of anatomical relevance, but availability and infection risks limit their practical use. Bench models are inanimate interactive tools that are readily available, reusable, and free of ethical drawbacks. There exists a wide range of bench models, from foam bricks for practicing injection to laparoscopic box trainers. Sawbones Worldwide offers over 2,000 bench models of different orthopedic pathologies, which are designed to be cut, drilled, or tapped with actual surgical tools (Sawbones Worldwide, December 15, 2011, http://www.sawbones.com/default.aspx). Best used to teach discrete, mechanical skills, bench models have been shown to possess training capabilities similar to cadavers (Anastakis *et al.*, 1999). Table 1 (adapted from Rosen *et al.*, 2009) compares the strengths and weaknesses of these simulators.

Modern computer simulators offer a solution to many of the limitations of these preliminary simulators. They are reusable, they display relevant patient-specific anatomy, they can accurately reflect the consequences of various surgical choices, they can provide feedback to the user, and they raise no ethical issues. Computer-based simulators used in medicine have built upon the example set by the aviation industry, which has been using flight simulators to train pilots and increase safety for over 50 years (Satava, 2007).

Today, a main focus of computer simulation development is to augment the authenticity of the simulated experience. Haptic feedback, for example, is being pursued to add a realistic sense of touch to simulators, so that a surgeon-in-training can feel (and not just see) when her simulated tool has entered an organ, cut into a blood vessel or crossed any anatomical boundary. Developers are also working to model specific environments, such as the battlefield or a disaster site, that have particular challenges and considerations. The development of surgical simulators for plastic surgery residents must take into account the needs of the trainee, which include patient specificity, anatomical variations, a range of pathologies, and both ideal conditions and unexpected complications.

Simulator Types: Comparison	Bench Models	Animal	Cadaver	Mannequin	Computer Simulation
Description/ Use:	Foam, basic skills (i.e., injections, suturing)	Microsurgery MIS-gallbladder	Entire anatomy	Anesthesia, resuscitation	Virtual, software visual-haptics-computer
Examples:	"Brick," IV insertion, catheterization, anastomosis, endoscopy/ laparoscopy, stent placement	Primate, sheep, pig, dog, cat, rat, many others	N/A	ePelvis, Virgil	Lap Mentor, GI Mentor, ES3, Virtual Environment
Advantages:	Inexpensive, portable, multiple use, safe	Closer to human anatomy than blocks, "living" physiology	Accurate anatomy	Multiple use	Multiple use, patient-specific, no ethical concerns, performance feedback
Dis-advantages:	Limited realism, finite use	Anatomical differences, ethical concerns, availability, cost, no multiple use	Ethical concerns, availability, cost, no multiple use, tissue compliance, infection risk	Limited realism, no "living" physiology	Realism varies, cost often increases with fidelity
Costs:	Low to medium	High	High	Varies	Varies
Sources:	Immersion Medical, SimQuest, Simulution, Mentice, Energid, Touch of Life	Various animal-sales laboratories	Donations to medical schools	METI, Laerdal, CIMIT	Simbionix, METI, Lockheed Martin

Table 1. **Comparison of simulators used in medical education.** *Table adapted from* Rosen, J. M., Long, S. A., McGrath, D. M., & Greer, S. E. (2009). Simulation in plastic surgery training and education: the path forward. *Plastic and Reconstructive Surgery*, Vol. 123, No. 2, (Feb 2009), pp. 729-740, 1529-4242. Used with permission.

3. Use of simulation in medical education

The efficacy of simulation as a training tool in the medical field has been validated in numerous studies. Okuda *et al.* conducted a thorough search of original papers relating to simulation in medical education, from undergraduate training to continuing medical education. They found numerous studies demonstrating that simulation is an effective tool to teach basic science, clinical knowledge, procedural skills, teamwork, and communication. Measurable clinical improvements were demonstrated in a number of studies that focused on simulation-based training in two particular areas of medicine. In the field of laparoscopy, residents who trained on a simulator performed better in the operating room than those who did not train on the simulator (Duncan *et al.*, 2007, as cited in Okuda *et al.*, 2009). Another study demonstrated that simulation training increased residents' adherence to advanced cardiac life support protocol, compared to residents who received traditional instruction (DeVita *et al.*, 2005, as cited in Okuda *et al.*, 2009). Though these results are encouraging, additional studies are needed to establish that ultimately patient outcomes also improve as a result of simulation.

In recognition of the benefits of simulation, several mandates have been put in place for the incorporation of simulation into general surgery residency training. In 2008, the Residency Review Committee (RCC) of the Accreditation Council for Graduate Medical Education required that all surgical residents have access to a simulation center with certain specifications (ACGME Program Requirements for Graduate Medical Education in Surgery, December 15 2011, http://www.acgme.org/acwebsite/rrc_440/440_prindex.asp). In 2009, the American Board of Surgery (ABS) added the requirement of successful completion of the Fundamentals of Laparoscopic Surgery simulation course in order to sit for the General Surgery Qualifying Examination (ABS Booklet of Information for Certifying Exam, December 15 2011, http://home.absurgery.org/xfer/BookletofInfo-Surgery.pdf). The American College of Surgeons (ACS), in response to these mandates, initiated the development of a simulation center certification process. The ACS Program for Accreditation of Education Institutes aims to create a network of training centers that incorporate bench models, virtual reality, simulators and simulation, with the ultimate goal of improving patient safety. A consortium of the accredited centers meets annually to develop a more uniform approach to simulation center training. A second objective of the program has been to develop a standardized residency curriculum that meets the requirements of the RCC and ABS and maximizes the utility of the simulation centers. It was from this objective that the three-phase strategy described earlier arose. The curricula developed under this initiative can serve as a starting platform for training programs developed by the ACS-Accredited Education Institutes (AEI) consortium (Satava, 2010).

In addition to a network of like-minded centers and a standard curriculum, measures of assessment are needed in order for simulation to be truly effective as a training tool. Current methods in use can be divided into qualitative and quantitative systems of evaluation. Qualitative measures are based on assessor observations and checklists. One such system is the Objective Structured Assessment of Technical Skills (OSATS), in which a variety of skills are performed on benchtop models during timed rotations. Educators grade residents' performances using checklists of global measurement standards (Martin *et al.*, 1997). The main drawback to OSATS, as with other qualitative tools, is the time requirement of the assessors, who must be physically present during training sessions in order to evaluate trainees. Jensen *et al.* found that OSATS could also be used as a valid tool to evaluate video-recorded surgical performance. While using OSATS following a procedure may ease scheduling conflicts and difficulty ensuring assessor blindness, the system does not minimize the assessor's time requirement (Jensen *et al.*, 2009). Quantitative evaluations avoid the need for an assessor by incorporating performance measurements into the training tools themselves. Such systems evaluate movement velocity and magnitude of forces imposed, among other metrics. Haptica's ProMIS is an example of a laparoscopic simulator with built-in motion tracking technology, which assesses and provides quantitative feedback in real time. It has been validated in a number of studies, though confirming improvements in real-life surgical skills remains a gap in the literature (Pellen *et al.*, 2008). The Electronic Data Generation for Evaluation (EDGE) is a laparoscopic simulator currently in development by Simlab Corporation, as a successor to their BlueDRAGON system. EDGE measures time, path, and force exerted for haptics-enabled laparoscopic instruments and allows trainees to see the collected metrics as they proceed through an exercise (Products in Development, December 15 2011, http://www.simulab.com/products-development).

4. Implementing simulation in plastic surgery training

This section of the paper focuses on adapting the ACS simulation initiative to plastic surgery training. ACAPS, together with the American Society of Plastic Surgeons (ASPS), recently launched the online Plastic Surgery Education Network (PSEN). Modules corresponding to divisions of plastic surgery (such as upper extremity, breast, and trunk) present a variety of learning tools, including case reports, clinical courses, procedural videos, and self-assessments (Plastic Surgery Education Network, December 15 2011, http://www.psenetwork.org/REC/Default.aspx). The wide range of educational materials offered by PSEN may be augmented in the future by the inclusion of simulated procedures, interactive animations, or virtual patients. PSEN is but one platform upon which simulation can be used to supplement traditional training. Below, we describe a strategy for incorporating simulation into plastic surgery education by following the three-phase plan set by the ACS.

4.1 Phase 1- Skills training

The first phase of the ACS's strategy uses simulation to teach the twenty surgical skills, outlined in Table 2, required of postgraduate year 1 and year 2 general surgery trainees. The list, compiled by the National Simulation Committee, includes skills from both general surgery and plastic surgery, though competence in all twenty skills is required for the completion of a general surgery residency. These skills are primarily technical and were chosen to establish in trainees a solid foundation of the motor function and visuospatial coordination that is necessary for more complex procedures learned later in training. For example, suturing skills must be mastered in Phase 1 before the successful completion of cleft-palate surgery is possible. Module templates, developed for each of the twenty skills, will present the trainee with objectives, assumptions, step-by-step instructions, common errors, and error-prevention strategies.

In the ever-changing field of surgery, simulators can be instrumental in updating training curricula in response to new surgical innovations. With the advent of laparoscopic surgery,

Skill	Relevance to:		
	General Surgery	Plastic Surgery	Both
Advanced laparoscopy skills	+		
Advanced tissue handling: flaps, skin grafts		+	
Airway management	+		
Asepsis and instrument identification	+	+	+
Basic laparoscopy skills	+		
Bone fixation and casting		+	
Central line and arterial line insertion	+		
Chest tube and thoracentesis	+		
Colonoscopy	+		
Hand-sewn gastrointestinal anastomosis	+		
Inguinal anatomy	+		
Knot tying	+	+	+
Laparotomy opening and closure	+		
Stapled gastrointestinal anastomosis	+		
Surgical biopsy	+	+	+
Suturing	+	+	+
Tissue handling, dissection, wound closure	+	+	+
Upper endoscopy	+		
Urethral and suprapubic catheterization	+		
Vascular anastomosis		+	

Table 2. **List of 20 skills required of postgraduate year 1 and year 2 general surgery trainees**. The skills on this list were included because of their importance to junior residents as well as their application in at least two specialties (as determined by the National Simulation Committee). (Information on skills in left column reprinted with permission from ACS/APDS Surgical Skills Curriculum for Residents, December 15 2011, http://www.facs.org/education/surgicalskills.html). Table adapted by Dr. Rosen.

the McGill Inanimate Systems for Training and Evaluation of Laparoscopic Skills (MISTEL) was developed to teach surgeons and trainees the new skills. The development of MISTEL provides a pathway to follow in the creation of future goal-specific simulators: first the discrete skills needed are identified, then these skills are modeled in a simulator, a set of metrics is established, and finally validity of the simulator is evaluated (Vassiliou *et al.*, 2006). MISTEL was incorporated into the Fundamentals of Laparoscopic Surgery curriculum to teach mechanical skills. In a study by Sroko *et al.*, residents performing laparoscopic cholecystectomy scored higher on the Global Operative Assessment of Laparoscopic Skills after completing the FLS course. This study indicates that training with the MISTEL system can positively affect OR performance (Sroko *et al.*, 2009).

In plastic surgery, several systems have emerged following the example set by MISTEL. Mimic Technologies (Seattle, WA) has responded to the introduction of surgical robots by adapting their simulation platform MSim™ to train surgeons on the use of Intuitive Surgical's *da Vinci*® robot system. Mimic's dV-Trainer™, released in 2007, is a tabletop

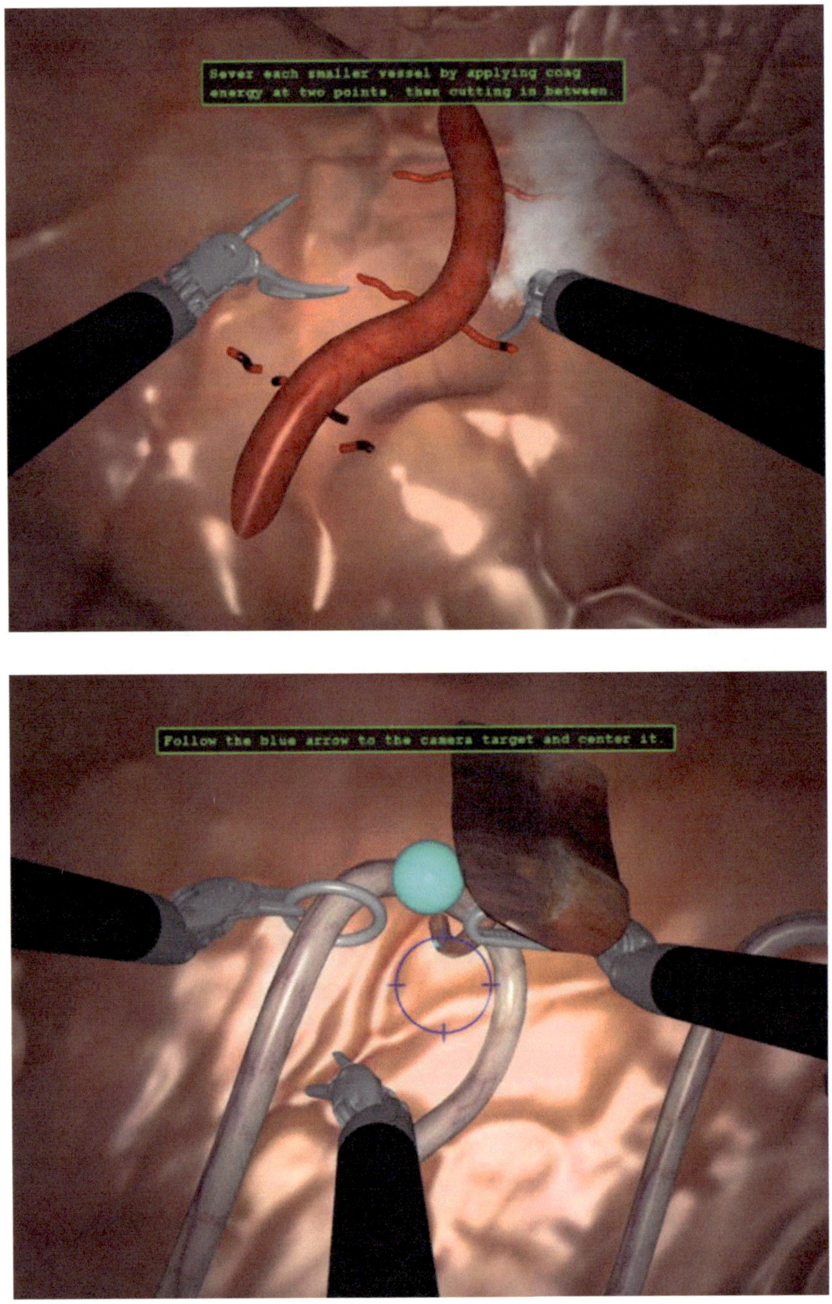

Fig. 1. **The Mimic Technologies dV-Trainer™ Simulator for Robotic Surgery** is designed to allow surgeons to practice the mechanical skills needed to operate Intuitive Surgical's *da Vinci®* robotic surgery system, including manipulating instruments and needles. Images courtesy of Jeff Berkley, PhD; copyright 2012, Mimic Technologies, Inc.

system that provides a realistic representation of the *da Vinci* experience, including Intuitive's EndoWrist™ instruments, foot pedals, and robot kinematics. The system includes a comprehensive set of metrics, MScore™, by which trainees can track their progress (dV-Trainer–Skills Training for Robotic Surgery, December 15 2011, http://www.mimic.ws/products/). The face, content, construct, and concurrent validity of the dV-Trainer have been confirmed in several studies (Lerner *et al.*, 2010; Kenney *et al.*, 2009).

Brown *et al.* have developed a virtual environment in which real surgical tools mounted on trackers can be used to interact with and manipulate models of tissue. The software system, which integrates a deformable object simulator, a tool simulator, and a collision-detection module, has been applied as a microsurgery simulator that allows trainees to practice suturing blood vessels. The microsurgery simulator demonstrates novel features of the software system that will make further applications of this software valuable in simulating additional skills and, potentially, procedures (Brown *et al.*, 2010).

Other research has focused on improving the software required for accurate virtual representation of skin. Lapeer *et al.* conducted a number of experiments with the aim of developing a deformable soft-tissue model that responds in real time to user manipulation. Tensile stress tests were carried out on human skin samples, and the resulting data were incorporated into a hyperelastic computer model. Ultimately this lab anticipates coupling the software with a haptic feedback device to create a real-time plastic surgery simulation in an interactive virtual environment (Lapeer *et al.*, 2010). Alteration of the geometry and topology of skin is central to plastic surgery; another new simulator accurately models these changes in response to surgical intervention. Sifakis *et al.* have used finite-element modeling to create a comprehensive real-time virtual surgical environment, enabling the surgeon to practice tissue cutting and manipulation. With incision, retraction, and suturing tools, trainees can practice current techniques for closing defects, while experts can experiment with and assess the efficacy of new techniques (Sifakis *et al.*, 2009).

Though many surgical skills are taught during general surgery residencies, there remain skills specific to plastic surgery that could benefit from simulation. By applying the ACS's plan for integrating simulation into curricula to plastic surgery, we can address those skills in a safe, efficient, and effective training environment.

4.2 Phase 2- Procedure training

In procedure training, there are many applications for plastic surgery-specific simulation. In post-graduate years 3, 4 and 5, competency in several procedures is expected of plastic surgery residents. Table 3 outlines these procedures, as defined by the Accreditation Council for Graduate Medical Education.

In 2008 the American College of Academic Plastic Surgeons (ACAPS) established an *Ad Hoc* Committee on Virtual Reality and Simulation for Plastic Surgery Education. The goal of this committee is to adapt virtual reality technology to standardize teaching, specifically with respect to procedures in four main areas of expertise: craniofacial, reconstructive, cosmetic and hand surgery. Cognitive task analysis, defined as "the process of deconstructing an expert's knowledge of a task and adapting it to the needs of the educational model," can be used to break procedures into steps weighted according to their relevance to outcomes, which can then become the basis of a computer simulation (Grunwald *et al.*, 2004). Cognitive task analysis has been demonstrated to be an effective training tool; one study showed that residents who had received a curriculum based on cognitive task analysis for flexor tendon repair were better equipped to make appropriate surgical decisions than those who had not received such training (Luker *et al.*, 2008).

PGY3	**PGY4**	**PGY5**
-Metacarpal fracture	-Mandible fracture	-Rhinoplasty
-Skin graft	-Tissue expander/implant	-Cleft palate repair
-Z-plasty	-Pressure ulcer coverage	-Cleft lip repair
-Harvest of iliac crest bone graft	-Microtia	-Iliac bone graft
-Extensor tendon repair	-Flexor tendor repair	-Face lift
-Excision of skin malignancy	-Abdominoplasty	-Otoplasty
-Local flap coverage of soft-tissue defect	-Breast augmentation	-Blepharoplasty
	-Reduction mammaplasty	-Lower extremity coverage
		-Autologous breast reconstruction

Table 3. **Procedures required of plastic surgery residents in post-graduate years 3, 4 and 5.** Table from Rosen, J.M., Long, S. A., McGrath, D. M., & Greer, S. E. (2009). Simulation in plastic surgery training and education: the path forward. Plastic and Reconstructive Surgery, Vol. 123, No. 2, (Feb 2009), pp. (729-740), 1529-4242. Reprinted with permission.

Several simulators that model plastic surgery procedures are currently available. BioDigital has partnered with SmileTrain to develop a cleft lip simulator that can be run on a standard PC or laptop (Figure 2). Their simulator, which uses data from CT scans to model unilateral or bilateral cleft lips, allows the user to navigate the anatomy and explore each layer of tissue. The user is also able to create and transpose tissue flaps, as the computer can accurately model tissue properties (Oliker and Cutting, 2005). BioDigital's Cleft Lip and Palate simulator is currently available for download as a beta version (SmileTrain Cleft Lip and Palate Viewer, December 15 2011, http://www.biodigital.com/smiletrain/download.htm).

BioDigital's simulators for other specialized procedures include a simulator for latissimus dorsi myocutaneous flap with tissue expander for breast reconstruction following mastectomy. Their newest and most comprehensive product, the BioDigital Human, was released in 2011. This simulator models the full human anatomy and also incorporates motion (a beating heart) and biomechanics (a golf swing). It can now be run directly from the web from any computer. Sample images are shown in Figure 3, although this product is best viewed interactively on the website (BioDigital Human, December 15 2011, http://www.biodigitalhuman.com).

BioDigital has also developed a library of animations, which are highly realistic, non-interactive computer models that illustrate procedures for educational purposes. Table 4 presents the procedures for which BioDigital has already built animations.

Joseph McCarthy, MD, professor of plastic surgery at the NYU Langone Medical Center, has spearheaded the creation of the Interactive Craniofacial Surgical Atlas, a collection of simulators ranging from a frontal orbital advancement simulator to the Le Fort III advancement/distraction simulator. The computer simulations are supplemented with features such as videos of live surgeries, audio voiceover animations, and 3D visualization to better illustrate the procedure and facilitate learning. (Flores et al., 2010, Parts I and II.)

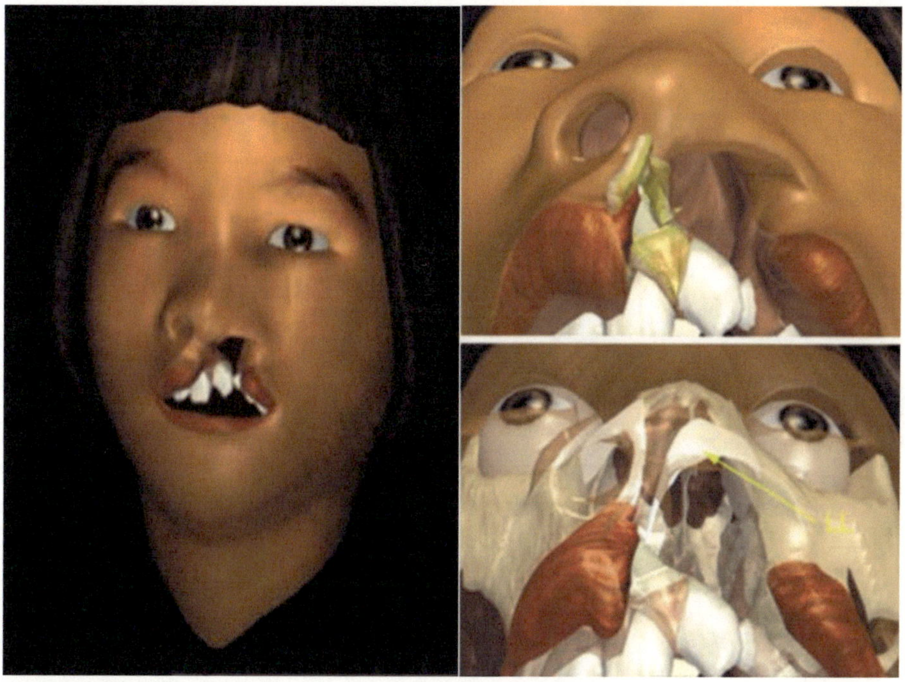

Fig. 2. **(left). BioDigital/SmileTrain; Cleft Lip Simulator Image. (right). 3D graphic animations to illustrate cleft lip and palate surgery.** Courtesy of SmileTrain, Court Cutting, MD, and BioDigital Systems, LLC. Copyright 2012 BioDigital Systems.

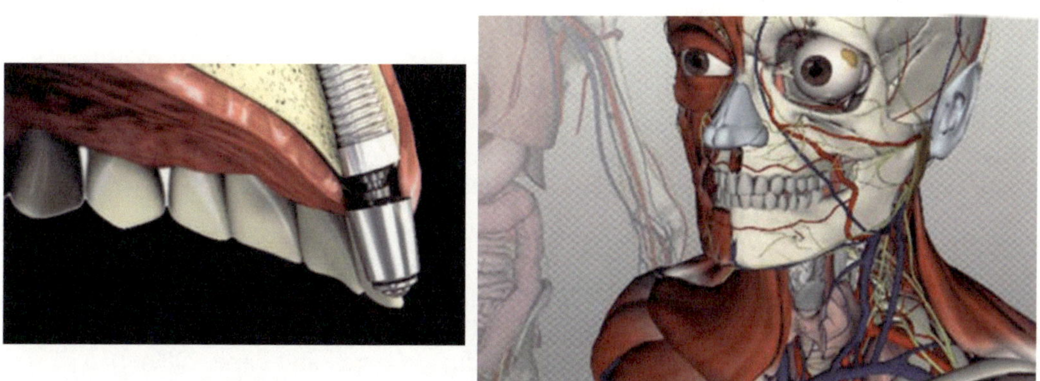

Fig. 3. **BioDigital human 3D animated simulator. Images of mouth anatomy with implant and craniofacial anatomy.** Courtesy of BioDigital Systems, LLC. Copyright 2012 BioDigital Systems.

SimQuest has recently developed the first platform for simulation of open surgical procedures (as opposed to the relatively more simple laparoscopic procedures). Their SurgSim Trainers will offer an anatomically precise model of tissue and tissue behavior, which can be manipulated with real surgical instruments attached to a haptics interface. The platform will also allow for trainers to create scenarios and content specific to their needs (Simquest SurgSim Trainers, December 15 2011, http://www.simquest.com/opensurgery.html).

<table>
<tr><th>Condition</th><th colspan="2">Animated Procedure</th></tr>
<tr><td>Genoplasty</td><td colspan="2">Genoplasty-Sliding</td></tr>
<tr><td rowspan="2">Prognathia</td><td colspan="2">Bilateral Saggital Split Osteotomy</td></tr>
<tr><td colspan="2">Vertical Ramus Osteotomy</td></tr>
<tr><td rowspan="3">Micrognathia</td><td rowspan="3">Mandibular Distraction</td><td>V-Vector</td></tr>
<tr><td>H-Vector</td></tr>
<tr><td>O-Vector</td></tr>
<tr><td>TMJ Ankylosis</td><td colspan="2">Transport Distraction</td></tr>
<tr><td>Maxillary Hypoplasia</td><td colspan="2">Le Fort I</td></tr>
<tr><td>Midface Hypoplasia</td><td colspan="2">Le Fort III</td></tr>
<tr><td>Upper 2/3 Hypoplasia</td><td colspan="2">Monobloc</td></tr>
<tr><td>Craniosynostosis</td><td colspan="2">Cranial Vault/Frontal Orbital Advancement</td></tr>
<tr><td rowspan="5">Breast Reconstruction</td><td colspan="2">Pedicle TRAM Reconstruction</td></tr>
<tr><td colspan="2">DIEP Flap Reconstruction</td></tr>
<tr><td colspan="2">Latissimus Dorsi Flap Reconstruction</td></tr>
<tr><td colspan="2">Free TRAM Reconstruction</td></tr>
<tr><td colspan="2">Tissue Expander</td></tr>
</table>

Table 4. **BioDigital has completed animations for these plastic surgery procedures.** Courtesy of BioDigital Systems, LLC. Copyright 2012 BioDigital Systems.

Simulation has been applied as a useful tool for minor, office-based procedures. In one approach to hybrid simulation, Kneebone *et al.* combined an inanimate mechanical model with a human actor posing as a patient to integrate the teaching (and practice) of technical and non-technical skills. Trainees interacted with the patient actor as they performed a procedure on the anatomical model, which was positioned over the actor to maximize realism. Initial trials indicated that covering the junction between patient and model with a simple drape offered a surprisingly high level of realism (Kneebone *et al.*, 2010).

Schendel and Lane designed the Patient-Specific Anatomic Reconstruction (PSAR), a fusion of CT, MRI, and surface-image scans combined with relevant biomechanical properties, which results in an anatomically valid 3D virtual patient that will help simulate the effects of surgical manipulation during procedures. The PSAR is intended for procedure planning, and could be a valuable addition to resident training (Schendel and Lane, 2009). In a similar vein, Kim *et al.* have developed a novel template-based facial muscle prediction program for computationally efficient simulation of soft-tissue deformation following surgery (Kim *et al.*, 2010). Such advances will increase the potential for high-fidelity simulations required for teaching more nuanced, subtle procedures.

4.3 Phase 3- Team training

In addition to proficiency in surgical skills and procedures, the success of an operation depends on organized and coordinated teamwork among all participants involved. The third and final phase in ACS's strategy introduces simulators to team training. In a team that may include a senior surgeon, a resident, a scrub nurse, a circulating nurse, and an anesthesiologist, efficient teamwork can help avoid medical errors while elevating staff morale. Simulation is now beginning to be recognized as a valuable tool for improving communication, leadership, and distribution of work in various areas of medicine. As surgical teams are often multi-disciplinary, the priorities and considerations of team training are quite similar across specialties. As such, the success of simulators in team training within one field of medicine is predictive of similar success within the realm of plastic surgery.

The simulators currently in use for team training primarily employ patient mannequins or live actors. Gaba *et al.* have developed the Anesthesia Crisis Resource Management (ACRM), which is based on aviation's Crew Resource Management training of cockpit teams. Emphasizing decision-making and teamwork principles, the ACRM curriculum advances mannequin-based patient simulators and has resulted in more realistic anesthesia training (Gaba *et al.*, 2001). Recently the ACRM program has been adapted for *in situ* simulation training for otolaryngology teams at Children's Hospital Boston (Volk *et al.*, 2011). While the ACRM curriculum appears to be effective in team training, there remains a need for objective, measurable indicators of team performance. Mica Endsley developed the Situation Awareness Global Assessment Technique (SAGAT) to fill this void (Endsley, 2000). Situational awareness, defined by Hogan *et al.* as "the perception of elements in the environment...the comprehension of their meaning, and the projections of their status in the near future," is a crucial dimension of performance (Hogan *et al.*, 2006). Using SAGAT, educators can "freeze" simulated actions in the middle of procedures to assess, debrief, and ask participants about their perceptions and comprehension. This method of assessment is more direct than traditional checklists, which can only infer data from participants' actions or secondary measures. This technique has been applied to many fields of medicine, from trauma life support (Hogan *et al.*, 2006) to otolaryngology (Volk *et al.*, 2011).

TeamSTEPPS, the product of collaboration between the Agency for Healthcare Research and Quality (AHRQ) and the US Department of Defense, is a relatively new multimedia curriculum designed to improve teamwork and communication. Standing for Team Strategies and Tools to Enhance Performance and Patient Safety, TeamSTEPPS offers a flexible, evidence-based toolkit with four key areas of competency: leadership, situation monitoring, mutual support, and communication (Clancy and Tornberg, 2007). Recently, Riley *et al.* presented a study in which perinatal morbidity at one community hospital decreased by 37% following a didactic TeamSTEPPS program with several simulation sessions. In contrast, a second hospital receiving no training intervention and a third that received only the didactic program both showed no improvement. This study is among the first to demonstrate a positive correlation between simulation training and patient outcomes (Riley *et al.*, 2011). Since the initial release of TeamSTEPPS, AHRQ and the Department of Defense have teamed with the American Institutes for Research to create a training and support network called the National Implementation of TeamSTEPPS project (Agency for Healthcare Research and Quality, December 16 2011, http://teamstepps.ahrq.gov/).

Currently, investigators under Eugene Santos at Dartmouth's Thayer School of Engineering are involved in research aimed at enhancing communication and ensuring patient safety. The goal is to develop a computational team-training simulation that will seamlessly monitor medical operations (Santos *et al.*, 2011). Santos's team is using Baysian Knowledge Bases (BKB) to simulate clinical decision-making prior to, during, and after surgical interventions, with the goal of detecting and alerting the team of any discrepancies. By measuring gaps in perception between physicians, nurses, and patients, errors caused by miscommunication and misaligned intent can be predicted and thus avoided. To analyze how accurately the simulations predict participants' decisions, BKBs have been built to model completed medical procedures. One such scenario involved a case in which the plastic surgeon and general surgeon had different understandings of the procedure to be done (whether a simple or subcutaneous mastectomy), and the patient's nipple was mistakenly discarded. In another case, a patient underwent a circumferential panniculectomy in which both a plastic surgeon and a general surgeon were involved. Once home, the patient experienced significant pain at the site of the surgery. Disagreement between the plastic and general surgeons over readmission versus home care was not resolved, and as a result diagnosis of the infected wound was delayed by several days. This case introduces another layer of complexity, in that the patient's condition is dynamic within the timeframe of interest. By integrating gap analysis and intent inferencing, the Santos team hopes to contribute to team training in health care by supplying individuals involved in complex situations the targeted information that will help them make the best decision for the patient (Santos *et al.*, In press).

5. Looking to the future

The American College of Surgeon's initiative to integrate simulation into general residency programs is an excellent demonstration of the recognized power of the technology. Accordingly, this paper proposes that Plastic Surgery follow their model. But this is just the beginning. Simulation has the power to change not merely education, but the entire paradigm of health care delivery. In order to take advantage of its full potential, it is essential to regard simulation as an environment in which the provider understands the disease process and life cycle of the patient, dealing with interruptions in health as they arise. In 1910 Flexner redefined the contract of service between physicians and society with his modifications to the education system. Today, we have the opportunity to reinstate this contract using information technology, namely simulation, applied from research to education to service. This change is not to be seen as an addition to our current system, but as in 1910, a fundamental transformation of the process, delivery, and business of medicine. In this new model of health care, the patient and provider will exist in a mobile, flexible network.

The paradigm shift will start in medical schools, with an integrated curriculum that features a more natural relationship between what is learned in medical schools and the delivery of care. As simulators are being used as training tools in residency and beyond, so too should they be used in medical school. The University of Central Florida College of Medicine, established in 2006, boasts a fully integrated curriculum in which web portals, immersive experiences, and computerized cases demonstrate the school's commitment to innovative technology. Students are assigned virtual families to follow through four years of medical school - just one example of simulation's role in the UCF curriculum. In the future, it is likely that more medical schools will follow the example set by UCF and will incorporate simulation heavily into their programs.

Outside of education, simulation can also help on a larger scale both nationally and internationally. At the population level, integrated large-scale simulation can be an epidemiological tool to anticipate the spread of a disease. Such a model could have been instrumental during 2010-2011 in containing the cholera outbreak in Haiti. At the level of the individual, simulation can facilitate a model of a human body that will predict the effect of a new medication or the combinations of treatments on a patient. Work toward this end has already begun in the placement of abdominal aortic aneurysm grafts by M2S, Medical Data and Image Management Services. The company can make patient-specific models of anatomical parts to predict the success of endovascular grafts (Medical data and image management services, access date: December 16 2011. http://www.m2s.com/). In the future, we will be able to include genetic markers in these models to anticipate susceptibility to disease based on individuals' genomes (Figure 4). Electronic medical records may soon include virtual patient holomers and behavioral models to assist physicians in following patient lifecycles (Satava, 2011).

Simulation will facilitate the transition from a past-oriented to a future-focused health care system. Today, evidence-based medicine (EMB) is seen as a standard to strive for, yet in its quest to extract information from completed interventions, EBM is rooted in the past. With simulation, we can predict, prepare for, and plan the future on the level of the cell, the body, or the population and with regard to physical, behavioral, and genetic response. Figure 4 displays the range over which simulation will one day have predictive power.

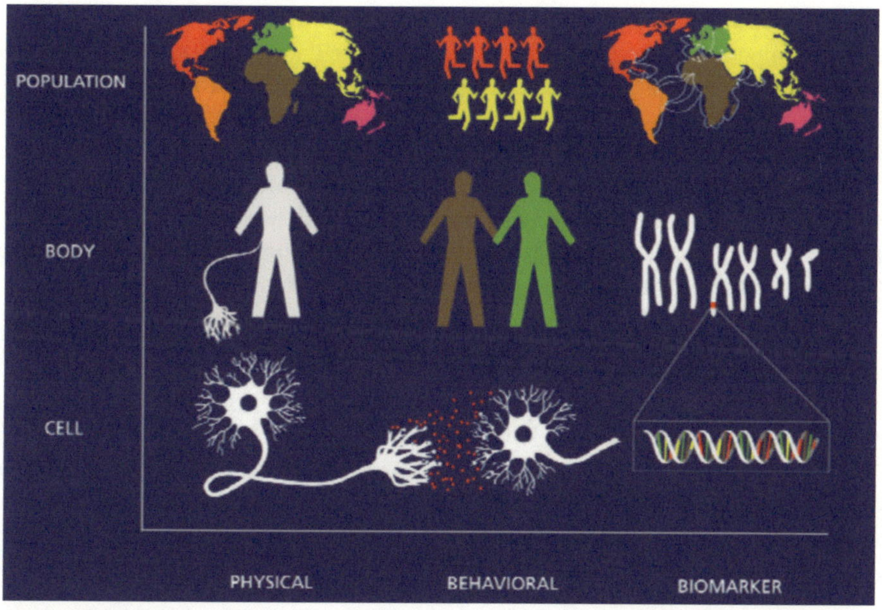

Fig. 4. **Physical-Behavioral-Genomics Model.** Dr. Joseph Rosen and colleagues are developing a model that would contain data on the physical body, behavior, and genetic information of an individual. This model could potentially include a person's cells, tissues and organs, vital signs, biomechanics, physiology, behavior and genetic traits, and link to epidemiological data of the population. It is hoped that such a model will simulate and predict the individual's behavior and health. Image courtesy of Joseph Rosen, MD, copyright 2012, used with permission.

Simulation will be instrumental in shifting health care from a platform-based to a network-based structure, in which the provider is removed from the patient and thus convenience, accessibility, and pathogen control are increased. A key role of simulation will be training physicians to practice in an increasingly digital world. When a new technology like a robotic surgical assistant is developed, there is initially an understandable shortage of experts. In the absence of experts, the apprenticeship model of training breaks down. A virtual expert must be simulated and built into or alongside the new device. Similarly, when distributing current technology to rural or underdeveloped areas, there may be no one to fill the role of expert *in situ*. The device then must act as the expert, training novices to competency through simulation (Aggarwal *et al.*, 2010). The idea that technology itself can instruct the trainee on its use opens the door to training at the point of care. Inclusion of the expert within the technology may enable a shift in the time, in addition to the manner, of medical education.

The US Army's combat philosophy of "train as you fight" can be applied to medicine as simulators become capable of turning surgical instruments into performance machines, providing targeted, organized, accessible information to surgeons as they operate. The recently launched Plastic Surgery Education Network website has the potential to move in this direction; already it demonstrates a centralization of relevant information specific to the plastic surgeon. With the proper organization and user interface, such a website could become a tool inside the operating room, walking a surgeon through a procedure with spoken instruction. While it may sound far-fetched and unrealistic to rely on a "train as you fight" model in medicine, the automated external defibrillator (AED) is a shining example of point-of-care training with enormous success. AEDs are designed to be used by non-medical personnel (i.e., first-time users with minimal training). All AEDs approved in the US have spoken prompts to instruct the user on how to safely deliver electric charges in order to restore a regular heartbeat in a patient, and many also include visual displays. Most models record the patient's ECG data, along with the number and strength of the shocks delivered. This information can be downloaded to a computer after the event to debrief responders and assess the efficacy of the device.

As simulators continue to be incorporated across medicine, they will become more advanced, more powerful, and more realistic. The training environment will become a closer replication of the actual environment until, eventually, the simulation is indistinguishable from reality and passes the "Virtual Turing Test". Introduced by Alan Turing in 1950, the Turing Test is a measure of a machine's ability to imitate human behavior. A human judge engages in a conversation with two hidden "partners", one human and one machine. If the judge cannot correctly identify the computer, the computer is said to have passed the Turing test (Turing, 1950). See Figure 5.

Low-fidelity simulators will continue to be useful for novices looking to practice generic skills, but experts will benefit from hyper-realistic models capable of accurately representing nuances of a procedure, from tissue interactions to potential complications. (Aggarwal *et al.*, 2010). See Figure 6.

Modern innovation needs to prepare physicians for the future, not the past. In order to train physicians today, we need to anticipate how medicine will look in thirty years. As the best way to predict the future is to invent it, our focus today should be on using simulation to

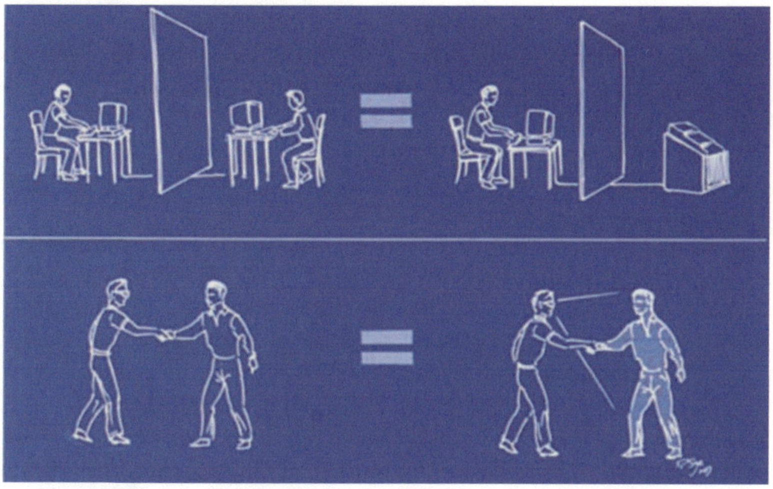

Fig. 5. **Virtual Turing Test.** A human observer (seated at left in each diagram in the top row) engages in a conversation with two hidden "partners", one human and one machine. If the human judge cannot correctly identify the computer, the computer is said to have passed the Turing Test (Turing, 1950). Image courtesy of Joseph Rosen, MD, copyright 2012, used with permission.

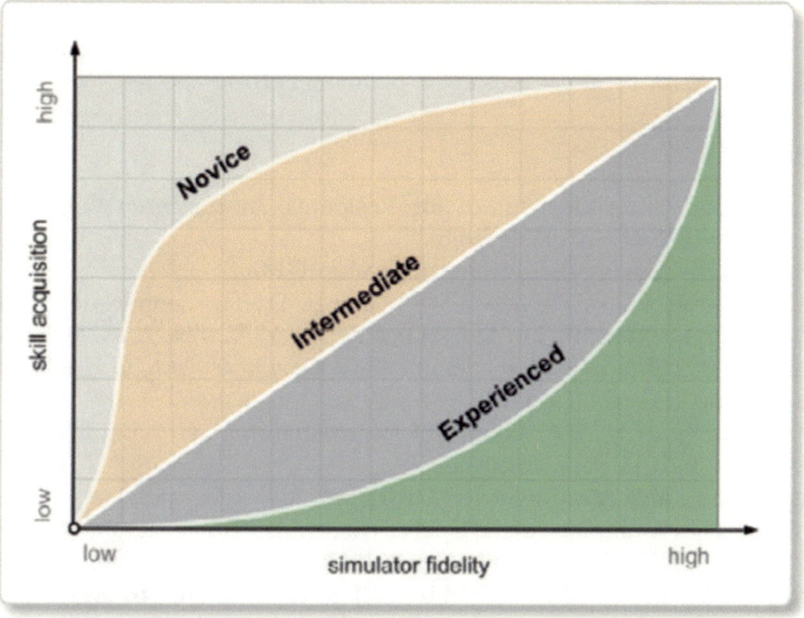

Fig. 6. **Relationship between fidelity of simulator and acquisition of skill at three levels of expertise.** Novices experience the most rapid skill acquisition at a lower level of fidelity, while experts require high fidelity simulators to improve their skills. Reproduced from [Quality and Safety in Health Care, Aggarwal, R., Mytton, O. T., Derbrew, M., Hananel, D., Heydenburg, M., Issenberg, B., MacAulay, C., Mancini, M., Morimoto, T., Soper, N., Ziv, A., & Reznick, R.Vol. 19, Suppl 2, pp. (i34-i43), 1475-3898, Copyright 2010] with permission from BMJ Publishing Group Ltd.

move towards a more functional, less expensive, network-based health care system rooted in telemedicine. By implementing simulation, we can shape a future of medicine in which patients are safe, education is cost-efficient and time-efficient, and the right care is delivered at the right time in the right place.

6. Conclusion

The American College of Surgeons has outlined a proactive and comprehensive plan to improve general surgery training with simulation in three phases: skills training, procedure training, and team training. In this paper, we have proposed to adapt this three-phase strategy for plastic surgery residency, modifying it to address challenges specific to the field. Already, considerable simulation technology exists to augment plastic surgery training at all levels. What is still needed is a unified commitment by medical educators to use simulation to simultaneously standardize the training curriculum, individualize the method of acquiring information, and objectively evaluate the training process. This methodology need not be restricted to residency; simulation has a role to play in medical education from the undergraduate level to the senior physician's maintenance of certification. The incorporation of innovative technology into today's curriculum will be an essential step in not only preparing for the future, but shaping it as well.

7. Acknowledgement

The authors would like to thank Robyn Mosher, M.S. for her invaluable editing expertise and Sarah Long, B.A. for her assistance in the planning of this paper.

8. References

ACS/APDS Surgical Skills Curriculum for Residents, In: *American College of Surgeons*, December 16 2011, Available from: http://www.facs.org/education/surgicalskills.html)

Aggarwal, R., Mytton, O. T., Derbrew, M., Hananel, D., Heydenburg, M., Issenberg, B., MacAulay, C., Mancini, M., Morimoto, T., Soper, N., Ziv, A., & Reznick, R. (2010). Training and Simulation for Patient Safety. *Quality & Safety in Health Care*, Vol. 19, Suppl 2, pp. (i34-i43), 1475-3898

American Board of Surgery (ABS) Booklet of Information for Certifying Exam (2009). p. 14. December 16 2011, Available from: http://home.absurgery.org/xfer/BookletofInfo-Surgery.pdf

American Council on Graduate Medical Education (ACGME) Program Requirements for Graduate Medical Education in General Surgery: Common Program Requirement, Effective: January 1, 2008, Section II D (2). p. 10. December 16 2011, Available from: http://www.acgme.org/acwebsite/rrc_440/440_prindex.asp

Anastakis, D. J., Regehr, G., Reznick, R. K., Cusimano, M., Murnaghan, J., Brown, M., & Hutchison, C. (1999). Assessment of Technical Skills Transfer from the Bench Training Model to the Human Model. *American Journal of Surgery*, Vol. 177, No. 2, (February 1999), pp. (167-170), 0002-9610

Brown, J., Montgomery, K., Latombe, J.-C., & Stephanides, M. (2001). A Microsurgery Simulation System. In: *Medical Image Computing and Computer-Assisted Intervention –*

MICCAI 2001 Vol. 2208, W. J. Niessen & M. A. Viergever, pp. (137-144), Springer Berlin Heidelberg Berlin, 978-3-540-42697-4, Berlin

Clancy, C. M., & Tornberg, D. N. (2007). TeamSTEPPS: Assuring Optimal Teamwork in Clinical Settings. *American Journal of Medical Quality: The Official Journal of the American College of Medical Quality,* Vol. 22, No. 3, (May-June 2007), pp. (214-217), 1062-8606

DeVita, M., Schaefer, J., Lutz, J., Wang, H., & Dongilli, T. (2005). Improving Medical Emergency Team (MET) Performance Using a Novel Curriculum and a Computerized Human Patient Simulator. *Quality & Safety in Health Care,* Vol. 14, No. 5, (Oct 2005), pp. (326-331) 1475-3898

Dunkin, B., Adrales, G. L., Apelgren, K., & Mellinger, J. D. (2007). Surgical Simulation: A Current Review. *Surgical Endoscopy,* Vol. 21, No. 3, (Mar 2007), pp. (357-366) 1432-2218

dV-Trainer–Skills Training for Robotic Surgery, In: *Mimic Technologies,* December 16 2011, Available from:
http://www.mimic.ws/products/

Endsley, M. (2000). Direct Measurement of Situation Awareness: Validity and Use of SAGAT, In: *Situation Awareness: Analysis and Measurement,* Endsley, M. and Garland, D., Chapter 7, Psychology Press, 9780805821345

Flexner, A. (1910). *Medical Education in the United States and Canada: A Report to the Carnegie Foundation for the Advancement of Teaching,* Carnegie Foundation for the Advancement of Teaching

Flores, R. L., Deluccia, N., Grayson, B. H., Oliker, A., McCarthy, J. G. (2010). Creating a Virtual Surgical Atlas of Craniofacial Procedures: Part I. Three-dimensional Digital Models of Craniofacial Deformities. *Plastic and Reconstructive Surgery,* Vol. 126, No. 6, (December 2010), pp. (2084-2092)

Flores, R. L., Deluccia, N., Oliker, A., McCarthy, J. G. (2010). Creating a Virtual Surgical Atlas of Craniofacial Procedures: Part II. Surgical Animations. *Plastic and Reconstructive Surgery,* Vol. 126, No. 6, (December 2010), pp. (2093-2101)

Gaba, D. M., Howard, S. K., Fish, K. J., Smith, B. E., & Sowb, Y. A. (2001). Simulation-Based Training in Anesthesia Crisis Resource Management (ACRM): A Decade of Experience. *Simulation & Gaming,* Vol. 32, No. 2, (June 2001), pp. (175-193)

Grunwald, T., Clark, D., Fisher, S. S., McLaughlin, M., Narayanan, S., & Piepol, D. (2004). Using Cognitive Task Analysis to Facilitate Collaboration in Development of Simulator to Accelerate Surgical Training. *Studies in Health Technology and Informatics,* Vol. 98, pp. (114-120), 0926-9630

Hogan, M. P., Pace, D. E., Hapgood, J., & Boone, D. C. (2006). Use of Human Patient Simulation and the Situation Awareness Global Assessment Technique in Practical Trauma Skills Assessment. *The Journal of Trauma,* Vol. 61, No. 5, (Nov 2006), pp. (1047-1052), 0022-5282

Jensen, A. R., Wright, A. S., Calhoun, K. E., Lillard, S., McIntyre, L. K., Mann, G. N., Kim, S., Anastakis, D., & Horvath, K. (2009). Validity of the Use of Objective Structured Assessment of Technical Skills (OSATS) with Videorecorded Surgical Task Performance. *Journal of the American College of Surgeons,* Vol. 209, No. 3 Supp 1, pp. (S110-S111), 1072-7515

Kenney, P. A., Wszolek, M. F., Gould, J. J., Libertino, J. A., & Moinzadeh, A. (2009). Face, Content, and Construct Validity of dV-Trainer, a Novel Virtual Reality Simulator for Robotic Surgery. *Urology*, Vol. 73, No. 6, (June 2009), pp. (1288-1292) 00904295

Kim, H., Jürgens, P., Weber, S., Nolte, L.-P., & Reyes, M. (2010). A New Soft-Tissue Simulation Strategy for Cranio-Maxillofacial Surgery Using Facial Muscle Template Model. *Progress in Biophysics and Molecular Biology*, Vol. 103, No. 2-3, (Dec 2010), pp. (284-291) 0079-6107

Kneebone, R. (2010). Simulation, Safety and Surgery. *Quality & Safety in Health Care*, Vol. 19, No. Suppl 3, (Oct 2010), pp. (i47-i52), 1475-3898

Lapeer, R. J., Gasson, P. D., & Karri, V. (2010). Simulating Plastic Surgery: From Human Skin Tensile Tests, Through Hyperelastic Finite Element Models to Real-Time Haptics. *Progress in Biophysics and Molecular Biology*, Vol. 103, No. 2-3, (Dec 2010), pp. (208-216) 1873-1732

Lerner, M. A., Ayalew, M., Peine, W. J., & Sundaram, C. P. (2010). Does Training on a Virtual Reality Robotic Simulator Improve Performance on the da Vinci Surgical System? *Journal of Endourology / Endourological Society*, Vol. 24, No. 3, (Mar 2010), pp. (467-472), 1557-900X

Luker, K. R., Sullivan, M. E., Peyre, S. E., Sherman, R., & Grunwald, T. (2008). The Use of a Cognitive Task Analysis-based Multimedia Program to Teach Surgical Decision Making in Flexor Tendon Repair. *American Journal of Surgery*, Vol. 195, No. 1, (Jan 2008), pp. (11-15), 1879-1883

Martin, J. A., Regehr, G., Reznick, R., Macrae, H., Murnaghan, J., Hutchison, C., & Brown, M. (1997). Objective Structured Assessment of Technical Skill (OSATS) for Surgical Residents. *British Journal of Surgery*, Vol. 84, No. 2, pp. (273-278), 1365-2168

Medical Data and Image Management Services, December 16 2011., Available from: http://www.m2s.com/

Morgan, B. (1984). The Planning of Local Plastic Operations on the Body Surface: Theory and Practice. *British Journal of Surgery*, Vol. 71, No. 11, (Oct 1984), pp. (920-920) 1365-2168

Okuda, Y., Bryson, E. O., DeMaria, S., Jr, Jacobson, L., Quinones, J., Shen, B., & Levine, A. I. (2009). The Utility of Simulation in Medical Education: What is the Evidence? *The Mount Sinai Journal of Medicine, New York*, Vol. 76, No. 4, (Aug 2009), pp. (330-343), 1931-7581

Oliker, A., & Cutting, C. (2005). The Role of Computer Graphics in Cleft Lip and Palate Education. *Seminars in Plastic Surgery*, Vol. 19, No. 4, (Oct 2005), pp. (286-293) 1535-2188

Pellen, M. G. C., Horgan, L. F., Barton, J. R., & Attwood, S. E. (2008). Construct Validity of the ProMIS Laparoscopic Simulator. *Surgical Endoscopy*, Vol. 23, No. 1, pp. (130-139), 0930-2794

Plastic Surgery Education Network, December 16 2011. Available from: http://www.psenetwork.org/default.aspx

Riley W., Davis, S., Miller, K., Hansen, H., Sainfort, F., Sweet, R. (2011). Didactic and Simulation Nontechnical Skills Team Training to Improve Perinatal Patient Outcomes in a Community Hospital. *Joint Commission Journal on Quality and Patient Safety*, Vol. 37, No. 8, (Aug 2011), pp. (357–364), 1553-7250

Rosen, J., Burdette, T., Donaldson, E., Mosher, R., Katona, L., & Long, S. (In press). Robotics, Simulation and Telemedicine in Plastic Surgery, In: *Plastic Surgery, 3rd Edition Vol. 1: Principles,* G. C. Gurtner, Chapter 36, Elsevier, London

Rosen, Joseph M, Long, S. A., McGrath, D. M., & Greer, S. E. (2009). Simulation in Plastic Surgery Training and Education: The Path Forward. *Plastic and Reconstructive Surgery,* Vol. 123, No. 2, (Feb 2009), pp. (729-740), 1529-4242

Santos, E., Kim, K., Yu, F., Li, D., Arbogast, P., Jacob, E., & Rosen, J., (In press). Modeling and Simulating Dynamic Health Care Practices. *Proceedings of International Defense and Homeland Security Simulation Workshop,* Rome, Italy, September 2011

Santos, E., Rosen, J., Kim, K., Yu, F., Li, D., Guo, Y., Jacob, E., Shih, S., Liu, J., & Katona, L., (2011). Reasoning About Intentions in Complex Organizational Behaviors: Intentions in Surgical Handoffs, In: *Theories of Team Cognition: Cross-Disciplinary Perspectives,* E. Salas, S. Fiore, & M. Letsky, Routledge Academic, 0415874130

Satava, R. M. (2007). The Future of Surgical Simulation and Surgical Robotics. *Bulletin of the American College of Surgeons,* Vol. 92, No. 3, (Mar 2007), pp. (13-19), 0002-8045

Satava, R. M. (2010). Emerging Trends that Herald the Future of Surgical Simulation. *The Surgical Clinics of North America,* Vol. 90, No. 3, (June 2010), pp. (623-633), 1558-3171

Satava, R. (2011). Future of Modeling and Simulation in the Medical and Health Sciences, In: *Modeling and Simulation in the Medical and Health Sciences,* John Sokolowski & Catherine Banks, pp. (175-194), Wiley, 0470769475

Sawbones Worldwide, December 16 2011., Available from: http://www.sawbones.com/default.aspx

Schendel, S. A., & Lane, C. (2009). 3D Orthognathic Surgery Simulation Using Image Fusion. *Seminars in Orthodontics,* Vol. 15, No. 1, (Mar 2009), pp. (48-56), 10738746

Sifakis, E., Hellrung, J., Teran, J., Oliker, A., & Cutting, C. (2009). Local Flaps: A Real-Time Finite Element Based Solution to the Plastic Surgery Defect Puzzle. *Studies in Health Technology and Informatics,* Vol. 142, pp. (313-318) 0926-9630

SimQuest, SurgSim trainers, In: *SimQuest,* December 16 2011., Available from: http://www.simquest.com/opensurgery.html

SimuLab Corporation, Products in Development: EDGE. December 16 2011., Available from: http://www.simulab.com/products-development

SmileTrain Cleft Lip and Palate Viewer, In: *BioDigital Systems,* December 16 2011., http://www.biodigital.com/smiletrain/download.htm

Sroka, G., Feldman, L. S., Vassiliou, M. C., Kaneva, P. A., Fayez, R., & Fried, G. M. (2010). Fundamentals of Laparoscopic Surgery Simulator Training to Proficiency Improves Laparoscopic Performance in the Operating Room--A Randomized Controlled Trial. *The American Journal of Surgery,* Vol. 199, No. 1, (Jan 2010), pp. (115-120), 0002-9610

TeamSTEPPS National Implementation, In: *Agency for Health care Research and Quality,* December 16 2011., Available from: http://teamstepps.ahrq.gov/

Turing, A.M. (1950). Computing Machinery and Intelligence. *Mind,* Vol. 59, No. 236 (Oct 1950), pp. (433-460), 0026-4423

Vassiliou, M. C., Ghitulescu, G. A., Feldman, L. S., Stanbridge, D., Leffondré, K., Sigman, H. H., & Fried, G. M. (2006). The MISTELS Program to Measure Technical Skill in

Laparoscopic Surgery. *Surgical Endoscopy*, Vol. 20, No. 5, (Feb 2006), pp. (744-747), 0930-2794

Volk, M. S., Ward, J., Irias, N., Navedo, A., Pollart, J., & Weinstock, P. H. (2011). Using Medical Simulation to Teach Crisis Resource Management and Decision-Making Skills to Otolaryngology Housestaff. *Otolaryngology -- Head and Neck Surgery*, Vol. 145, No. 1, (July 2011), pp. (35 -42)

13

Prevention of Microsurgical Thrombosis

S.M. Shridharani, M.K. Folstein,
T.L. Chung and R.P. Silverman
University of Maryland, School of Medicine
USA

1. Introduction

Free tissue transfer is a safe and reliable mode of tissue reconstruction. Though it is the highest rung on the reconstructive ladder, this method of reconstruction is utilized by a multitude of surgical specialties including: plastic and reconstructive, orthopaedic, otolaryngology, and oral maxillofacial. There are multiple indications for free tissue transfer. A few examples are: skeletal defects after debridement for osteomyelitis, breast reconstruction, various trunk and extremity defects, and most recently composite tissue allotransplantation - primarily face and hand transplantion. Despite employing perfect microsurgical technique, flap failure caused by anastomotic thrombosis continues to occurs in complicated and uncomplicated microvascular anastomosis. Many pharmacologic agents have been studied experimentally and clinically both in the treatment and prophylaxis of microvascular thrombosis; however, there still remains no consensus as to what the optimal pharmacologic regimen should be. In this chapter, we discuss the reported incidence of flap failure caused by microvascular thrombosis, review the pathophysiology of thrombus formation, review the anti-thrombotic pharmacologic agents commonly used for prophylaxis, and overview the current methods of flap monitoring.

2. Complications of free tissue transfer

The most common and feared complication of microvascular anastomosis is graft failure secondary to arterial or venous thrombosis. It is reported that this occurs in five to ten percent of cases[1]. Thrombosis is the body's natural defense mechanism to prevent blood loss. When a vascular insult occurs, the body employs platelets and fibrin to seal the defect. The physiologic process is initiated by the presence of tissue factor when injury to the vascular intima occurs. This results in the extrinsic pathway of the coagulation cascade to begin. Tissue factor activates factor X, which in turn activates thrombin, eventually leading to the activation of fibrinogen. When discussing free tissue transfer, the vascular intima has been injured as a result of the microsurgical anastomosis. It is imperative that the inherent process of coagulation be prevented. The use of pharmacologic anticoagulation has been a point of contention in free tissue transfer with no clinical study yielding conclusive evidence that it is the most effective means to prevent thrombosis.

In the vascular surgery literature, the use of pharmacologic anticoagulation has been shown to improve outcomes and patency rates. It has been described in the microvascular literature that three main pharmacologic agents exist and are used as an adjunct to preventing thrombosis. They are heparin, aspirin, and dextran. A multitude of pharmacologic protocols exist. Nearly all are based on anecdotal data Various doses of aspirin, heparin at subtherapeutic levels without titration to partial thromboplastin time, and intraluminal irrigation prior to completion of the anastomosis are a few examples. The authors explore the various pharmacologic agents and the evidence that exists in the literature. In addition, we review the methods for monitoring and protecting the fragile initial uncomplicated microsurgical anastomosis in order to prevent complication and reoperation.

3. Pharmacologic agents

ASPIRIN

Aspirin (acetylsalicylic acid) is part of the non-steroidal anti-inflammatory drug group (NSAIDs) and a well known medication for analgesia, antipyretic, and anti-inflammatory purposes. Its mechanism of action was described in 1971 by the British pharmacologist John Robert Vane[2] from the Royal College of Surgeons in London, and noted to prevent the production of thromboxanes and prostaglandins. It was shown that aspirin irreversibly inactivates the cyclooxygenase (COX) enzyme which is required for the synthesis of both thromboxane and prostaglandin. Aspirin functions differently when compared to other NSAIDs in that it acetylates the serine residue in the active site of the COX enzyme, whereas other NSAIDs bind reversibly. This property affords aspirin the ability to inhibit platelet aggregation, the primary role of thromboxane A_2, for the life of the platelet. Furthermore, aspirin decreases endothelial production of prostacyclin which acts as a vasodilator and inhibitor of platelet aggregation. It has been shown that low doses (40-80mg) selectively inhibit platelet-derived thromboxane by 95% while only slightly decreasing endothelial derived prostacyclin (35%). However, the aspirin dose of 325mg decreases prostacyclin production by 75%. The side effect profile for aspirin includes bronchospasm, peptic ulcers, gastritis, risk of gastric hemorrhage with concurrent use of alcohol of warfarin, hemolytic anemia in glucose-6-phosphate dehydrogenase deficiency[3], gout exacerbation, and Reye's syndrome[4](potentially fatal disease affecting the brain, liver, and other organs in children with concurrent viral illness). Despite the side effect profile, surgeons performing vascular anastomosis and free tissue transfer take advantage of the platelet aggregation inhibition properties of aspirin.

HEPARIN

Heparin was discovered in 1916 and noted to be a highly sulfated glycosaminoglycan with the highest negative charge density of any known biological molecule[5]. Heparin as well as enoxaparin (a low molecular weight derivative) has been shown to be effective in preventing deep venous thrombosis (DVT) and pulmonary embolism (PE) in at risk patients[6]. The primary function of heparin is the binding of antithrombin III (ATIII) which renders it active due to increased flexibility of the reactive site loop of the enzyme as a result of a conformational change[7]. Due to this, ATIII inactivates thrombin induced activation of factors V and VIII as well as factor Xa, which are all important factors in the coagulation cascade. Heparin can be administered as a once or multi daily dose for prevention/prophylaxis of DVT and/or PE in at risk hospitalized patients. The dose depends on the formulation/preparation of heparin, patient renal function, and patient weight. The side effect profile of heparin most notably includes heparin-induced thrombocytopenia (HIT) with or without thrombosis (HITT). In this phenomenon, antibodies are produced against heparin when it is bound to a protein (platelet factor 4) which forms a complex that attaches to a receptor on the surface of a platelet resulting in activation of platelet microparticles leading to the formation of a thrombis[8]. As a result, thrombocytopenia ensues and the patient is also at risk of hemorrhage. Additionally, other side effects include elevation of serum aminotransferases which is not a result of liver dysfunction, but rather a drug effect, and hyperkalemia as a result of heparin-induced aldosterone suppression. As a result of heparin's mechanism and proven effects, systemic therapy has been employed by cardiothoracic and vascular surgeons to maintain patency of vascular anastomosis.

DEXTRAN

Dextran is a complex branched glucan with weights ranging from 3 to 2000 kilodaltons made from the polysaccharide fermentation of sucrose. The use of dextran in microsurgery revolves around its ability to decrease vascular thrombosis by reducing blood viscosity. This effect is hinged on dextran's binding of platelets, vascular endothelium, and erythrocytes which increases the overall negative charge thereby reducing aggregating properties. As a result, low molecular weight dextrans impair platelet function, prolong bleeding time, destabilize fibrin polymerization, act to expand blood volume by acting as potent osmotic agents, and decreased stability of platelet thrombus. The side effect profile of dextran is relatively small yet severe. The list includes anaphylaxis, pulmonary edema, cerebral edema, platelet dysfunction, and volume overload. Occasionally, acute renal failure has been described as a result of dextran

4. Anticoagulation use in free tissue transfer

In a study by Davies[9] in 1982, a questionnaire was dispersed to 73 microsurgery centers worldwide. In the responses, 825 free flaps were evaluated which showed that 691 surgeons used varying methods of anticoagulation, and 161 surgeons used no form of anticoagulation including no intraluminal heparin irrigation. In the anticoagulation group, it was found that there was an 89% success rate of free flap survival versus an 88% success rate in the non-anticoagulation group. This study was flawed by a lack of control for anticoagulation protocol which made inferences difficult to determine from the results.

In 1997, a study by Glicksman[10] surveyed microsurgeons' practices over a four year period and administered a retrospective questionnaire to investigate anticoagulation regimens. From these findings, 96% of respondents used some form of antithrombotic treatment. The various regimens employed by surgeons included: dextran, heparin, and aspirin. Of these surgeons who used dextran, 75% gave dextran intraoperatively and continued treatment for three to seven days. Other surgeons used heparin as an intraoperative bolus of 3000U to 5000U. Additionally, aspirin at a dose of 325mg once a day for up to fourteen days postoperatively was also documented. It is notable that this type of variety exists in that there is no empirical evidence in the literature to support these various protocols.

5. Evidence for aspirin

In 2005, a study by Chien[11] showed that in 216 head and neck reconstruction cases a post operative anticoagulation regimen of aspirin 325mg daily and administering heparin at 5000U subcutaneous twice a day showed similar flap survival and hematoma rates versus other anticoagulation protocols. This study however was limited by a lack of an internal control.

6. Evidence for heparin

A prospective multi-institutional study by Khouri[12] in 1998, which included 23 centers over a six month period, yielded 493 free tissue transfers to be evaluated. The results of the study showed a 4.1% flap failure rate, 8.3% intraoperative thrombosis, and 9.9% postoperative thrombosis requiring reexploration. It was found that administering only postoperative subcutaneous heparin therapy was responsible for a statistically significant decrease in the incidence of thrombosis. Further, it was concluded that intraluminal heparin, intraoperative systemic heparin, aspirin, and dextran had no impact on thrombosis rates and overall outcome. Unfortunately, this study was limited by the diversity of anticoagulation protocols used by each participating center.

In an animal model conducted by Ritter[13] in 1998, these authors investigated whether unfractionated heparin, low molecular weight heparin, could improve the patency of microvascular anastomoses. They concluded that due to the hematoma rate being present only in the unfractionated heparin group, that low molecular weight heparin is the anticoagulant of choice to both maintain vascular anastomotic patency and minimize hemorrhage.

7. Evidence against heparin

Pugh[14] in 1996 conducted a retrospective study evaluating the use of anticoagulants during surgery. It was determined that of the 15 patients who underwent microvascular free flap reconstruction for wound coverage, the use of heparin in addition to other anticoagulants had a higher associated hematoma rate versus the use of dextran and aspirin, both separately and together. This finding confirms the current regimen employed by most surgeons that the use of a single anticoagulant is necessary.

8. Evidence against dextran

While heparin, aspirin, and dextran all have pharmacologic properties making them wonderful agents to prevent anastomotic thrombosis and flap failure, they each have a side effect profile that is not benign. Many of the side effects are quite rare, and they each have the ability to cause bleeding and possibly overwhelming hemorrhage. Further, dextran has the ability to cause devastating systemic complications including anaphylaxis and volume overload leading to cerebral and/or pulmonary edema.

Disa[15] in 2003 found that patients receiving dextran had up to a 7.2 times increased rate of developing a systemic complication versus patients receiving aspirin. As a result, low molecular weight dextran was removed from use at that institution as an option for anticoagulation after head and neck reconstruction.

Further, in a study from 2003 by Sun[16], it was concluded that dextran was not necessary for microvascular anastomosis thrombosis prevention as the dextran free arm of their review had a 100% patency rate versus 96% in the dextran use group. Additionally, they mention the serious side effects of dextran and note that they can be prevented by not using this pharmacologic agent.

9. No evidence of efficacy

In a study from 1994, Kroll evaluated 517 free tissue transfers[17]. It was shown that the relationship between the use of anticoagulants and prevention of flap loss or prevention of thrombosis could not be established. Further, it was also concluded that low-dose (bolus heparin) in the perioperative period did not significantly increase the risk of hematoma.

Deutinger[18] in 1998 conducted a study evaluating the influence of dextran versus heparin as well as the technique of the anastomosis in free tissue transfer. In the study, 81 patients received dextran and heparin postoperatively, and 123 patients received heparin alone. It was found that there was no statistically significant difference in the rate of thrombosis in these two groups. However, an 8.9% ($p < 0.02$) higher rate of thrombosis was found with end-to-end anastomosis as compared with end-to-side.

In 2004, Veravuthipakorn[19] conducted a study to determine whether a pharmacologic agent is necessary to prevent anastomotic thrombosis and flap failure. They discussed 40 cases of free tissue transfer and replantation in which no antithrombotic agent was instituted intraoperatively or postoperatively. Their results showed one partial flap loss and two replantantion losses due to severe crush injuries. They state that technique is paramount in microvascular anastomosis. It was concluded that antithrombotic agents alone do not play a significant role in anastomotic patency.

Ashjian[20] in 2007 looked at 505 microvascular free tissue transfers to reconstruct oncologic defects, in which they allocated 260 patients to receive postoperative aspirin for five days whereas 245 patients received low molecular weight heparin. It was concluded that postoperative anticoagulation choice has no statistically significant effect on the incidence of free flap complications in terms of the following outcome variables: microvascular thrombosis, partial or total flap loss, hematoma, bleeding, deep venous thrombosis, pulmonary embolism, and death. They stated that aspirin and low molecular weight heparin therapy demonstrate equivalent outcomes when used as a single-agent in the posoperative period. The authors also concluded that intraoperative systemic heparin had no statistically significant effect on prevention of microvascular thrombosis, and a single dose of intraoperative heparin does not prevent thrombosis. They believe that intraoperative anticoagulation does not affect flap survival.

In 2010, Brands[21] conducted a review of the literature which showed that there is currently no consensus in the literature to prevent thrombosis after microvascular free flap reconstruction. Conclusions were drawn that non-pharmacologic means such as smoking cessation and meticulous microvascular surgery plays a crucial role in the outcome. The authors stated that it has not been determined as to which preoperative, intraoperative, or postoperative protocol for pharmacologic anticoagulation regimen is most effective to prevent thrombosis, and that the decision should be made based on the individual patient and the risk profile for the development of thrombosis.

10. Conclusions

From these powerful studies in the current literature, it is evident that surgeons utilize preoperative, intraoperative, and postoperative anticoagulation to prevent the catastrophic negative outcome of vascular thrombosis leading to flap failure and necrosis. The specific method used by surgeons thus far is based upon operator preference. These highlighted studies provide evidence that there is no definitive protocol in microsurgery to prevent thrombosis; although there are some important insights that can be agreed upon after a careful review of the literature.

First and foremost, the rate of flap failure in microvascular surgery is very low, with success rates generally >95%. When flaps fail, it is not always a result of vascular thrombosis, but rather can be for a variety of other reasons as well, including improper flap inset, systemic hypotension, or perhaps even as a result of certain medications that causes severe vasoconstriction (which is certainly occasionally necessary as a life saving measure). When rates of flap failure are so low, and when they have multiple causes, it requires an extremely large study in order to show a statistically significant difference in any type of intervention. Thus far, such a study does not exist in regards to anticoagulation.

It is fair to say, based on one of the largest prospective studies (REF 12), that at the very least, subcutaneous heparin injections should be considered, if no other anticoagulant is to be used. Although this was certainly a flawed study, it was one of the largest studies, drawing upon the experiences of many of the most reputable microsurgery centers at that time. Because of the well established benefit of subcutaneous heparin in DVT prophylaxis, along with the long period of immobilization that these patients invariably experience at least during surgery, subcutaneous heparin does appear to be a prudent option. Currently, in our own institution, low molecular weight heparin injections has generally replaced regular heparin for DVT prophylaxis. It is also the opinion of the authors, that the risk of Dextran prophylaxis, as pointed out by the Disa study (REF 15), is enough evidence to preclude its use in our practice, particularly considering the lack of any other clinical data to support its use in preventing thrombosis in microvascular surgery. In summary, although anticoagulation may have a limited benefit in preventing thrombosis in microvascular surgery, it is far more important to perform a technically perfect operation, with painstaking attention to detail along every step of the procedure, including patient selection, pre-operative behavior modification (such as smoking cessation), flap selection and design, flap inset, and post-operative flap monitoring and care. The use of the venous coupling systems, as well as the recently available intra-operative fluoresence imaging system using indocyanine green dye are two technological advances that may prove to be quite beneficial in improving outcomes in microvascular surgery.

11. References

[1] Khouri RK. Avoiding free flap failure. Clin Plast Surg. 1992;19:773- 781.
[2] John Robert Vane (1971). "Inhibition of prostaglandin synthesis as a mechanism of action for aspirin-like drugs". Nature - New Biology 231 (25): 232–5.

[3] Frank B. Livingstone. (1985). Frequencies of hemoglobin variants: thalassemia, the glucose-6-phosphate dehydrogenase deficiency, G6PD variants, and ovalocytosis in human populations. Oxford University Press.

[4] Macdonald S (2002). "Aspirin use to be banned in under 16 year olds". BMJ 325 (7371): 988.

[5] Cox, M.; Nelson D. (2004). Lehninger, Principles of Biochemistry. Freeman. p. 1100. ISBN 0-71674339-6.

[6] Agnelli G, Piovella F, Buoncristiani P, et al. (1998). "Enoxaparin plus compression stockings compared with compression stockings alone in the prevention of venous thromboembolism after elective neurosurgery". N Engl J Med 339 (2): 80–5

[7] Chuang YJ, Swanson R. et al. (2001). "Heparin enhances the specificity of antithrombin for thrombin and factor Xa independent of the reactive center loop sequence. Evidence for an exosite determinant of factor Xa specificity in heparin-activated antithrombin". J. Biol. Chem. 276 (18): 14961–14971

[8] Ahmed I, Majeed A, Powell R (September 2007). "Heparin induced thrombocytopenia: diagnosis and management update". Postgrad Med J 83 (983): 575–82.

[9] Davies, D. M. (1982). "A world survey of anticoagulation practice in clinical microvascular surgery." Br J Plast Surg 35(1): 96-99.

[10] Glicksman, A., M. Ferder, et al. (1997). "1457 years of microsurgical experience." Plast Reconstr Surg 100(2): 355-363.

[11] Chien, W., M. A. Varvares, et al. (2005). "Effects of aspirin and low-dose heparin in head and neck reconstruction using microvascular free flaps." Laryngoscope 115(6): 973-976.

[12] Khouri, R. K., B. C. Cooley, et al. (1998). "A prospective study of microvascular free-flap surgery and outcome." Plastic and Reconstructive Surgery 102(3): 711-721.

[13] Ritter, E. F., J. C. Cronan, et al. (1998). "Improved microsurgical anastomotic patency with low molecular weight heparin." J Reconstr Microsurg 14(5): 331-336.

[14] Pugh, C. M., R. H. Dennis 2nd, et al. (1996). "Evaluation of intraoperative anticoagulants in microvascular free-flap surgery." Journal of the National Medical Association 88(10): 655-657.

[15] Disa, J. J., V. P. Polvora, et al. (2003). "Dextran-related complications in head and neck microsurgery: Do the benefits outweigh the risks? A prospective randomized analysis." Plastic and Reconstructive Surgery 112(6): 1534-1539.

[16] Sun, T. B., S. H. Chien, et al. (2003). "Is dextran infusion as an antithrombotic agent necessary in microvascular reconstruction of the upper aerodigestive tract?" Journal of Reconstructive Microsurgery 19(7): 463-466.

[17] Kroll, S. S., M. J. Miller, et al. (1995). "Anticoagulants and hematomas in free flap surgery." Plastic and Reconstructive Surgery 96(3): 643-647.

[18] Deutinger, M., T. Rath, et al. (1998). "The influence of postoperative medical treatment and type of microvascular anastomosis on free tissue transfer." European Journal of Plastic Surgery 21(6): 273-276.

[19] Veravuthipakorn, L. and A. Veravuthipakorn (2004). "Microsurgical free flap and replantation without antithrombotic agents." Journal of the Medical Association of Thailand 87(6): 665-669.

[20] Ashjian, P., C. M. Chen, et al. (2007). "The effect of postoperative anticoagulation on microvascular thrombosis." Annals of Plastic Surgery 59(1): 36-39.
[21] Brands, M. T., S. C. van den Bosch, et al. (2010). "Prevention of thrombosis after microvascular tissue transfer in the head and neck. A review of the literature and the state of affairs in Dutch Head and Neck Cancer Centers." Int J Oral Maxillofac Surg 39(2): 101-106.